Nihil Obstat: Rev. Lorenzo M. Albacete, S.T.D.

Imprimatur: Bernard Cardinal Law
Dated: April 13, 1987

The Nihil Obstat and Imprimatur are a declaration that a book or pamphlet is considered to be free from doctrinal or moral error. It is not implied that those who have granted the Nihil Obstat and Imprimatur agree with the contents, opinions, or statements expressed.

Library of Congress Cataloging-in-Publication Data

Griese, Orville N.
 Catholic identity in health care.

 Includes bibliography references and index.
 1. Catholic health facilities—Standards. 2. Medical ethics. 3. Medicine—Religious aspects—Catholic Church. I. United States Catholic Conference. Ethical and religious directives for Catholic health facilities. 1987. II. Title.
RA975.C37G75   1987   241'.642   87-2270
ISBN 0-935372-19-9

The intellectual nature of the human person is perfected by wisdom and needs to be. . . Our era needs such wisdom more than bygone ages if the discoveries made by man are to be further humanized. For the future of the world stands in peril unless wiser men are forthcoming.

Vatican II: *Constitution on
The Church in the Modern World*, n.15

THE ILLUSTRATION ON THE OPPOSITE PAGE projects the persuasion that religious faith, if alive and responsive to divine grace, must have consequences. St. Paul provides three examples of such consequences in his *Epistle to Philemon*:

+ Although St. Paul himself was a prisoner of the authorities in Rome, he just had to welcome the young runaway slave, Onesimus, to his prison quarters and extend comfort and guidance. Faith has consequences . . .

+ + St. Paul received Onesimus into the Catholic faith and insisted that, as a Christian, he just had to return to his master, Philemon, and accept whatever Christian justice might require of him for running away and even stealing from his master. Faith has consequences . . .

+ + + St. Paul addressed his epistle to his convert and friend, Philemon, and reminded him diplomatically that, as a Catholic master, he just had to welcome back Onesimus and forgive him (now a convert) as a brother in Christ. Faith has consequences . . .

In like manner, all who are engaged in the Catholic mission of healing must face the challenge of manifesting the depth and sincerity of their Catholic faith by exercizing their responsibilities in full accord with approved Catholic standards and values, for the salvation of souls and for the Glory of God:

"In the same way, your light must shine before men so that they may see goodnes in your acts and give praise to your Heavenly Father" (Matthew, 5:16).

Catholic Identity in Health Care:
Principles and Practice

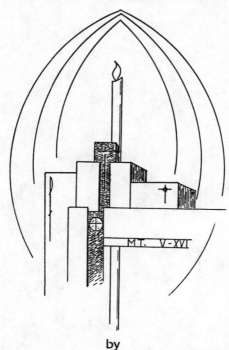

by
Rev. Msgr. Orville N. Griese, STD, JCD
Director of Research, Pope John Center

Foreword By

✝ Lawrence J. Riley, S.T.D., Auxiliary Bishop of Boston

1987
THE POPE JOHN CENTER
186 Forbes Road, Braintree, Massachusetts 02184

Foreword

Catholic Identity in Health Care: Principles and Practice is a timely volume, embodying Catholic values and standards, so direly needful in a contemporary society whose approach to serious problems is often marked by a merely pragmatic attitude. Even the most cursory contact with the field of health care will reveal that today moral and ethical problems are rampant, many of which touch upon life and death. Perhaps never in the past was it so necessary to stress the sanctity and the sacredness of human life and the dignity of the human person. How regrettable it is that in large measure our society seems to have abandoned these truths, which are founded on the fact that all human beings have been made in the image and likeness of God, and have been redeemed by the Precious Blood of Jesus Christ, the Son of God.

The rapidity of scientific developments in the area of health care during the past half century is unparalleled in human history. In consequence there have arisen exceedingly serious problems which, left unaddressed, might lead to an apparent conflict between scientific research and ethical standards. We must never lose sight of the fact, as the Second Vatican Council has insisted, that it is our obligation to incorporate the new findings of the sciences and the understanding of new scientific discoveries into Christian morality and thought, in such wise that, constantly keeping abreast of the facts of science and technology, we will be able to evaluate and interpret them from the viewpoint of an authentically Christian sense of values (cf. *Gaudium et spes,* n.62). We can be certain that "methodical research . . . provided it is carried out in a truly scientific manner and does not override moral laws, can never conflict with the faith, because the things of the world and the things of faith derive from the same God" (*ibid.,* n. 36).

I am delighted that Monsignor Orville Griese has written *Catholic Identity in Health Care: Principles and Practice.* A careful perusal of this impressive volume will reveal how brilliantly it reflects his outstanding qualifications as a learned scholar and a caring pastor. Expert in the fields of moral theology and canon law, and with a doctorate in each, he has had a wealth of varied experience in his priestly ministry. Now as Director of Research of the Pope John XXIII Medical-Moral Research and Education Center, he has produced a work of great value, which is scholarly, thorough, insightful, up-to-date, carefully balanced and uncompromisingly loyal to the teaching of the Church. The book is appropriately titled. It is indeed marked by a Catholic identity in its explanation of issues regarding health care; and it is concerned both with principles and with practice. As a matter of fact, many of the cases which are discussed in the volume pertain to actual problems submitted over the years to the Pope John Center for advice and counsel. There is no doubt that Monsignor Griese's work will be immeasurably helpful to those who are in any way involved in health care.

In mentioning Catholic identity we are brought face to face with the fact that not only the responsibility of the Church to teach, but the very teaching office of the Church—the magisterium—are under attack today. It is essential, then, to emphasize that down through the centuries the Church has consistently vindicated her right and her obligation to teach in all times and in all places the divine message revealed to the human race by Almighty God. One recent instance is to be found in the new Code of Canon Law, where it is succinctly stated: "The Church, to whom Christ the Lord entrusted the deposit of faith so that, assisted by the Holy Spirit, it might reverently safeguard revealed truth, more closely examine it and faithfully proclaim and expound it, has the innate duty and right to preach the gospel to all nations . . ." (Canon 747, #1).

This responsibility on the part of the Church does not refer to doctrinal matters only. It includes also matters pertaining to the moral law, as the same canon points out (cf. Canon 747, #2).

Nor is the Church's authority with respect to the moral law restricted to truths of divine revelation. Rather it extends likewise to issues that pertain to the natural order. Such is the explicit teaching of the Second Vatican Council, for example: "It is her [the Church's] duty to proclaim and teach with authority the truth which is Christ and, at the same time, to declare and confirm by her authority the principles of the moral order which spring from human nature itself" (Dignitatis humanae, n. 14).

Since the Second Vatican Council this teaching has many times been reaffirmed. Thus Pope Paul VI declared: "No believer will wish to deny that the teaching authority of the Church is competent to interpret even the natural moral law. It is, in fact, indisputable, as our predecessors have many times declared, that Jesus Christ, when communicating to Peter and to the Apostles His divine authority and sending them to teach all nations His commandments, constituted them as guardians and authentic interpreters of all the moral law, not only, that is, of the law of the Gospel, but also of the natural law, which is also an expression of the will of God, the faithful fulfillment of which is equally necessary for salvation" (Pope Paul VI, *Humanae vitae,* July 25, 1968, n. 4).

Monsignor Griese is not afraid to propose new solutions to problems confronting practitioners in the field of health care, which have never received fully satisfactory answers. This is done in a tone of sensitivity and understanding. Where his answers are tentative, he clearly so indicates,—and with a deference and a respect toward the magisterium of the Church that reflect a total willingness to abide by any decisions that may be forthcoming from the Church in the future.

In summary, *Catholic Identity in Health Care: Principles and Practice* is a very timely and valuable contribution to medico-moral literature. We are deeply indebted to its author and to the Pope John XXIII Medical-Moral Research and Education Center.

✝Lawrence J. Riley, S.T.D.
Auxiliary Bishop of Boston

Preface

The forty-three *Ethical and Religious Directives for Catholic Health Facilities* cover a broad spectrum of medical-moral situations and problems. Responding to the challenge of providing commentary on the full range of subjects results in a fairly comprehensive course in moral theology. The effort to provide such a commentary reminded me again and again of the medieval author/canonist who entitled his manuscript: *De Omnibus Rebus et De Quibusdam Aliis (About All Things, and a Few Others Besides)*. In this case, the "Few Others Besides" department might be considered as including very contemporary concerns and challenges such as the AIDS infection, innovative means of overcoming human infertility, prenatal testing and treatment, etc. Moral theology must keep pace with the advances in medical technology.

The readership in mind throughout the prolonged preparation of this publication has been concentrated on two groups in particular: health facility professionals, and pastoral personnel. Attention to the responsibilities of the first group (physicians, nurses, administrators) is revealed by the fact (as apparent in the index) that references to "physician" and "physician/patient relationship" outnumber by far any other individual references. Attention to the ministrations of the second group (chaplains, pastors and associate pastors, pastoral care personnel, deacons) has been buttressed by frequent references to the present Code of Canon Law and to authoritative decrees and declarations from the Holy See. The reasons for a divergence of opinion among theologians and ethicists on medical-moral issues are apparent, in many cases, from an explanation and an evaluation of the Theory of Proportionalism (Chapter VII, pp. 255ff.).

Expressions of gratitude are due to The Reverend William M. Gallagher, President of the Pope John Center, for assigning me to this research/writing project, and to the members of the Pope John Center staff for their challenging suggestions and comments. Three gracious scholars have reviewed the entire manuscript. The list begins with the Most Reverend Lawrence J. Riley,

DD, STD, Auxiliary Bishop of Boston, who completed his review of the manuscript by writing the splendid Foreword to this publication. The two other experts who reviewed the entire manuscript were the Reverend Albert S. Moraczewski, O.P., Ph.D., Regional Director of the Houston office of the Pope John Center, and the Reverend Monsignor Sylvester F. Gass, JCD, former Vicar General of the Archdiocese of Milwaukee, Wisconsin, and a past president of the Canon Law Society of America. A candidate for the Society of Jesus, William Stempsey, MD, also reviewed most of the chapters. Comments and suggestions from these scholars were incorporated into the composition and revision process.

The many obstetrical procedures discussed in Chapter VII required review by medical experts. That service was provided by the Reverend Thomas J. O'Donnell, S.J., author of *Medicine and Christian Morality* (1976) who was Professor of Medical Ethics and Regent of the School of Medicine of Georgetown University for many years; and by Richard T. F. Schmidt, MD, Director of the Department of Obstetrics and Gynecology at Good Samaritan Hospital, Cincinnati, Ohio, and a past president of the American College of Obstetricians and Gynecologists. A sincere "God bless" to all of these generous collaborators. The same fond wish must be extended to the Very Reverend Ralph F. Firneno and to the community of the Immaculate Conception Province of the Pallotine Fathers (S.A.C.) who financed the publication of this book.

The *Ethical and Religious Directives for Catholic Health Facilities* are presented throughout this book as applications of accepted medical-moral principles, beginning with the Principle of Human Dignity. That master principle, which promotes primary concern for "The total good of the patient, which includes his higher spiritual as well as his bodily welfare," is singularly emphasized in the Preamble of these *Directives* (paragraph two) as a distinctive, identifying mark of every Catholic health facility. Assurance of maintaining the witness and luster of that distinctive, identifying mark can be guaranteed, however, only if the trustees and administrators of Catholic health facilities are inspired to exercise leadership in promoting respect and reverence for human dignity. The world has a right to look to Catholic health facilities for such leadership. By virtue of historical background, teaching tradition and spiritual motivation, the Catholic Church stands above any other agency in human history in her record of respecting, promoting and defending the highest ideals of the inherent dignity of each and every human individual.

Rev. Msgr. Orville N. Griese, STD, JCD

Extended Table of Contents

CHAPTER I

Origin and Development of a Catholic Hospital Code of Ethics, 1921–1971

The Catholic Hospital Association of the United States and Canada (now known as the Catholic Health Association, but for the U.S.A. only) traces its origin to the leadership and persistence of Father Charles B. Moulinier, S.J. This association became a reality at a meeting of about 200 concerned men and women during their first assembly in the hall of St. Francis School, Milwaukee, Wis. (Fourth and Harmon Streets), June 24 to 26, 1915.[1] The American College of Surgeons, founded just two years earlier, had adopted a document known as "Minimum Standard" for approved hospitals, and courted the support of the newly-formed Catholic Hospital Association in their campaign for appropriate professional standards particularly in surgical procedures. With the encouragement of Cardinal Gibbons of Baltimore and with the hearty approval of Archbishop Messmer of Milwaukee, a resolution

---

[1]"The Catholic Hospital Association of the United States and Canada" by B.F. McGrath in *Hospital Progress,* June, 1922, p. 214.

to "approve of the work being done by the American College of Surgeons for the standardization of hospitals, and (to) assure the College of our fullest cooperation" was passed at the third annual convention of the Catholic Hospital Association at Chicago in 1918.[2]

This resolution met with a stormy reaction from two quarters; from Father Joseph C. Straub, spiritual director of the Hospital Sisters of St. Francis (owners of 14 hospitals in Illinois and Wisconsin), and from an organized group of members of the medical profession. The opposition felt strongly that "outside agencies were not competent to deal with a Catholic hospital," and that "compliance with the dictates of a secular crediting agency threatened the nature of a Catholic institution." They insisted that the Catholic Hospital Association should discontinue their support of the American College of Surgeons' Standardization Program and should take steps to set up their own standardization program.[3] The association's support of the American College of Surgeons' program was not discontinued, but some semblance of harmony was restored at the 1921 convention of the Catholic Hospital Association when a code of ethics previously drawn up by the Rev. Michael P. Bourke of St. Joseph Sanatorium, Ann Arbor, Michigan, was presented and accepted as a suitable code for the Catholic Hospital Association.[4]

This code by Father Bourke, who was also Director of Hospitals for the Diocese of Detroit, was printed in the very first issue of *Hospital Progress* (May, 1920) for the expressed purpose of stimulating "thought and discussion" among both hospital staff members and members of the clergy and hierarchy with regard to the need of a more extensive code. That first issue of *Hospital Progress* also announced a firm purpose of organizing a "National Board of Experts on Ethics and Surgery to handle all the ethical questions that arise in connection with surgical and medical practice."[5] Father Bourke was named as chairman of a permanent committee of three members at that 1921 convention.[6] This was not the "National Board of Experts" as proposed in the first

---

[2] *The History of the Catholic Hospital Association* by Robert J. Shanahan, S.J. (St. Louis, Mo.: The Catholic Hospital Association, 1965), p. 32.

[3] *Ibid.*, pp. 36–45.

[4] *Ibid.*, p. 43.

[5] *Hospital Progress*, May, 1920, p. 36.

[6] *Hospital Progress*, June, 1922, p. 230. Father Bourke's code as presented in the first issue of *Hospital Progress* (May, 1920, p. 36) consisted of two listings of unethical operations. The first listing, "involving the destruction of foetal life," included 6 operations. The second listing included "all operations involving the sterilization or mutilation of men or women, except where such follows as the indirect and undesired result of necessary interference for the removal of diseased structures" (7 are listed). The code then insists on "previous competent consultation" in determining "the question of the presence of life, and the necessity for the removal of the reproductive organs or interfering therewith, by surgery or medicine."

issue of *Hospital Progress*. It should also be added that the handy but brief surgical code prepared by Father Bourke never was regarded as the official code for Catholic hospitals.

Ten years later, the tireless Father Alphonse Schwitalla, S.J. undoubtedly was referring to the "Bourke Code" when he said in a formal report as president of the Catholic Hospital Association:[7] It is true that in 1921 a surgical code was adopted by the association. This code has been in general use in the Catholic hospitals since that date and has done incalculable good." He added that many Catholic hospitals printed this code "either in their staff constitution or as a part of the agreement with their staff members," while other Catholic hospitals required all staff members to "subscribe to the code before these members were given staff appointments or are allowed to use the operating room." He then expressed the hope that "through the carrying out of extensive studies which have already begun it may be possible in the not too distant future to reformulate an ethical code."

That "not too distant future" turned out to be 15 years later. In his "Historical Reflections" talk at the annual convention of the Catholic Hospital Association in Atlantic City in June, 1971, Monsignor Harrold A. Murray, Director of the Department of Health Affairs of the United States Catholic Conference, stated that between 1920 and 1930, despite the fact that "this matter was brought up again and again" at board meetings, no further progress was made with regard to the development of a code of ethics.[8] Presumably he was referring to the "Bourke Code" when he said: "For many years, this simple mimeographed page called a 'surgical code' was used widely." He then added:

With the development of theology and medicine with the newer surgical techniques, several dioceses drew up their own codes. Most important of these were the Hartford Code, the Toledo Code, the Grand Rapids Code and the Los Angeles Code. Since the Catholic Hospital Association was not ready to come out with its suggested code, the National Catholic Welfare Conference distributed or suggested the Toledo Code to some dioceses and a good many hospitals.

---

[7]*Hospital Progress,* June, 1931, p. 244.

[8]This informative report, entitled "Historical Reflections," is taken from the files of United States Catholic Conference (USCC), Department of Health Affairs, Washington, D.C., p. 1.

1.1 EFFORTS TO ESTABLISH A NEW CODE OF CATHOLIC HOSPITAL DIRECTIVES, 1946–1954

Beginning in July, 1946, the Executive and Administrative Boards of the Catholic Hospital Association pressed for action. At a meeting in St. Louis on July 9, 1946 (Executive Committee), the names of Father John Clifford, S.J. (Mundelein Seminary, Chicago) and of Father T.L. Bouscaren, S.J. (West Baden, Ind.) were suggested for membership on a Committee of Medical Ethics. It was also agreed that the clerical members of the Executive Board would constitute a steering committee for the drafting of the general objective of this Committee. At a meeting in Washington, D.C. on Sept. 11, 1946 (Administrative Board), a suggestion was made to have the Bishops' Representatives (also known as Diocesan Directors of Hospitals) discuss a code of ethics for Catholic hospitals at their meeting in February, 1947.[9]

In April, 1946, the Administrative Board of Bishops had appointed an Episcopal Commission to study ethical problems facing Catholic hospitals. The members of this commission (with indication of episcopal jurisdiction as of 1946) were Bishops Bryan J. McEntegart of Ogdensburg, N.Y., Michael J. Ready of Columbus, Ohio, and Karl J. Alter of Toledo, Ohio. The following theologians had been designated as consultants to the Episcopal Commission: Monsignor James O'Brien (Mt. St. Mary's Seminary, Cincinnati, Ohio), Father John J. Clifford, S.J. (Mundelein Seminary, Chicago), Father Francis J. Connell, C.SS.R. (Catholic University, Washington, D.C.), Father T.L. Bouscaren, S.J. (West Baden, Ind.), and Father Walter Farrell, O.P. (Dominican House of Studies, Washington, D.C.). At a meeting in St. Louis on Sept. 20, 1947 (Administrative Board), Bishop Alter reported on the work of the Episcopal Commission. A formal report was also prepared by Bishop Alter for the Conference of Bishops' Representatives (Diocesan Directors of Hospitals).[10]

At the time of Bishop Alter's report at the Sept. 20, 1947 meeting, Father John J. Flanagan, S.J. had succeeded Father Alphonse Schwitalla, S.J. as Executive Director of the CHA as of June, 1947. A very significant decision was made at the December 4, 1947 meeting of the Administrative Board of the CHA in St. Louis: the Executive Board concurred with the Administra-

---

[9]*Ibid.*, p. 1. At a meeting of the Council on the Constitution of the Catholic Health Association on June 12, 1933, the decision was made to give the Diocesan Directors of Hospitals the status of ex officio associate membership. Later, in 1942 (then an organization separate from the CHA) they gained representation on the Administrative Board of the CHA. Cf. Shanahan, Robert J., *The History of the Catholic Hospital Association* (cf. note 2), pp. 97 and 110–112.

[10]Murray, Msgr. Harrold A., "Historical Reflections" (cf. note 8), p. 2.

tive Board in the appointment of Father Gerald Kelly, S.J. to prepare a Code of Ethics.[11] Since 1928, Father Schwitalla had been Dean of the St. Louis University School of Medicine, President of the Catholic Hospital Association and editor of its official journal, *Hospital Progress*. As editor of that publication, he had made regular contributions on medical-moral questions. When he retired from all of these positions in 1947, Father Gerald Kelly assumed the task of making regular contributions to *Hospital Progress* on medical-moral questions.[12]

At the March 1, 1948, meeting of the Executive Committee of the Catholic Hospital Association in St. Louis, Father Flanagan outlined the progress that was being made in preparing a Code of Ethics under the authorship of Father Kelly.[13] At a meeting of the Executive Board in Cleveland, Ohio, from June 5 to 10, 1948, the publication of responses to ethical problems in *Hospital Progress* was authorized. The possibility of compiling reprints of such responses was also discussed.[14] Six months later, at a meeting of the Executive Board in Chicago, Ill., December 12 and 13, Father Flanagan unveiled a plan to publish two booklets: the Code itself, and publication of Father Kelly's responses (articles) in *Hospital Progress*.[15] The President of the Catholic Hospital Association, Monsignor George Lewis Smith, was pleased to announce the completion of both publications (the "Code of Ethics—1948," and separate commentary) at the CHA meeting in St. Louis on June 13, 1949:

> During the year Father Gerald Kelly, S.J. completed drafting the text of the Code of Ethics formulated under the sponsorship of the Catholic Hospital Association entitled: "Ethical and Religious Directives for Catholic Hospitals" and we have published it, together with the commentary entitled "Medico-Moral Problems" in booklet form. As I pointed out in the foreword, it is distinctly understood that these Directives do not constitute the official Code of Medical, Surgical or Hospital Ethics, and have no authoritative status in any diocese unless and until the Most Reverend Ordinary so directs, but we hope that the Code and Commentaries will be of service in explaining and promoting the

---

[11]*Ibid.*, p. 2.

[12]*The Historical Context and Sources of Moral Theology in the Writings of Gerald A. Kelly, S.J.*, a doctoral dissertation by Edwin L. Lisson, S.J. (Rome: Gregorian University, 1975), p. 167.

[13]Murray, Msgr. Harrold A., "Historical Reflections" (cf. note 8), p. 2.

[14]*Ibid.*, p. 2.

[15]*Ibid.*, p. 2.

observance of the Moral Law of God in our Catholic institutions.[16]

In the appendix of his excellent doctoral dissertation entitled *A Theological Analysis of the Ethical and Religious Directives For Catholic Health Facilities In The United States,* the late Father Clarence Deddens of the Archdiocese of St. Louis, Mo. included a copy of the *second* edition of these *Ethical and Religious Directives for Catholic Hospitals* (second printing, April, 1957; imprimatur by Archbishop Joseph E. Ritter, November 16, 1955). The Preface to the Second Edition provides valuable historical information:

> This booklet was first published by the Catholic Hospital Association of the United States and Canada in 1949. It was originally intended to serve as a code for the Catholic hospitals in these countries. Subsequently, however, it became clear that in the United States there was a widespread desire for a briefer code that could be conveniently printed in the form of a chart. To satisfy this desire the *Code of Medical Ethics for Catholic Hospitals* was published in chart and pamphlet form in 1954. At approximately the same time the Catholic Hospital Association of Canada published its own *Moral Code* in pamphlet form in both English and French. This latter publication has been officially adopted by the entire Canadian hierarchy. In the United States the new code is official in most dioceses. Although *Ethical and Religious Directives for Catholic Hospitals* is the basis for both the new Codes, it is not itself an official code in any diocese unless the bishop adopts it.[17]

The reasons for rewording some of the directives in this second edition of the Code, and for the addition of some entirely new directives (regarding professional secrecy, experimentation, ghost surgery, psychotherapy, shock-therapy, unnecessary surgery, and the spiritual care of non-Catholics) were stated as follows:

> . . . to include some important points from recent statements of the Holy See; secondly, to clarify some matters that were found to

---

[16]*Ibid.,* p. 3.
[17]Cf. *A Theological Analysis of the Ethical and Religious Directives for Catholic Health Facilities in the United States* (Rome, Italy: Pontifical University Angelicum, 1980), p. 186. For comparison purposes, the earlier version of the 1954 code (published in 1949) is found in *Medical Ethics* by Father Charles J. McFadden, O.S.A., 2nd ed. (Philadelphia, Pa.: F.A. Davis Co., 1952), pp. 419 ff.

be somewhat obscure in the first edition; and, finally, to establish greater conformity between this booklet and the new Codes that are based on it.[18]

A noteworthy feature of the second edition of the 1954 Code was that the directives were numbered consecutively as in the Code of Canon Law. This edition listed 60 directives, and 59 footnotes.

Following this historical note on the relationship between what sometimes was called the Code of Ethics—1948, and the Code of 1954, it is important to point out that only the 1954 version received the official approval of the U.S. Bishops as a group. At the Thirty-Sixth Annual Meeting of the Bishops of the United States in November, 1954, Bishop William A. O'Connor presented the report of the Bureau of Health and Hospitals. After referring to Father Kelly's involvement, since 1948, in the compilation and editing of the *Ethical and Religious Directives for Catholic Hospitals* and in the publication of the pamphlet reprints of his articles in *Hospital Progress* (eventually five pamphlets) in one volume entitled *Medico-Moral Problems,* he spoke of the wide distribution given to those two publications: 47,800 copies of the *Directives,* and 30,000 copies of *Moral-Medical Problems.* The minutes of this report conclude with the following testimonial of approval:

> It was moved by Archbishop Alter, seconded by Bishop Ready that the "Code of Medical Ethics for Catholic Hospitals" published by the Catholic Hospital Association of the United States and Canada proposed by Bishop O'Connor, be approved by the Bishops as the official medical code subject to the approval of the authorities for use in their dioceses. The motion carried.[19]

At the January 11, 1955 meeting of the Administrative Board in Boston, Father Flanagan reported on the "development of [a] condensed version of "Ethical and Religious Directives for Catholic Hospitals" recommended at the May, 1951, convention—both in booklet and chart form. Letters were sent to Bishops' Representatives to ascertain their wishes with respect to the adoption of the revised Code in their respective dioceses. At the May 15, 1955, meeting of the same board in St. Louis, it was reported that of 127 dioceses, 29 had accepted the Code with little change (usually involving the

---

[18]Deddens, Clarence, *Doctoral Dissertation* (cf. note 17), p. 186.
[19]Murray, Msgr. Harrold, "Historical Reflections" (cf. note 8), pp. 3–4.

use of the imprimatur of the local Ordinary), and that 80 dioceses made no objections whatever.[20]

The Extent of Father Kelly's
Contribution to Moral-Medical Theology

When Father John Ford, S.J. left the Weston Jesuit Theologate in Massachusetts in 1946 to accept a teaching assignment at the Jesuit Gregorian University in Rome, Father Gerald Kelly assumed the task of writing the "Notes on Moral Theology" in *Theological Studies*. He continued to perform this valuable service until he suffered his first heart attack in 1953. At this time (1946), he began to write on specifically medical topics.[21] He was not only a regular contributor to *Hospital Progress* (succeeding Father Schwitalla in that task in 1947), but also wrote extensively for the official journal of the National Federation of Catholic Physicians' Guilds, the *Linacre Quarterly*.

These contributions to two moral-medical publications were practical and concrete responses to problems presented by medical personnel and hospital administrators. At the end of his first year as the moral-medical correspondent for *Hospital Progress,* the Catholic Hospital Association assembled twelve of Father Kelly's articles into a pamphlet entitled *Medical-Moral Problems* (Vol. I). Each successive year for the next four years, his articles in *Hospital Progress* and *Linacre Quarterly* were bound in pamphlet form. After 1954, as mentioned previously, the five pamphlets were bound into book form with the title *Medical-Moral Problems.* In the "Explanatory Preface" of the 1958 edition of *Moral-Medical Problems,* Father Kelly states that he had omitted some discussions from the pamphlet series which had become obsolete (for example, on the Eucharistic fast); that he reorganized other materials so that everything about a given topic is treated under a single chapter; that he brought all of the old material up to date insofar as possible and added much completely new material.[22]

Father Kelly was more than the compiler and editor of the *Code of Ethical and Religious Directives for Catholic Hospitals.* After describing the Code which was published in 1949 (presumably the one referred to sometimes as the "code of 1948," for it was prepared in 1948), Father Edwin Lisson, S.J. in his doctoral dissertation on the writings of Father Kelly, makes the following statement:

---

[20]*Ibid.,* pp. 4–5.

[21]Deddens, Clarence, *Doctoral Dissertation* (cf. note 17), p. 8.

[22]*Medico-Moral Problems* (St. Louis, Mo.: Catholic Hospital Association, 1958), Introduction, p. VII.

Although the document is unsigned, from the fact that twenty-six of the twenty-eight footnotes refer to Kelly's articles, it would not be unreasonable to infer that the composition of this code was largely his work.[23]

In the second edition of this same Code (discussed on pages 5 and 6), the 59 footnotes abound with references to Father Kelly's writings in *Moral Medical Problems* and in his contributions to *Hospital Progress* and the *Linacre Quarterly*. Again, Father Lisson is justified in concluding:

Again, insofar as each of the sixty directives [except directive n.60] is footnoted with an article by Kelly, it would appear to be largely his work. This one work of Kelly's directly affected 840 member hospitals of the Catholic Hospital Association and the more than five million patients they served each year.[24]

1.2 "RUMBLINGS OF CONCERNS," 1965–1971 AND THEREAFTER

Monsignor Murray reported that "nothing of substance" appeared in the archives of the Catholic Hospital Association or of the National Catholic Welfare Conference regarding the Code of Ethics from the middle 50's to the middle 60's. He does speak of "a few rumblings of concerns" for restudy and revision of the directives as of 1965–1966.[25] This rising crescendo of concerns focused primarily on the question of material cooperation. The task, however, of sketching the personalities, issues and events which led to the formal approval of the present revised version of the *Ethical and Religious Directives for Catholic Health Facilities* by the Bishops of the United States in November, 1971, has been reserved for chapter X on the *Principle of Material Cooperation*. Due to the fact that the rising clamor for change concerned above all the preamble to the Code with only minimal attention to the directives themselves, however, the present Code still stands in large part as a valued legacy of a moral theologian of prestigious intellectual acumen, remarkable foresight and inspiring dedication—Father Gerald Kelly, S.J.

The approval of the present Code of Hospital Directives by the American

---

[23]Lisson, Edwin, S.J., *Doctoral Dissertation* (cf. note 12), p. 169.
[24]*Ibid.*, p. 170.
[25]Murray, Msgr. Harrold, "Historical Reflections" (cf. note 8), p. 5.

hierarchy in November, 1971, did not signal the end of the "rumblings of concerns." As Archbishop John F. Whealon of Hartford, Conn. (Chairman of the Bishops' Committee on Doctrine in 1971) said in a June, 1971 address to the convention of the Catholic Hospital Association, the "real issue" was not the directives themselves but rather the "quite complex philosophical and theological questions which undergird this subject."[26] As the debate both before and after November, 1971 revealed, those issues focused on controverted questions such as an appeal to the right to dissent from the non-infallible teachings of the Church, a more liberal application of the principle of material cooperation, a more realistic understanding of the fact and facets of pluralism in America, and a more tolerant recognition of the right to freedom of conscience.[27]

Beginning early in 1972, reports of problems with the new Code of 1971 began to come in from various dioceses—the Diocese of Baker, Oregon, the Archdiocese of Detroit, Mich., the Diocese of Green Bay, Wis., the Diocese of Juneau, Alaska. At a meeting of the Committee on Health Affairs on Feb. 9, 1972, the members voted for the establishment of a special committee to study such reports and reactions and to convey their concerns and possible solutions to the Committee on Health Affairs. In due time, 17 members were appointed to serve on that special committee including two bishops, three theologians, and representatives of various professions such as medicine, health-care administration, psychiatry, nursing, sociology, etc., as well as representatives of Diocesan Directors of Hospitals (Bishops' representatives for hospital affairs).[28]

The first meeting of this Special Committee on Ethical and Religious Directives on Jan. 25, 1973, at the United States Catholic Conference under the chairmanship of Archbishop John Quinn, was a challenging introduction to sensitive and complicated problems of the present and future. The proceedings of this meeting included a discussion of an alarming case of civil

---

[26]"Questions and Answers on the Ethical and Religious Directives for Catholic Hospitals," *Hospital Progress*, October, 1971, p. 70.

[27]Cf. Deddens, Clarence, *Doctoral Dissertation* (cf. note 17), pp. 40–44, for a review of the adverse comments of the three theologians originally designated to write a revision of "code of 1958," namely Father John Connery, S.J. (mild comments), Father Richard McCormick, S.J. (strong comments) and Father Paul McKeever (mild comments). The more extensive adverse comments of Father Warren Reich are also presented.

[28]*Ibid.*, pp. 108–116. The committee members are listed on p. 116, note 10. The two members of the hierarchy were Archbishop John Quinn (then of Oklahoma City, Okla.) and Bishop Walter Curtis of Bridgeport, Conn. The theologians were Father Thomas O'Donnell, S.J., Father Austin Vaughan (later Auxiliary Bishop of the Archdiocese of New York) and Father Anthony Kosnik.

litigation against two Catholic hospitals in Montana which had denied a patient's demand for a tubal ligation following a cesarean section; an extremely lengthy discussion of the confusion caused by either misunderstanding of or dissent from the directive on sterilization procedures (Directive 20); and a brief discussion of the principle of material cooperation.[29] The reports on the work of this committee provide an excellent opportunity to gain insights into the theological issues as encountered in their discussions.

1) The Problem of Direct Sterilization by Tubal Ligation

The core of confusion could be traced to the fact that some hospital authorities and theologians were disposed to make a distinction between procedures *done primarily for contraception* and *directly-contraceptive sterilization*. The truth is that procedures done primarily for contraception (as stated in Directive 20: contraception IS the purpose) are all examples of directly-contraceptive sterilization. When the Principle of the Double Effect (or the "indirect voluntary") is applied to a sterilization procedure which is chosen uniquely because another pregnancy might pose a danger to a woman with a serious heart condition or chronic kidney disease (a serious pathological condition outside of the generative system), it is clear that the desired objective (freedom from conception) is realized through the sterilizing procedure (hysterectomy, tubal ligation, vasectomy, etc.). This is directly-contraceptive sterilization.

In resolving value conflicts in any procedure which involves the generative system, the Principle of Double Effect must be applied.[30] This statement is based on the fact that the blessing of human procreation is subordinated primarily not to the good of the individual, but to the good of society. Hence (as will be emphasized in following chapters) the individual has only a limited domination over the generative or reproductive function. A procedure may be allowed only if any consequent sterilization is willed *indirectly* as a foreseen but unintended and merely permitted side effect of a procedure required for the cure of some serious pathological condition *of the generative system* (for example, hysterectomy for a woman in early pregnancy who is a victim of advanced uterine cancer).

In defense of their contention that some procedures done primarily for contraceptive purpose should be considered as *indirect* sterilization, some theologians have proposed that a distinction be made between sterilizations made

---

[29]*Ibid.*, pp. 116–117.

[30]*Ibid.*, pp. 118–120. The problem was submitted by the Cardinal-Archbishop of the Archdiocese of Los Angeles, Cal.

for *medical reasons* (for example, for serious heart or kidney condition) and sterilization for *non-medical reasons* (simply the determination NOT to have another child). These theologians considered the latter to be directly contraceptive and prohibited whereas they would allow the former (for medical reasons) as indirectly contraceptive. Jesuit Fathers John Connery and Thomas O'Donnell were asked to draft a response to this line of thought. Their response states in part:

> Admittedly, Directive #20 makes reference to a pathological condition, and in this sense calls for a medical reason. But the presence of a medical reason does not make the procedure non-contraceptive, nor does the directive imply this in any way. If the procedure achieves its goal by preventing a pregnancy, it is directly contraceptive, whether that goal be medical or not. And if it is directly contraceptive, it does not meet the requirement of the directive.[31]

2) The Importance of a Canonical and a Civil Law Review of the Directives

As early as June 1st, 1972, the Catholic Hospital Association had issued a memorandum to all member health facilities, advising sponsoring groups of Catholic health facilities to:

> . . . take a canonical stand by their Provincial Councils and/or General Council, as well as by their respective Corporations and to formulate a RESOLUTION OF statement of policy, reaffirming and adopting the revised ETHICAL AND RELIGIOUS DIRECTIVES FOR CATHOLIC HEALTH FACILITIES as promulgated by the United States Catholic Conference.

The recommended form of resolution stated that such health facilities "shall require that all persons associated with the health facility agree to adhere to the *Ethical and Religious Directives for Catholic Health Facilities* as promulgated by the United States Catholic Conference and implemented by the local ordi-

---

[31]*Ibid.*, pp. 120–121. Cf. *Medicine and Christian Morality* by Father Thomas O'Donnell, S.J. (New York, N.Y.: Alba House, 1976), p. 115, for the significant observation that the word "ordinarily" is used in directive 6 ("ordinarily the proportionate reason . . .") precisely to indicate that the principle of totality cannot be used to justify direct sterilization.

nary."[32] Without such corporate evidence of adherence to the values and principles underlying the Code of 1971, both on the part of Catholic health facilities and their sponsoring groups, the Church could well become embroiled in protracted cases of civil litigation.

Nine months later (March 7, 1973), John Cardinal Krol of Philadelphia, then President of the National Conference of Catholic Bishops, addressed the same urgency in a letter to all of the bishops of the United States. The letter began as follows:

> As you know, the law suit in Billings, Montana, involving a sterilization operation in a Catholic hospital is a most serious matter. Because of the far-reaching implications of litigation such as this, the USCC Administrative Board, last November, asked the USCC Committee on Law and Public Policy to give consideration to the matter.

Cardinal Krol then listed the recommendations of that Committee on Law and Public Policy (promulgation of the Code of 1971 by the local ordinary; adoption of that Code by a formal vote of the Board of Directors or Trustees of each hospital; dissemination of knowledge of the directives of the Code among staff and patients; and the creation of medical committees within the hospital organization). He also recommended recourse to legal safeguards against civil litigation as follows:

> . . . passage of appropriate local legislation immunizing the personnel of hospitals and kindred institutions from civil and criminal liability for refraining from performing medical and surgical procedures contrary to their religious and ethical convictions.[33]

This important subject will be discussed briefly in Chapter X on the *Principle of Material Cooperation.* Its significance for now is to point to the obvious arguments for an early promulgation of the Directive by local ordinaries and its adoption by Catholic health facilities.

3) Eventual Clarification of Sterilization and Material Cooperation

At the Sept. 19, 1973, meeting of the Special Committee for the Ethical and Religious Directives (of the United States Catholic Conference) it was

---

[32]From the files of the Catholic Health Association, St. Louis, Mo. as well as the files of the Pope John Center, Braintree, Mass.

[33]Deddens, Clarence, *Doctoral Dissertation* (cf. note 17), p. 123.

moved, seconded and passed (as this advisory committee had recommended to the Committee on Health Affairs) that Catholic hospitals cannot provide abortion services based on the principle of material cooperation. The same motion could not be reached at that meeting, however, with regard to sterilization. When this recommendation on abortion was accepted by the Committee on Health Affairs at their Oct. 17, 1973 meeting, it was the first time that an official interpretation of the directives was made in terms of material cooperation.[34]

A significant turn of events unfolded at the May 15, 1974 meeting of the Committee on Health Affairs. The Chairman, Bishop Edward Head of Buffalo, N.Y., read the following resolution which had been passed by the Administrative Board of the United States Catholic Conference on Feb. 13th, 1974.

> Be it resolved that for the benefit of the Catholic health apostolate, commentaries be developed by the Committee on Health Affairs in the form of interpretations, clarifications and other specific information concerning the *Ethical and Religious Directives*. Any matter touching doctrine or morality is to be submitted to the National Conference of Catholic Bishops' Committee on Doctrine for approval . . .[35]

By virtue of this new mandate, Father John Connery, S.J. prepared a draft on the Principle of Material Cooperation for the Nov. 22, 1974 meeting of the special advisory committee. Father Deddens states that it was the committee's decision to consider the topic of material cooperation both as a directive and as a commentary. Due to the fact that Father Connery was to be in Rome for the next two months, however, Father Thomas O'Donnell, S.J. was asked to review the proposed directive and commentary.

The fact is that the review of the proposed directive and commentary on cooperation was held in abeyance. A likely explanation of this change of tactics is that Bishop Maurice Dingman of Des Moines, Iowa, succeeded Bishop Head as Chairman of the Committee on Health Affairs at the Feb. 13, 1975 meeting of the special committee not only as Chairman of the Committee on Health Affairs but as Chairman of the Special Committee for Ethical and Religious Directives as well. In all probability, Bishop Dingman may have allowed the matter to remain "on hold" pending a very important event

---

[34]*Ibid.*, pp. 124–125.
[35]*Ibid.*, p. 126.

which was to take place within the next few months—an official decision and clarification from Rome on the subject of material cooperation and sterilization.[36]

The fact that many Catholic hospitals were performing sterilizations based on the views of some theologians (that this was in accord with the Principle of Material Cooperation) indicated that the hospital directives on the subject of sterilization were in need of clarification. Archbishop Quinn and several other bishops had an audience with Pope Paul VI as well as a meeting with members of the Sacred Congregation for the Doctrine of the Faith in early 1975. Father Deddens provides evidence that an effort was made to impress upon the Holy Father the pluralistic character of health care in the United States.[37] The Holy See's response entitled *Reply of the Sacred Congregation of the Faith on Sterilization in Catholic Hospitals,* was dated March 13, 1975. There will be ample opportunities throughout this book to comment adequately on this historic document. It may suffice to say for now that the reply specifically confirmed the traditional doctrine of the Church on contraceptive sterilization as expressed in Directive 20 of the revised *Ethical and Religious Directives for Catholic Health Facilities.*[38]

1.3 COMMENTARY (1977) AND STATEMENT (1980) OF THE AMERICAN HIERARCHY

The reference to the application of the *Principle of Material Cooperation* emphasized the need for some type of official commentary from the American Bishops. Although Archbishop Bernardin, then President of the National Conference of Catholic Bishops, informed the American Bishops of the substance of the Roman reply by letter of April 14, 1975, the bishops still did not have the actual text as of late October, 1975. The efforts to prepare a proper commentary began with the Committee on Health Affairs as early as May, 1975 when Bishop Dingman announced that the *Special Committee on Ethical and Religious Directives* (sometimes referred to as the "Advisory Committee") was working on a paper on material cooperation which would be brought to the Committee on Health Affairs in due time. Despite diligent efforts on the part of the Committee on Health Affairs and the Advisory Committee to arrive at unanimity of thought in producing that commentary on the Roman

---

[36]*Ibid.*, pp. 127–128.

[37]*Ibid.*, pp. 128–129.

[38]*Canon Law Digest*, VIII (Mundelein, Ill.: St. Mary of the Lake Seminary, 1978), pp. 924–926.

Reply of March 13, 1975, their report to the Administrative Committee incorporated also minority positions as expressed by those participants who wished to have such positions reported.[39]

The solution to this delay came from the Administrative Committee of the USCC. The task of writing the commentary was assigned to the Committee on Doctrine. The finished product, entitled *Commentary on the Reply of the Sacred Congregation For the Doctrine of the Faith on Sterilization in Catholic Hospitals* was published on September 15, 1977. The "Guidelines for Hospital Policy" as presented in this *Commentary* stress the conditions under which material cooperation might be justified in a Catholic hospital—conditions which will be discussed at length in several chapters of this book. Since a certain degree of confusion continued to persist even after the publication of the Commentary of September 15, 1977, especially with regard to tubal ligations, the National Conference of Catholic Bishops issued a further clarification on July 3, 1980 entitled *Statement on Tubal Ligation.*[40]

Additions to the Hospital Directives in 1975

The current edition of the *Ethical and Religious Directives for Catholic Health Facilities* as approved by the American hierarchy in Nov., 1971 bears a small notation: "Revised—1975." First, there was the need of incorporating the recommendation with regard to abortion services in Catholic hospitals as accepted by the Committee on Health Affairs on Oct. 17, 1973 (cf.page 12). As of the 1975 printing, therefore, the directive on abortion (n.12) ends with the following: "Catholic hospitals are not to provide abortion services based upon the principle of material cooperation." This marked the first and only mention of the phrase "material cooperation" in the present directives.

The longest addition to the "revised-1975" version of the hospital Code concerns the "Sacraments of the Sick" as they are called in Directive n.41 of the November, 1971 version, which was formulated as follows:

> When possible, one who is seriously ill should be given the opportunity to receive the Sacraments of the Sick, while in full possession of his rational faculties. The chaplain must, therefore, be notified as soon as an illness is diagnosed as being so serious that some probability of death is recognized.

---

[39]Deddens, Clarence, *Doctoral Dissertation* (cf. note 17), pp. 130–133.
[40]For the *Commentary,* as well as the *Statement on Tubal Ligation,* cf. appendix, lines 68 ff. (commentary) and lines 181 ff. (statement).

Due to the significant changes and refinements with regard to the sacramental care of the sick as elaborated in the documents of the Second Vatican Council and implemented in the *Revised Roman Ritual,* the revised-1975 version of the *Ethical and Religious Directives for Catholic Health Facilities* made a substantial addition by treating the subject of the "Sacraments of the Sick" as follows:

–The administration of the Sacrament of the Anointing of the Sick, *Directive 41*

–The administration of Viaticum, *Directive 41a*

–The administration of the continuous rite (penance, anointing, and the Eucharist as viaticum in one service), *Directive 42b*

These were the last additions to the present hospital directives. The *Commentary* on sterilization of September 15, 1977, and the *Statement* on tubal ligations of July 3, 1980, were relevant to the interpretation and observance of the regulations but were not incorporated into the directives. At the general meeting of the bishops in May, 1977, a decision was made to consolidate the Committee on Health Affairs with the Department on Social Development. At the general meeting of the U.S. Catholic Conference in November, 1985, the bishops authorized the creation of a new position in the Department of Social Development and World Peace (formal title: "Specialist in Catholic Health Care Sponsorship"). The major responsibility of this official will be to assist the bishops and diocesan staff on issues arising from changing conditions in the administration or sponsorship of Catholic health care institutions.[41] The primary agency for regularly receiving "suggestions and recommendations from the field" on moral-medical problems, and for periodically discussing "any possible need for an updated version of these *Directives*" (preamble, paragraph 7), however, will continue to be the Committee on Doctrine of the United States Catholic Conference.

1.4   DIRECTIVES PRESENTED AS APPLICATIONS OF ACCEPTED PRINCIPLES

Rules and regulations, especially if they are both normative and binding, usually are accepted more readily if they are seen as applications of general principles which are accepted and observed widely among moral theologians and ethicists in seeking solutions to moral-medical problems. The *Ethical and*

---

[41]Letters to this writer from Rev. Robert N. Lynch, Associate General Secretary, USCC, July 29, 1985, and from Rev. J. Bryan Hehir, Secretary of the Department of Social Development and World Peace, Feb. 19, 1986 and March 3, 1986.

Religious Directives for Catholic Health Facilities remind all Catholic health facilities of their "responsibility to reflect in [their] policies and practices the moral teachings of the Church, under the guidance of the local bishop" (preamble, paragraph 4). They were approved at the annual meeting of the National Conference of Catholic Bishops and the United States Catholic Conference in November, 1971, "as the national code, subject to the approval of the bishop for use in the diocese" (prefatory note on the inside front cover of the publication: *Ethical and Religious Directives for Catholic Health Facilities*).

As an additional means of presenting the following nine principles as responding to contemporary needs in the solution of moral-medical problems, a special effort has been made throughout this book to base or fortify these principles with quotations from one of the documents of the Second Vatican Council. Most of these quotations are from the *Pastoral Constitution on the Church in the World Today* (Gaudium et Spes). The nine principles which will be presented and discussed to provide a working basis for the understanding, interpretation and application of the *Ethical and Religious Directives for Catholic Health Facilities* (to be referred to in most instances throughout this book as *Catholic Hospital Directives*) are the following:

Chapter II—The Principle of Human Dignity
Chapter III—The Principle of the Right to Life
Chapter IV—The Principle of Religious Freedom
Chapter V—The Principle of Informed Consent
Chapter VI—The Principles of Integrity and Totality
Chapter VII—The Principle of the Double Effect
Chapter VIII—The Principle of the Common Good
Chapter IX—The Principle of Confidentiality
Chapter X—The Principles of Material Cooperation

Each one of the nine principles will be stated but once at the head of each chapter. The reader will note, however, that successive sections of each chapter will correspond to another portion of the principle as stated at the head of the chapter. The objective has been to permeate each discussion, insofar as possible, with the basic meaning of the principle. Finally, after each major discussion of one of the 43 *Catholic Hospital Directives,* the actual wording of the directive will be presented in "boxed in" format.

Fortunately the discussions throughout all chapters can be integrated with reference to and interpretation of canons of the new *Code of Canon Law* as they apply to moral-medical issues. Unfortunately, the effort to trace the moral implications of all contemporary medical-societal challenges and of the advances in medical technology must, of necessity, leave something to be desired. This effort is circumscribed not only by the near-impossibility of keeping "up to date" with progress on the medical technology front, but also by the subject matter as limited to the parameters of the 43 Directives of the *Ethical and Religious Directives for Catholic Health Facilities*.

CHAPTER II

The Principle of Human Dignity

An outstanding cause of human dignity lies in man's call to communion with God. From the very circumstances of his origin, man is already invited to converse with God. For man could not exist were he not created by God's love and constantly preserved by it. And he cannot live fully according to truth unless he freely acknowledges that love and devotes himself to his creator (*Pastoral Constitution on the Church Today*, n.19).

PRINCIPLE: HUMAN DIGNITY, GROUNDED AS IT IS ON MANKIND'S CALL TO COMMUNION WITH GOD, REQUIRES THAT HUMAN INSTITUTIONS BOTH PRIVATE AND PUBLIC MUST MINISTER TO THE PHYSICAL, PSYCHOLOGICAL, SOCIAL, AND ABOVE ALL, THE SPIRITUAL NEEDS OF EVERY HUMAN PERSON. BECAUSE OF THAT SUBLIME DIGNITY, THE HUMAN PERSON STANDS ABOVE ALL THINGS WITH RIGHTS AND DUTIES THAT ARE UNIVERSAL AND INVIOLABLE, INCLUDING THE RIGHT TO HAVE READY ACCESS TO ALL THAT IS NECESSARY FOR LIVING A GENUINELY HUMAN LIFE (Adapted from *The Church Today*, nn.19,26,27,29).

As stated in the *Pastoral Constitution on the Church Today* (to be referred to hereafter as *The Church Today*): "Since all men possess a rational soul and are created in God's likeness, since they have the same nature and origin, have been redeemed by Christ, and enjoy the same divine calling and destiny, the basic equality of all must receive increasingly greater recognition" (n.29). It is that equality based on human dignity which makes the command of love of God and neighbor and the "golden rule" intelligible. That golden rule, enshrined in the cultures of ancient peoples well before the time of Christ, was proclaimed by Christ in the Sermon on the Mount: "Treat others the way you would have them treat you: this sums up the law and the prophets" (Matthew,7:12). He proclaimed it, however, on the basis of love of neighbor (Matthew 19:19). On an even higher level, He proposed this regard for human dignity as a *manifestation* of our love of God: "I assure you, as often as you did it for one of my least brethren, you did it for me" (Matthew,25:40).

That same Vatican II document (*The Church Today*) states, in effect, that we are to love people and use things, and not love things and use people (n.26), quoting Mark,2:27: "The sabbath was made for man, not man for the sabbath." That is why the human person stands above all things. That hierarchy of values is violated whenever, by intention or by deed or attitude, the principal motive behind any action or any relationship with another person is some utility to be realized or some pleasure to be gained. It is in large part because many who call themselves Christians have put **things** before persons, or have *used* persons to acquire things, that Christianity has lost much of its appeal among the working classes, the intellectuals, and others in our contemporary world.[42] The Catholic faith, with its emphasis on a fundamental call to communion with God, guarantees men and women a dignity which no other agency can provide.

2.1 "COMMUNION WITH GOD" THROUGH BAPTISM

The first two paragraphs of the preamble to the Catholic Hospital Directives establish witnessing "to the saving presence of Christ and His Church" and concern for the spiritual and physical welfare of every patient, as the

---

[42]As Cardinal Koenig pointed out in remarks to the Fathers of Vatican II, atheism has its root not in Asia or Africa, but in the western world where Christianity has been preached for 2,000 years. Cf. *Commentary on the Documents of Vatican II,* 5 vols., V, Herbert Vorgrimler, ed. (New York, N.Y.: Herder and Herder, 1969), p. 147.

distinctive mark of every Catholic health facility. To quote the second paragraph of the preamble:

> The total good of the patient, which includes his higher spiritual as well as his bodily welfare, is the primary concern of those entrusted with the management of a Catholic health facility. So important is this, in fact, that if an institution could not fulfill its basic mission in this regard, it would have no justification for continuing its existence as a Catholic health facility. Trustees and administrators of Catholic health facilities should understand that this responsibility affects their relationship with every patient, regardless of religion, and is seriously binding in conscience.

The baptism of infants in emergency situations is a special concern in the Church's mission of healing. Through baptism an individual "is constituted a person in the Church" (*Code of Canon Law*, to be referred to hereafter as Can. and number, in this case, Can.96) as a member of the "People of God" (Can.204,1) and becomes "fully in communion with the Catholic Church" (Can.205). The standard precaution is: "If the fetus is not certainly dead, it should be baptized" (Directive n.13).

The situations which require quick action in administering baptism include spontaneous abortions (miscarriages), hysterectomies when pregnant women are victims of a serious pathological condition of the uterus, premature and/or difficult deliveries, etc. If time allows, doubtful cases as to how, when, and even "what" to baptize should be referred to the hospital chaplain. Precious time should not be wasted in looking for signs of life. The only certain sign of death is corruption as indicated by easily-detected factors such as putrefaction, decomposition, offensive odor, discoloration of flesh, etc. If the fetus is not "certainly dead," baptism should be administered *conditionally* ("If you are alive, I baptize you . . ."). If such words of conditional baptism should be omitted for whatever reasons (nervous, in doubt, simply forgot) the validity of the baptism is not in question as long as the words of baptizing are pronounced as the water is being poured and provided that it is done with the desire or intention (at least implicit) of baptizing "according to the mind of the Church."[43] A small embryo may be baptized by immersion. The membranes of the amniotic sac are separated with thumb and forefinger and the words of baptism are pronounced as the embryo is immersed in a bowl of water a *second* time (a *first* immersion is required to wash the amniotic fluid from the embryo). With this precaution, the water will come in direct contact with the fetus or embryo.

The Necessity of Baptism

The current trend in some quarters to minimize the importance of baptism cannot be reconciled with the constant tradition of the Church. The *Instruction on Infant Baptism* as issued by the Holy See on October 20, 1980, strongly reiterates the traditional teaching of the Church on the necessity of baptism for salvation. With regard to infants who die without baptism, there is no inference that they will be denied salvation. The *Instruction* simply states: "the Church can do nothing more than to commit them to the mercy of God."[44] Other recent declarations on the necessity of baptism are found in Canon 849 of the *Code of Canon Law,* and in Vatican II's *Dogmatic Constitution on the Church* (n.14) which refers to Mark,16:16 and to John,3:5.

Canon 868,2, states that in danger-of-death cases, the baptism of the infant *even* of non-Catholic parents (as in the case of an infant of Catholic parents) is licitly administered even though the parents are unwilling ("etiam invitis parentibus"). Due to the overriding priority of eternal salvation, the phrase "etiam invitis parentibus" can be interpreted to mean "even if one or both parents are opposed to the baptism,"—provided that the baptism can be administered unobtrusively without incurring resentment or bitterness to-

---

[43]Kelly, Gerald, S.J., *Medico-Moral Problems* (cf. note 22), p. 299, suggests that there is no harm done if, when flustered as in emergency or doubtful situations, the phrases "if you are alive," or "if you have not been baptized" (in conditional baptisms) are unintentionally omitted: "The main thing is to say the essential words and pour the water (or immerse) correctly, with the desire to baptize according to the mind of the Church." Even if the baptism is administered in emergency cases by non-Catholics or ministers of other Christian denominations, the baptism is NOT to be presumed to be invalid "because of the lack of the requisite intention on the part of the minister to do what the Church does or what Christ instituted" unless the contrary is proved in a particular case. If the right *matter* (pouring of water) and *form* (words of baptism) are used, the baptism is to be presumed to be valid unless there is evidence to the contrary. Cf. *Canon Law Digest,* III (Milwaukee, Wis.: Bruce Publishing Co., 2nd printing, 1956), p. 423. This response of the Holy Office of Dec. 28, 1949, referred to baptisms administered by the Disciples of Christ, the Presbyterians, the Congregationalists, the Baptists and the Methodists insofar as these denominations were mentioned expressly in the question submitted to the Holy Office.

[44]*Canon Law Digest,* IX (Mundelein, Ill.: St. Mary of the Lake Seminary, 1983), p. 515.

wards the Church."[45] It can be done unobtrusively without detection by the parents by placing a water-soaked piece of cotton batting on the forehead of the infant (who is in danger of death) so that the water trickles along the skin of the infant as the words of baptism are pronounced (even inaudibly if necessary). Since these "little ones" often do not live long, the procedure does not amount to "signing them up" as members of the Catholic Church. Hence the non-Catholic parents could not accuse the hospital authorities of proselytism or of having usurped their parental rights.

In other words, unless there are definite reasons to presume that one or both of the non-Catholic parents or the non-Catholic of a mixed marriage is strongly opposed to the baptism, it is proper ("the supreme law is the salvation of souls") NOT to wait for the parents to ask for the baptism of their infant or to object to the baptism in such emergency cases, but to take advantage of an occasion to baptize the fetus or infant unobtrusively. If the parents spontaneously express strong opposition to baptism, and there simply is no occasion to administer the baptism unobtrusively, the only solution is to omit the baptism so as to avoid resentment or hostility towards the Church. The Church "commits [such infants] to the mercy of God." If both parents are Catholics, it can be presumed that they are willing to have the baptism administered. If the parents are non-Catholics and indicate an interest in having the infant baptized, it is right and proper to invite them to contact their minister to "do the honors." In most cases, however, the emergency will be such that time will not allow an ecumenical gesture of that nature.

The Minister of Baptism

The general rule is that baptism is not to be administered in hospitals "except in case of necessity or for some other pressing pastoral reason"

---

[45]The *Instruction on Infant Baptism* of Oct.20,1980(cf.p.23) speaks of the mission the Church has received from God of offering to all who can be baptized, rebirth "out of water and the Holy Spirit" . . ., "and adds that "[The Church] does not, outside of danger of death, admit an infant except with the consent of the parents . . ." *Ibid.*, pp. 515, 516. The inference is that in a danger of death situation, an infant could be baptized *without* the consent of the parents. The baptism should be omitted, however, if it would lead to hatred or bitterness towards the Church. It must be noted, however, that the argument for omitting baptism in a situation which would involve the danger of hatred towards the Church was not adopted in the study-group consultation in finalizing the wording of Can.868,2. Cf."Canons 867 and 868 and Baptizing Infants Against the Will of Parents," by John W. Robertson, *Jurist,*45(1985):2, pp.631–638. Cf. also *Commentary: The Code of Canon Law,* ed. by James A. Coriden, Thomas J. Green, Donald E. Heintschel (New York, N.Y.: Paulist Press, 1985), p. 627. To be referred to hereafter as *CLSA Commentary, 1985.*

(Can.860,2). Likewise due to the urgency of the situation, ". . . only those elements which are required for the validity of the sacrament must be observed" (Can.850). The elements for validity are expressed in *Directive 36* as quoted below. Only "true" water may be used (Can.849). Liquids such as milk, wine, fruit juice, amniotic fluid, saliva, etc., would make the baptism invalid. If a sponsor is not present at an emergency baptism (not necessary and usually not possible), an effort should be made to have at least one witness standing by "who can prove that the baptism was conferred" (Can.875). This would be important for survivors of any emergency baptism who later present themselves for the reception of other sacraments (confirmation, marriage, etc.). Additional proof of baptism might be required if that person is involved in a declaration of nullity of marriage later on. The reason is because the rights of another person may be adversely affected.

The hospital chaplain should be informed of all emergency baptisms. He is not only in charge of all spiritual and sacramental ministrations and responsible for supervising the administration of sacraments by others, but also has the obligation of attending to the registration of baptisms in accord with Canon 878.

Special Situations in Emergency Infant Baptisms

Some of the procedures mentioned below were specified in the former *Code of Canon Law,* but are not included in the new and shorter code which went into effect in 1983. Even though such former canons are considered as abrogated (Can.6,1), the directives contained therein still apply as time-tested applications of sound theological principles.

Baptism in the Womb: No one is to be baptized while still in the womb as long as there is a probable hope that baptism can be conferred in proper form after delivery. In danger of death cases, the necessity of baptism can provide a proportionate reason for inducing labor so as to hasten the delivery of a viable infant (cf.*Directive* 23). If the head emerges at the time of delivery and the danger of death is imminent, the infant is to be baptized on the head. There would be no need to re-baptize the infant conditionally later on if he or she survives. If some other member of the body emerges first (arm, leg, shoulder, breech presentation) and death is imminent, baptism should be administered conditionally ("If you are alive . . .") with re-baptism on the head later on ("If you have not been baptized . . .") in the event of survival.

If there is danger that the infant might die before delivery, it should be baptized in the womb if at all possible. Due to the danger of infection in the process, however, the baptism should be administered by a physician or a trained nurse. After making a small opening through the membranes surrounding the infant (amnion, chorion, decidua), the physician or nurse inserts a sterile bulb containing sterile water and directs the flow so that it touches the skin directly. The words of baptism should be pronounced by that same person while the water is flowing. Some authors would apply the *Principle of the Double Effect* to justify attempting such a baptism even if the fetus is not viable and there is some danger of causing an abortion.[46] It would be wrong, however, on the basis of "the end does not justify the means," to bring about an abortion precisely in order to baptize the infant. *Intrauterine* baptisms are doubtfully valid; hence they are to be repeated conditionally after the infant has been delivered, or if there is at least a head presentation (in a difficult delivery). It is the chaplain's responsibility to instruct physicians and nurses with regard to all "unusual situation" baptisms (as above, and as below).

When the Pregnant Mother has Died: The chaplain should make it his concern to urge the surviving parent to have a *living* infant extracted from the mother's womb as soon after death as the laws of the state permit. This would apply only if there is at least some probability that the infant is alive. In similar circumstances, a *living* infant could also be delivered by cesarean section. In order to avoid possible civil-law problems and/or hostility towards the Church, however, such a surgical alternative should not be attempted without the consent of the husband,[47]—and never without first checking the civil law in the matter. The danger of legal complications increases if the intent is to deliver a deceased mother of an *inviable* infant merely in order to administer baptism. In such a situation, the prudent course is to attempt an intrauterine baptism.

Baptism of Abnormal Infants: The general rule is that all abnormal fetuses (also known as "monstrosities") are to be baptized at least conditionally ("If you are capable . . ."). If there is doubt as to whether the fetus is one person or more than one person, one head should be baptized absolutely (that is, without the "If you are capable . . ." condition) and the others conditionally. Possibilities of abnormality include the following: two heads with two bodies, or two bodies with one head, or two heads with one body, or a double-faced head, or a headless body, etc. If the rule suggested above presents a difficulty

---

[46]Healy, Edwin F., S.J., *Medical Ethics* (Chicago, Ill.: Loyola University Press, 1956), pp. 364, 365.

[47]If the fetus is living *and viable,* a cesarean section may be performed even without the consent of the parent or guardian. If there is doubt as the the civil law in that regard, however, legal advice is recommended. Cf. Kelly, Gerald, S.J., *Medico-Moral Problems* (cf. note 22), p. 302.

(for example, no heads at all), Father Gerald Kelly's suggestion will be practical: simply pour water over the entire unit, or immerse it (moving it in the water) while pronouncing the words of baptism *with the intention of baptizing as many persons as are present.*[48]

Directive 13 (in part): . . . If the fetus is not certainly dead, it should be baptized.

Directive 35: Except in cases of emergency (i.e. danger of death), all requests for baptism made by adults or for infants should be referred to the chaplain of the health facility.

Directive 36: If a priest is not available, anyone having the use of reason and proper intention can baptize. The ordinary method of conferring emergency baptism is as follows: The person baptizing pours water on the head in such a way that it will flow on the skin, and, while the water is being poured, must pronounce these words audibly: *I baptize you in the name of the Father, and of the Son, and of the Holy Spirit.* The same person who pours the water must pronounce the words.

Directive 37: When emergency baptism is conferred, the chaplain should be notified.

2.2 OUR HIGHER SPIRITUAL WELFARE—PRIORITY OF SPIRITUAL NEEDS

Vatican II's document, *The Church Today,* refers to the Church's ministry of healing and reconciliation as having a "healing and elevating impact on the dignity of the person, by the way in which she strengthens the seams of human society and imbues the everyday activity of men with a deeper meaning and importance" (n.40). As a means of harmonizing contemporary culture with Christian teaching, there is the need to take note "not only of theological principles, but also of the findings of the secular sciences, especially of psychology and sociology" (n.62). The effort to meet psychological and social needs will be discussed more effectively in the final section of this chapter.

---

[48]*Ibid.,* pp. 302, 303.

The priority of spiritual needs extends to every patient in the hospital setting, regardless of age or religious affiliation or background. Pastoral care personnel play a vital role in advancing the mission of spiritual healing and reconciliation. In their visits with non-Catholic patients in an atmosphere of friendship and loving concern, the individual often volunteers information on his or her religious affiliation, on their family origins, and even on their spiritual needs. In many cases, especially if they have no religious affiliation or if their pastor is not readily available, they may indicate a willingness to pray with the chaplain or pastoral care person, or even to receive the blessing of the chaplain. This is all in keeping with the new ecumenical spirit. When it comes to sharing Catholic sacraments, however, an enlightened spirit of ecumenism requires caution and prudent guidelines.

Sacramental Inter-Communion: Catholics and Eastern-Rite Christians

The general rule is that Catholics may receive the sacraments licitly "only from Catholic ministers" (Can.844,1). Priests of the Eastern or Oriental Rites who are in union with the Catholic Church are listed in the annual *Catholic Directory* (1985 edition, p.991 ff.). Their priests are "Catholic ministers" in the true sense of the word. A recent publication entitled *The New Latin Code of Canon Law and Eastern Christians* lists 21 Eastern Rite jurisdictions in the United States and Canada.[49] Priests of the Eastern *Orthodox* Rites (NOT in union with the Catholic Church) do not rate as "Catholic ministers." Nonetheless, their ordinations as priests are regarded by the Catholic Church as valid. They are *non-Catholic ministers of the Orthodox Rites,* and the sacraments as administered by them are considered to be valid.

There are areas in the U.S.A. where there are no Catholic priests, but where a resident Eastern *Orthodox* priest may have charge of several congregations of his denomination. Catholics living in such areas (no Catholic priest for miles around) may approach such an Eastern Orthodox priest (valid sacraments, but not in union with the Catholic Church) to receive the sacraments of penance, Eucharist, and anointing of the sick "whenever necessity requires or genuine spiritual advantage suggests, and provided that the danger of error or indifferentism is avoided" (Can.844,2). Naturally such Catholics would not have to be in danger of death before taking advantage of the availability of a priest of the Eastern *Orthodox* Rites. Any doubt as to spiritual need or advantage in contacting such a priest should be settled in favor of the

---

[49] *The New Latin Code of Canon Law and Eastern Catholics* by Victor J. Pospishil, JCD, and John D. Faris, JC Orient. D (Brooklyn, N.Y.: Diocese of Saint Maron, 1984), pp. 46–49.

one who asks for one of those three sacraments. The "danger of error or indifferentism" can be interpreted in accord with the teaching of Vatican II's *Decree on the Eastern Churches* (n.26) as forbidding anything "which would damage the unity of the Church, or involve formal acceptance of falsehood or the danger of deviation in the faith, of scandal, or of indifferentism." In other words, a good Roman Catholic should not want to put himself in spiritual danger (for example, the *Orthodox* priest in question is definitely anti-Catholic) in order to fulfill a spiritual need.

A more delicate situation arises if members of an *Eastern Orthodox Rite* in a Catholic hospital request one of those sacraments (penance, Eucharist, anointing) from a Catholic priest. This would also apply to "members of other churches, which in the judgement of the Apostolic See are in the same condition as the oriental churches as far as these sacraments are concerned" (Can.844,3); that is, priests are validly ordained but the group is not in union with the Catholic Church. Requests for one of those sacraments from a Catholic priest can be honored provided that the person asks for the sacrament of his or her own volition ("sponte") and is properly disposed.

Such a request from a member of one of the *Eastern Orthodox Rites* could be a delicate matter. When this matter of inter-communion with Orthodox Christians was discussed by the Fathers of Vatican II, an attitude of caution was advised. In fact, the American Orthodox Bishops reacted unfavorably to such a concession from the Catholic Church at one of their meetings (in 1965).[50] This explains why Canon 844,5, states that in this matter of inter-communion with non-Catholics, the diocesan bishops or the Episcopal Conference of the area "is not to issue general norms except after consultation with the competent authority, at least at the local level, of the interested non-Catholic church or community." This legislation provides some protection against any accusation of proselytism from non-Catholic Christians. If such requests are likely to be made in a Catholic health facility, the chaplain or visiting priest should contact the diocesan bishop and the Eastern Orthodox priest or minister so as to assure ecumenical harmony.

Sacramental Inter-Communion: Catholics and "Our Separated Brethren"

Since the Catholic Church, as a general rule, does not regard the sacraments of "our Separated Brethren" as valid (Episcopalians, Lutherans,

---

[50]*Commentary on the Documents of Vatican II*, 5 vols., I, Herbert Vorgrimler, ed. (New York, N.Y.: Herder and Herder, 1967), p. 329. Cf. also *The Documents of Vatican II*, Walter M. Abbott, S.J., ed. (Piscataway, N.J.: New Century Publishers, Inc., 1966), p. 385, note 58.

Methodists, etc.), Catholic patients in hospitals may not request the sacraments of penance, the Eucharist, or the anointing of the sick from ministers of those denominations. If members of those non-Catholic denominations request any of these sacraments from a Catholic priest, however, the request may be granted in very specific cases. Before speaking of the four conditions which must be fulfilled in every case, it must be emphasized that favorable consideration can be given to such a request only if the non-Catholic petitioner is in danger of death OR in other cases of urgent necessity as may be determined by the diocesan bishop or by the Episcopal Conference of the area (in the U.S.A., that would be our National Council of Catholic Bishops). A reliable interpretation of this canon can be gleaned from several Catholic ecumenical documents. These documents reveal that "other cases of urgent necessity" could include times of persecution and of imprisonment, as well as situations when non-Catholics are in grave spiritual danger because they are scattered in Catholic regions and are "often deprived of the help of their own communion and unable to get in touch with it except at great trouble and expense." One document adds: "But it will be for the bishop to consider each case."[51]

It seems clear that the Church wants this matter of Catholics administering the sacraments to non-Catholics in urgent situations to be *strictly interpreted*. The same sources as quoted above rule out any general regulation "which makes a category out of an exception case," or which uses epikeia [that is, the reasonable moderation of a strict right] to turn an exceptional case into a general category. Again, as in cases of Catholics receiving these sacraments from ministers or priests of oriental churches (Can.844,2), and of Catholics administering these sacraments to members of oriental churches (Can.844,3), "neither the diocesan bishop nor the conference of bishops is to enact general norms except after consultation with at least the local competent authority of the interested non-Catholic church or community" (Can.844,5). Apparently these rather complicated regulations have been enacted in an effort to balance ecumenical Christian charity with the danger of offending the sensitivities of other denominations.

---

[51]Cf. two declarations from the Secretariate for the Promotion of Christian Unity: *The Declaration on the Position of the Catholic Church on the Celebration of the Eucharist In Common by Christians of Different Confessions,* Jan. 7, 1970, n. 7, and, *On Admitting Other Christians to Eucharistic Communion in the Catholic Church,* June 1, 1972, n. 55. Both documents are found in *Vatican Council II,* 1981 edition, Austin Flannery, O.P., ed. (Northport, N.Y.: Costello Publishing Co., 1980), pp. 505 and 559 respectively. A third document from the same Secretariate entitled, *Note Interpreting the Instruction on Admitting Other Christians to Eucharistic Communion in the Catholic Church Under Certain Circumstances,* issued on Oct. 17, 1973, n. 6., *Ibid.,* p. 561, is also quoted above.

The *four conditions* to be fulfilled (in addition to the pre-conditions of "danger of death" or "other cases of urgent necessity") are the following:
1) The non-Catholic patient is not able to have access to a minister of his or her own denomination. If the address or phone number of the minister is available and time allows, an effort should be made to contact the minister. Naturally this would not apply if the patient is dying ("in articulo mortis").
2) The non-Catholic makes the request of his or her own volition. The very spirit of ecumenism would be violated if the nurse said: "Shall I have the Catholic chaplain bring you Holy Communion?" There would be no objection if the request came spontaneously in answer to: "Is there anything I can do for you?"
3) The non-Catholic manifests a faith in these sacraments which is in conformity with that of the Catholic Church. This should involve more than an affirmation of the Real Presence. The requirement apparently would be fulfilled if the patient manifests a "serious spiritual need for Eucharistic sustenance."[52]
4) The non-Catholic patient is properly disposed. One of the sources referred to above states: "provided that they have proper dispositions and lead lives worthy of a Christian;" and adds that even if all conditions are fulfilled, "it will be a pastoral responsibility to see that the admission of these other Christians to communion does not endanger the faith of Catholics."[53] All of these precautions emphasize, regretfully but realistically, that our "separated brethren" are not in full communion with the Catholic Church.

Other aspects of the administration of the sacraments in a hospital setting (baptism, anointing, etc., outside of "danger of death" situations) will be discussed in chapter IV under the *Principle of Religious Freedom*.

Directive 34: The administration should be certain that patients in a health facility receive appropriate spiritual care.

---

[52]Documents of June 1, 1972 (n. IV, 2), and of Oct. 17, 1973 (n. 7), as in note above. *Ibid.*, pp. 557 and 562 respectively.
[53]*Ibid.*, pp. 557, 558.

2.3 THE PRIORITY OF PERSONHOOD

Based on human personhood and dignity, human rights are inviolable. Based on the equality of all human individuals, they are universal. No individual's rights are limited because of "quality of life" considerations. There is no diminution of rights because an individual may be retarded or physically incapacitated. It is only when human rights are fully respected that the individual is free to fulfill his or her obligations with regard to God and society. The phrase "the human person stands above all things" is of prime significance. The properly-guided will of the individual patient is the final determinant in decision-making and self-determination with regard to his or her welfare.

Among the "many subjects arousing universal concern today," Vatican II's document on *The Church Today* (n.46) assigns first place to marriage and the family. If there is any area of human endeavor where things are preferred to people and where people are used as things, it is in the critical area of marriage and human sexuality. Throughout Vatican II's *The Church Today*, the centrality of human love in Christian marriage is emphasized. Referring to conjugal love as "eminently human," and as "uniquely expressed and perfected through the sexual act," the document continues: "Expressed in a manner which is truly human, these actions signify and promote that mutual self-giving by which spouses enrich each other with a joyful and thankful will" (n.49). Just as the intrinsic ordination between the marital act and prospect of new life cannot be denied, so the procreative element (new life) cannot be excluded or separated positively from the unitive (conjugal love) without depriving Christian marriage of its God-given human dignity. It is noteworthy that the distinguished ethicist, Dr. Paul Ramsey (not of the Catholic faith) echoes similar sentiments: "Neither should there be among men and women (whose man-womanhood—and not their minds only—is in the image of God), any love set out of the context of responsibility for procreation, any begetting apart from the sphere of love."[54]

The positive *exclusion* of children in marriage (contraception) will be discussed in the next chapter under the *Principle of the Right to Life*. This chapter will focus on problems associated with efforts to *bring about* the creation of new life, with special emphasis on the Catholic Church's sympathetic concern for the plight of couples who are afflicted with infertility or subfertility in the togetherness of marriage.

---

[54] *Fabricated Man: The Ethics of Genetic Control* (New Haven, Conn.: Yale University Press, 1970), p. 38.

> *Directive 3:* Every patient, regardless of the extent of his physical or psychic disability, has a right to be treated with a respect consonant with his dignity as a person.

Attacking the Scourge of Infertility

Infertility is an obstacle to full marital bliss for millions of couples throughout the world. As to the U.S.A. alone, figures from the National Center for Health Statistics reveal that there are 4.3 million currently married women, ages 15–44, who experience impaired fecundity. Of this number, more than 2,000,000 want to bear a child. For 840,000 of those women, the desire is to bear a *first* child.[55] *The Merck Manual* has bad news and good news on the subject (1982 edition): Although infertility affects about 15% of married couples in the U.S.A., it is good to know that the causes of infertility can be identified in 90% of the cases. Of 100 subfertile couples, 40 will show a male factor, 20 a female hormonal defect, 30 a female tubal disorder, and 10 a "hostile cervical environment." Psychogenic influences must also be considered. The recommendation is that the husband should be the first to see the physician: "Because investigation of infertility in women is time-consuming and expensive, prompt evaluation of the male is essential."[56]

Strictly speaking, *infertility* in men is the inability to fertilize the ovum; in women, it is the absence of conception after a year or so of marriage without the use of contraceptives. *Sterility* in men is the lack of proper sperm production; in women, it is the inability to ovulate. Here the word "infertility" is being used in the comprehensive sense of "unable to have children." Naturally the infertility of one partner in marriage brings about "couple infertility." The fact remains that sterility can be reversed in many cases.

Causes of Infertility in the Male can be an *impaired ability to produce sperm* resulting from environmental toxins, undescended testicle or testicles, testicular atrophy, varicose condition of the veins of the spermatic cord, effects of drug use, prolonged fever, etc.;—or it can be an *obstruction of the seminal tract* resulting from congenital anomalies, inflammation of the testicles, inflammation of the prostate gland or other genital components, urethral stricture, etc.;—or it can

---

[55]Walters, LeRoy, Ph.D., Kennedy Institute, Wash. D.C., "Ethical Aspects of Surrogate Embryo Transfer," in *Journal of the American Medical Association*, Oct. 28, 1983, p. 2184.

[56]*The Merck Manual*, Robert Berkow, MD, ed., 14th edition (Rahway, N.J.: Merck, Sharpe and Dohme Research Laboratories, 1982), p. 1638.

be a matter of *defective delivery of the sperm* into the vagina resulting from surgery of the bladder neck, removal of the prostate gland, hypospadias, premature ejaculation, organic impotence, etc. Special attention must be given to a possible varicose condition of the spermatic cord known as "varicocele" which (among other effects) can raise the temperature of the scrotal and testicle area so as to impede the proper formation of sperm.[57]

Causes of Infertility in the Woman can be the *absence of ovulation* (often due to hormonal imbalance), a *sluggish pituitary gland* (sometimes called the "fertility pump"), *blocked or defective fallopian tubes* (often due to pelvic inflammatory disease), *endometriosis* (portions of the inner lining of the uterus growing outside the uterus), and *sperm allergy* (the woman's immune system attacks the husband's sperm).

In addition to these sources of infertility, there are many contributing causes which come under the heading of sexual dysfunction. Both men and women can be troubled by *inhibited sexual desire* (resulting from boredom in the relationship, depression, use of drugs, etc.). Particular afflictions for men are the following: *inhibited sexual excitement* (inability to attain or to maintain an erection satisfactory for normal intercourse), *inhibited orgiastic control* (could be premature or retarded ejaculation), or a *condition called "anhedonia"* (absence of a pleasure experience in erection and ejaculation). Particular afflictions for women include: *frigidity* (recurrent and persistent inhibition of sexual excitement during normal sexual activity), *inhibited orgasm* (probably applies to as high as 50% of all women), *painful intercourse* for various reasons (known as "dyspareunia"), and *"vaganismus" or spasms of the vagina* (conditional contraction of the lower muscles of the vagina resulting from an unconscious desire to prevent penetration).[58]

Finally, the diverse conditions which call for psychotherapy must also be included among the obstacles to fertility. It is encouraging to know that there is a light at the end of the tiresome regime of fertility-testing. To quote a respected author, Gerald Leach: "After all these tests and treatments, and also psychotherapy for impotent men or clinically frigid women, more than 50 per cent of younger couples and about a third of older ones (women over 30) will be likely to conceive normally.[59]"

---

[57] *Ibid.*, p. 1639.
[58] *Ibid.*, pp. 1631–1643.
[59] *The Biocrats: Ethics and the New Medicine*, rev. ed. (Baltimore, Md.: Penguin Books, Inc., 1972), p. 82.

Moral Considerations

Some of the tests and treatments for infertility must be rejected by Catholics because immoral practices are involved such as masturbation, the use of a surrogate sex partner, etc. The good end (desire to have a child) does not and cannot justify the evil means employed to realize that end. To add to the confusion, some Catholic authors would consider masturbation to be justified morally if it is done as a means of fulfilling a legitimate desire to have children.[60] The fact remains, however, that the long-standing and traditional teaching of the Church on the immorality of masturbation was reaffirmed by the Holy See as recently as Dec. 29, 1975, in the *Declaration On Certain Questions Concerning Sexual Ethics.* In this document, masturbation was condemned as "an intrinsically and seriously disordered act." The following quotation explains the "why" of this condemnation: "The main reason is that, whatever the motive for acting in this way, the deliberate use of the sexual faculty outside normal conjugal relations essentially contradicts the finality of the faculty."[61]

Throughout the centuries, the Church has warned the faithful about the error of "dualism,"—a philosophy which regards the human body and the human soul as separate and independent elements or realities of human personality. There is something of that error in the mindset of a person who might try to justify stealing, for example, by saying: "I didn't take it; my hand (my body) did the stealing." Human persons are not merely minds, but minds that think and act through bodies and in a world of bodies. Human bodies are not adjuncts to the self, but essential to it. Theologian William E.

---

[60]For example, Father Bernard Häring, C.SS.R. states in *Medical Ethics* (Notre Dame, Ind.: Fides, 1973): "There are no convincing arguments to prove either the immorality of ejaculation by the husband in view of fatherhood nor the immorality of introducing that sperm into the wife's uterus," p. 93. A surprising inconsistency is found in Dr. Karl Menninger's book entitled *Whatever Became of Sin?*. On the one hand, this well-known non-Catholic psychiatrist seems to bewail the fact that the approval of masturbation in contemporary life has "affected our attitude toward other disapproved behavior," (p. 36) . . . yet he says clearly (almost pontificating) on p. 140 that "there is no harm in masturbation, no evil in it, and no sinfulness in it, the former religious stipulations notwithstanding."

[61]Issued by the Sacred Congregation for the Doctrine of the Faith, Dec. 29, 1975; cf. *Love and Sexuality,* Consortium Series (Wilmington, N. Car.: McGrath Publishing Co., 1978), n. 9, p. 436. Cf. also, *Canon Law Digest,* I (Milwaukee, Wis.: Bruce Publishing Co., 1934), p. 156, for the response of the Holy Office of August 2, 1929; and *The Human Body* (Boston, Mass.: St. Paul Editions, 1960), pp. 391, 392, for Pope Pius XII's condemnation of masturbation, in his Allocution to the Second World Congress on Fertility and Sterility, May 19, 1956.

May of Catholic University, Washington, D.C. analyses this concept and concludes:

> To be a human being is to be an animal—to be an animal with a difference from other animals, to be sure—but it is still to be an animal. Our bodies are not instruments attached to ourselves, our persons. I am not one reality and my body another . . . and my body is an integral dimension of my self, my personhood. It is not subpersonal, subhuman, an element of physical nature that I can use apart from myself, now for one purpose, now for another. I believe that the apologia advanced to justify masturbation for artificial insemination for AIH [insemination by the husband] reflects a dualistic view of man which makes me a spirit dwelling in a body that I can "use" to secure "higher" values.[62]

If that "using" of the body is at variance with God's plan and design in the human function of sexuality (MY will vs God's plan), it amounts to not merely: "I abused my body," but "I abused MYSELF." A basic principle of scholastic philosophy comes to mind: "actions are attributed to the person." Thus St. Paul writes to the Corinthians (I Corinthians,6:20) referring to sexual sins: "You have been purchased, and at a price. So glorify God (that is you, as a person) in your body." Direct masturbation, for whatever reason, is a gross violation of that mandate.

1) Lawful Means of Fostering Human Fertility

In his encyclical letter, *Humanae Vitae*, Pope Paul VI expressed the wish that medical science might succeed in "providing a sufficiently secure basis for a regulation of birth, founded on the observance of natural rhythms" (n.24). Referring to Pope Pius XII's mention of the use of the infertile periods (1951), Paul VI adds also his approval as follows:

> If, then, there are serious motives to space out births, which derive from the physical or psychological conditions of husband and wife, or from external conditions, the church teaches that it is then licit to take into account the natural rhythms immanent in the

---

[62] *Human Existence, Medicine an Ethics* (Chicago, Ill.: Franciscan Herald Press, 1977), pp. 49, 50.

generative functions, for the use of marriage in the infecund periods only, and in this way to regulate birth without offending the moral principles which have been recalled earlier.[63]

Since the early 1930's, the Church has encouraged childless couples to use the so-called "Rhythm Method" in reverse, that is, to concentrate conjugal love-making on the days when the wife is most likely to conceive. In fact, one of the two pioneers in perfecting the "Rhythm Method," Dr. Kyusaku Ogino of Japan (the other was Dr. Hermann Knaus of Prague) pursued his studies as a labor of love so as to enable couples to *have children*. This method—sometimes referred to as the Ogino-Knaus method—was hailed as a method of *avoiding* the conception of children. It still remains a respected and reliable means of promoting conception, but has lost favor as a means of avoiding conception. In order to be effective for the latter purpose, couples must *count backward* in their efforts to determine the time most favorable for avoiding conception (the sterile periods). Due to the variability in the length of a woman's monthly cycle, too much had to be left to chance. Obviously, couples who have recourse to the "Rhythm Method" in order to *have children* take no chances, and encounter no imposed restrictions with regard to their conjugal rights in their search for the fertile days.

Two effective methods of family planning which (in the words of Paul VI, above) "take into account rhythms immanent in the generative functions" are the *Billings Ovulation Method,* which is based on the woman's awareness and detection of cervical mucus (which reaches a peak of clearness, stretchiness, and wetness about a day *before* ovulation), and the *Sympto-Thermal Method,* which is based on the woman's awareness and observation of mucus, cervix, basal temperatures and other secondary signs. Both methods are promoted by the *Natural Family Planning* movement (NFP) with worldwide publicity and promotion through the *International Federation for Family Life Promotion* (IFFLP, 1974). The Billings Ovulation Method has been promoted through the laudable efforts of a husband-wife team of physicians, Dr. John J. Billings and Dr. Evelyn L. Billings of Australia. The international group which is dedicated to the dissemination of this method is the *World Organization of the Ovulation Method* known as WOOMB. Abundant information on these fertility-control methods is found in a book entitled *The Art of Natural Family Planning.*[64]

---

[63]*Love and Sexuality* (cf. note 61), p. 339.

[64]Published by the Couple to Couple League International, P.O. Box 11084, Cincinnati, Ohio, 45211. Authors: John and Sheila Kippley. Revised, 5th printing, 1977.

The *moral* aspects of the use of the Rhythm Method, the Billings Ovulation Method and the Sympto-Thermal Method as means of *preventing* conception and/or of spacing children will be discussed in the following chapter on the *Principle of the Right to Life*. In all three methods, the search for *fertile* days implies no violation of conscience, and imposes no restrictive obligations beyond the need of calculated vigilance in the effort to pinpoint the peak days of fertility in the woman's cycle.

(a) The "Rhythm Method" and Anovulant Pills

There are reliable indications in medical practice that the Rhythm Method can be used more effectively as a means of *conceiving* a child if a pathologically abnormal menstrual cycle of a woman (should that be the case) can be brought within a more normal and regular range. The Rhythm Method dates back to 1929 (Dr. Knaus) and 1930 (Dr. Ogino). The advantage of a normal range in the menstrual cycle is of more importance in the search for the sterile days (in the effort to avoid conception) than in the search for the peak fertile days. Couples who are already discouraged in the failure to achieve a conception in the past are most anxious, however, to give the practice of the Rhymth Method every chance of success by pinpointing the peak of fertility as accurately as possible. One author interprets "normal range" to be "possibly no more than a two-day variation within the menstrual cycle" (that is, for example, cycles between the 30-day and 32-day range throughout the year). This author bases his opinion on the argument that regularity and predictability are of the essence of the natural law.[65]

The strictly anovulant or steroid "pill," so popular in preventing conception by preventing ovulation, is considered to have the side effect of regularizing the menstrual cycle. If the physician of the woman who desires to conceive is of the opinion, based on clinical experience, that her widely-ranging menstrual cycles could be brought within a more normal range so as to offer a better chance of conception, there would be no moral objection if she accepted his prescription of taking anovulant pills for six months or so. She would be following his advice not with contraception in mind, but as a possible means of assuring conception at the peak fertile period. The same would apply with regard to the contention of some physicians, based on clinical experience (not necessarily of that particular physician but of colleagues in the

---

[65] *The Dignity of Life*, by Father Charles J. McFadden, O.S.A., Ph.D. (Huntington, Ind.: Our Sunday Visitor, Inc., 1976), p. 89, 90. Cf. also *Contemporary Moral Theology*, by Fathers John C. Ford, S.J., and Gerald Kelly, S.J., II (Westminster, Maryland: The Newman Press, 1964), p. 359.

medical profession) that a woman is more likely to conceive if ovulation is suppressed over a prescribed period, through the use of the anovulant pill. This is known as "ovulation rebound," whereby sluggish ovaries are said to be activated through the temporary suppression of ovulation. In both cases, the temporary recourse to anovulant pills would be intended as "facilitating" or "assisting" in the normal, natural process of conception. In his address to the Fourth International Congress of Catholic Doctors Pope Pius XII said that he did not necessarily forbid the use of certain artificial means whose sole purpose is either to facilitate the natural act or to assist the natural act, placed normally, in attaining its purpose.[66]

This would apply, however, only to anovulant or "anti-ovulation" pills, and not to the pills which are prescribed as abortifacients. The "morning-after" pill, for example, is designed to affect the uterine lining in such a way as to render the uterus incapable of receiving and nurturing the fertilized ovum. Implantation in the lining of the uterus is rendered impossible. This is equivalent to an abortion (hence "abortifacient"). It must be admitted that many contraceptive pills on the market today contribute somewhat to reducing the likelihood of implantation. Again and again, in describing the effects of contraceptive pills, the *Physician's Desk Reference* describes the clinical pharmacology of the product as follows:

> Combination oral contraceptives act primarily through the mechanism of gonadotropin suppression due to the estrogenic and progestational activity of their components. Although the primary mechanism of action is inhibition of ovulation, alterations in the genital tract, including changes in the cervical mucus (which reduce sperm penetration) and the endometrium (which reduce the likelihood of implantation) may also contribute to contraceptive effectiveness.[67]

Through the application of the *Principle of the Double Effect,* the intended effect is the eventual normalization of ovulation through the temporary "inhibition of ovulation" (the "primary mechanism" of the pill as described above). That good effect (normal ovulation leading to conception) justifies the toleration of a *possible* evil side effect (reducing the likelihood of implantation). If an individual had to abstain from medicinal products because of possible

---

[66]*Canon Law Digest,* III (cf. note 43), p. 433. Statement repeated in address of May 19, 1956. Cf. *The Human Body* (cf. note 61), p. 389.

[67]The *Physicians' Desk Reference* (Oradell, N.J.: Medical Economics Co., 1986), p. 1680. The product described is "Enovid."

side effects of a bad or evil nature, it would be immoral to take many if not most prescribed medications. The popular medication for hypertension known as "Aldactazide," for example, could not be prescribed in good conscience because of the boxed-in *warning* in the *Physicians' Desk Reference* that one of the main ingredients of the product "has been shown to be a tumorigen in chronic toxicity of rats . . . Unnecessary use of this drug should be avoided."[68] A proportionate reason would justify the prescribing of such a medication.

If a contraceptive pill is prescribed, therefore, as a means of promoting normal ovulation and eventual conception, the physician would be obligated to choose a brand of contraceptive pill which was designed to inhibit ovulation—and NOT one of the abortifacient variety. It must be added, however, that if the good effect desired (normalizing ovulation with a view to eventual conception) could be promoted by some other treatment or medication which would not involve a temporary contraceptive effect (which must be regarded objectively as an evil effect) nor other serious physical or mental effects, that individual would be obliged to choose that alternative. The "availability" aspect should include consideration of the woman's financial status. Other alternatives could be far beyond her ability to pay.[69]

(b) Other Promising Approaches to Human Fertility

Contemporary solutions to the problem of human infertility such as "in vitro" fertilization, artificial insemination by donor, etc., will be discussed presently. These well-intentioned solutions to a pressing human problem (infertility) present serious moral problems. Yet, the mental anguish and deep disappointment of child-less couples must be met with more than expressions of sympathy on the part of the Church. If something can be done to overcome infertility which is not in conflict with Catholic moral standards, it should be heralded and promoted by the Church. For the more-or-less standard cases of infertility and sub-fertility (i.e., less than normal fertility), there is Natural Family Planning which offers various approaches as explained earlier in this chapter. Are there other approaches especially for the more difficult cases of infertility which would not conflict with Catholic moral principles? The answer to the question must be sought in a diligent effort to analyze the teachings of Pope Pius XII on the subject of artificial insemination.

---

[68]*Ibid.*, p. 1674.

[69]For confirmation of the liceity of using such steroids for worthy purposes, cf. O'Donnell, Thomas, S.J., *Medicine and Christian Morality* (cf. note 31), pp. 242–244.

Pope Pius XII On the Subject of Artificial Insemination

Pope Pius XII referred to the subject of artificial insemination in four scholarly addresses. For reference purposes, it might be well to list these addresses as follows (based on the composition of his audience): *Doctors* (Sept. 29, 1949); *Midwives* (Oct. 29, 1951); *Fertility Experts* (May 19, 1956); *Hematologists* (Sept. 12, 1958). For reasons best known to him alone (perhaps because he did not wish to *close* the question too definitely), he really did not give a clear definition of what he meant by artificial insemination. He rejected "artificial insemination outside matrimony" and artificial insemination "produced by means of the active element of a third person" (*Doctors*);—he spoke of bringing about the "mere union of two life-germs . . . artificially, that is, without the natural action of the spouses . . . when the performance of this function in its natural form is, from the beginning, permanently impossible . . ." (*Midwives*);—he states that artificial insemination "violates the natural law and is contrary to justice and morality" (*"contraire au droit et à la morale,"* apparently referring to the unmarried) in his address to the *Fertility Experts*;—he refers to his former condemnation of "all types of artificial insemination, on the ground that this practice is not included among the rights of married couples and because it is contrary to the natural law and Catholic morals" (*Hematologists*).[70]

It is clear that he condemned artificial insemination among the unmarried, as well as among married couples with donor-semen, as well as artificial insemination used by married couples outside of and as a substitute for the conjugal act. In the latter case, artificial insemination conceivably could be used either because of infertility, or because of impotence. He makes a clear distinction, however, between these examples of artificial insemination, and what might be called "facilitated insemination" or "assisted insemination" by artificial means. That distinction from Pope Pius XII mentioned previously (cf. p.39) was a statement in the context of an *open-ness* on the part of the pontiff to new methods of promoting human fertility which might be provided by medical science in the future:

> Although one cannot *a priori* exclude new methods because they are new, yet, as far as artificial fecundation is concerned, not only does it call for an extreme reserve, but it is absolutely to be re-

---

[70]His message to *Doctors* and to *Midwives*, cf. *Canon Law Digest*, III (cf. note 43), pp. 432–434; to *Fertility Experts*, cf. *The Human Body* (cf. note 61), p. 390; to *Hematologists*, cf. *The Pope Speaks*, 6 (1959–1960), p. 393.

jected. To say this is not necessarily to proscribe the use of *certain artificial means* designed only to *facilitate the natural act* or to *enable that act* [better translated as "to assist that act"], *done in the normal way, to attain its end"* (emphasis added).[71]

Hence a distinction must be maintained between "artificial insemination" as condemned by Pope Pius XII, and "assisted insemination" by artificial means.

It must be emphasized that Pope Pius XII insisted that any facilitating or assisting means to promote human fertility must be related to the conjugal act "done in the normal way, to attain its end," or within the context of a normal conjugal act. Well in advance of Pius XII's references to artificial insemination, however, an impressive list of theologians had approved of the practice of assisting the natural act to attain its purpose by retrieving the ejaculate of a particular act of human intercourse and simultaneously projecting or propelling it closer to the cervical canal so as to enhance the possibility of fertilization.[72] To claim that the pontiff had such a procedure in mind when he condemned homologous artificial insemination (AIH) in 1949 would be merely an assumption. It is true that on March 26, 1897, the Roman Congregation of the Inquisition had issued a simple "No" in response to the following inquiry: "May artificial insemination be applied to a woman?" The decree carried no reference to actual cases, "nor was mention made of the nuanced distinctions taught by the moral theologians."[73] In the spirit of Canon 18 of the present Code of Canon Law with regard to restrictive laws and regulations, it seems only right and proper to apply the canonical axiom: "a doubtful regulation is no regulation." It is also probable that the response was a definite "No" because of an assumption that the sperm would have been obtained by masturbation.

An argument for the morality of "assisted insemination" (but within the context of conjugal union) could be based on the right of the husband and wife to the act "in itself suitable for the procreation of offspring" (Can.1061,1). Just as that right is considered to include the right to a fairly-regular menstrual cycle for the woman, so that the use of steroid pills on a temporary basis to bring about that regularity is justified, so the right to

---

[71]*Canon Law Digest* (cf. note 43), III, p. 433

[72]Wakefield, John C., *Artful Childmaking* (St. Louis, Mo.: Pope John Center, 1978), p. 44, and footnote 81, p. 169. The 21 theologians listed were respected moralists of their day. Four of them approved of the practice, however, "only with the reservation that the seminal deposit was not withdrawn from the vagina." *Ibid.*

[73]*Ibid.*, p. 38. Father Vermeersch interpreted that decree of March, 1897, as applying if the semen is obtained by masturbation. Cf. note 81.

conjugal intercourse should include the right of the spouses to seek optimum means within the performance of the conjugal act, to assure the ability and potency of the natural components of human generation (human sperm and ova) to reach the natural and teleological site of human fertilization. It is precisely on this basis that various means of inducing ovulation or of enhancing the concentration, motility and maturity of human gametes are justified (for example, treatments with human chorionic gonadotropin, recourse to progesterone supplementation, etc.).

The following procedures for promoting human fertility are presented with the persuasion that they serve as examples of "facilitating" or "assisting" the natural act of conjugal intercourse, placed normally, in attaining its purpose. The proper parameters within which each procedure might be considered as in accord with Catholic moral standards will be emphasized in each case.

The Tubal Ovum Transfer Procedure (TOT)

On September 1st, 1983, the St. Elizabeth Medical Center of Dayton, Ohio issued a news release stating that a team of medical specialists, headed by David S. McLaughlin, MD would begin using a new procedure to help women with absent or blocked fallopian tubes to realize the blessing of motherhood. The news release added that Dr. McLaughlin, a reproductive gynecologist specializing in infertility and micro-laser surgery, had studied "in vitro" fertilization (cf.pp.46,47) under the tutelage of Carl Wood, MD at Monash University in Melbourne, Australia and at two American universities, and that much of the research on "in vitro" fertilization was applied to the research pool for his studies.[74] In an article in the March, 1984 issue of *Hospital Progress,* Father Donald McCarthy of the Pope John Center staff emphasizes the "in vivo" (within the living womb) aspect of the procedure, and explains why the procedure was known as "Low" tubal ovum transfer (then known as LTOT):

> LTOT attempts to overcome female infertility by bypassing blocked, diseased, or absent fallopian tubes. After the infertile couple have marital relations at the time of predicted ovulation, the mature egg or eggs are retrieved from the woman's ovary by laparoscopy and reinserted in the mid or lower portion of the tube

---

[74]*News Release*, St. Elizabeth Medical Center, Dayton, Ohio, Sept. 1, 1983, pp. 1-3.

or in the uterus. The couple are encouraged to repeat the marital act to increase their chances of pregnancy.[75]

Since the procedure failed to produce any pregnancies, however, Dr. McLaughlin and his associates modified the procedure so that both the retrieved ova (by laparoscopy) and the husband's sperm (obtained by using the *Silastic Seminal Fluid Collection Device*, cf. p.52) were introduced into the fallopian tube by means of laparoscopy. Similar to the GIFT procedure (to be discussed presently), the transfer of the ova and sperm, separated by a bubble of air, was accomplished by using a catheter. Out of six patients who received this modified treatment in the late summer of 1985, two women became pregnant.[76] The procedure now became known as "TOT." The "L" (formerly "LTOT") could be dropped presumably because the target area now is not the lower tube or the uterus, but rather a site as high as possible in the fallopian tube. In 1983, referring to the first version of this procedure (LTOT), Archbishop Daniel E. Pilarczyk of Cincinnati, Ohio wrote: "It is my opinion that the procedure as described is not contrary to Catholic moral teaching."[77] The same moral evaluation would apply to the "TOT" procedure.

It remains to establish that supplementing sperm obtained not through conjugal union preliminary to the TOT procedure, but by use of a perforated condom in previous conjugal acts, is a morally acceptable means of facilitating or assisting the "natural act, placed normally, in attaining its purpose." It must be admitted that a conception resulting from the TOT procedure rarely would be ascribed to the act of conjugal union preliminary to the re-positioning procedure. If the husband is capable of providing sperm of proper volume, concentration and motility, however, the *possibility* exists that sperm from that preliminary act of marital union *could* fertilize the re-positioned ova. It must be remembered, however, that the carefully-calculated retrieval of the woman's mature ova by laparoscopy would supplant the normal movement of ova in the ovulation process for that preliminary act of marital union. If conception does occur, it will be due in all probability to the facilitating (and

---

[75]"Should Catholic Hospitals Encourage Low Tubal Ovum Transfers?," in *Hospital Progress*, March, 1984, p. 55. Father McCarthy contrasts "in vitro" fertilization (literally "in glass") with the LTOT method as "in vivo" conception: "a couple 'love their child into existence'." *Ibid.*, p. 56.

[76]"Overcoming Infertility," by Father Donald McCarthy, in the *National Catholic Register*, Jan. 19, 1986. p. 9.

[77]"New Hospital Infertility Program Seen as a Blessing," by Peter Feuerherd, in *The Catholic Telegraph*, Cincinnati, Ohio., Sept. 9, 1983, p. 124.

supplementing) aspects of the TOT procedure in overcoming a natural weakness or defect of the reproductive system.

As mentioned previously, many theologians of the early 20th century saw no moral objection to a type of *assisting insemination* as a means of promoting fertility in a particular act of marital union. Father Healy explains this facilitating or assisting procedure as follows:

> It is permissible for a physician, however, after husband and wife have rightly performed the marital act, artificially to propel the semen deposited in the vagina into the uterus and Fallopian tubes, for the physician's act in this case would consist merely in aiding nature. To accomplish this he may use a syringe, syphon the semen from the vagina, and at once project it into the uterus and tubes. There is in the action momentary interference with the ordinary process of nature, it is true; but the interference is directly aimed at rendering that particular intercourse fruitful and in no sense may be viewed as a frustration of nature. This process is rightly called, not artificial, but assistant, insemination [sic].[78]

Father Otis Kelly, MD and obstetrician Frederick L. Good, MD, co-authors of *Marriage, Morals and Medical Ethics,* would allow the ejaculate, as in the quotation above, to be *removed* from the vagina in order to be "centrifuged to bring about a greater concentration of spermatazoa," and then injected into the vagina. They would consider such a procedure to be (in the presence of a sufficient reason) "not, strictly speaking, artificial, but . . . rather an aid to natural insemination."[79] Other theologians would allow accumulated amounts of the husband's sperm (obtained by legitimate means within the context of conjugal union), to be injected into the wife's vagina preliminary to

---

[78]*Medical Ethics* (cf. note 46), p. 154. Cf. also Kelly, Gerald, S.J., *Medico-Moral Problems* (cf. note 22), p. 240: "This practical rule may still be followed, because the pope made it clear that he wished to make no official statement either for or against assisted insemination . . ." O'Donnell, Thomas, S.J., *Medicine and Christian Morality* (cf. note 31), p. 269; McFadden, Charles, O.S.A., *Medical Ethics* (cf. note 17), p. 69, who mentions theologians Noldin, Ubach, Wouters and Vermeersch as "renowned writers who permit this act for a grave reason;" Wakefield, John, *Artful Childmaking* (cf. note 72), p. 44, and note 81, p. 169, who mentions 17 authors in addition to those mentioned by McFadden.

[79]*Marriage, Morals and Medical Ethics* (New York, N.Y.: P.J. Kenedy and Sons, 1951), p. 135.

conjugal intercourse "in order to mix with and fortify the husband's ejaculate." Father Thomas O'Donnell, S.J. writes as follows:

> An intriguing possibility presents itself in cases of sterility due to the husband's oligospermia. It is possible to collect amounts of the husband's ejaculate, by morally acceptable methods, in proper acts of intercourse. These amounts can be conserved and spun down, leaving a residue containing a heavy concentration of viable spermatazoa. There are several ways whereby this concentrated deposit of active sperm could be placed within the generative tract of the wife, immediately before a natural marital act, in order to mix with and fortify the husband's ejaculate.
>
> Although this type of procedure would undoubtedly give rise to some difference of opinion among theologians, we believe that, in view of the explicit papal distinction regarding "artificial means whose sole purpose is either to facilitate the natural act or to assist the natural act, placed normally, in attaining its purpose," it could be permitted in practice.[80]

Father Arthur Vermeersch, S.J. (1858–1936), one of the most influential and respected theologians of the early 20th century, won considerable support for his opinion that sperm obtained by licit means *outside* of the context of conjugal union (but *excluding* the use of a condom) could be used to promote fertility between husband and wife.[81] This opinion could be interpreted to mean that sperm obtained in a licit manner could be used to promote fertility *outside of the context of conjugal relations.* Such a practice would fall under Pope Pius XII's condemnation of artificial insemination (AIH) in the strict sense. Clearly it would be regarded as a *substitute* for conjugal union. The same opinion of Father Vermeersch can be interpreted, however, to mean that

---

[80]*Medicine and Christian Morality* (cf. note 31), p. 269. Dominican authors, Benedict M. Ashley and Kevin D. O'Rourke, would also approve: ". . . the child is begotten as the fruit of an actual expression of unitive love." Cf. *Health Care Ethics* (St. Louis, Mo.: Catholic Health Association, 1982), p. 289. These authors explicitly refer to Father O'Donnell's opinion.

[81]*De Castitate et De Vitiis Contrariis* (Rome, Italy: Gregorian University, 1921), p. 246, n. 241. After commenting on the response of the Holy Office of March 24, 1897, to the effect that artificial insemination is forbidden whenever the semen is obtained by masturbation ("praevia pollutione"), he states (paragraph 3): "Praeterea, si qua punctionis ratione semen (i.e., nemasperma) ex epididymo mariti sumatur ut in vas uxoris infundatur, haec ratio fecundationis artificialis damnanda non videtur, cum sine ullu abusu venereo, i.e., sine ulla sexuali commotione, finem matrimonii procuret." Father Gerald Kelly, S.J. writes (*Medico-Moral Problems*, cf. note 22, p. 224): "Father Vermeersch's opinion permitting this practice is still solidly probable."

sperm obtained in a licit manner (but NOT by the use of any type of condom) could be injected into the vagina of the wife either soon before or soon after an act of marital union—that is, within the context of conjugal union. Needless to say, such a mode of fertility-promotion would require a serious reason; for example, the lack of any other reasonable and available alternative to realizing the blessing of parenthood. This can be viewed as *supplementing* for some weakness or defect of nature in assisting and facilitating "the natural act, placed normally, in attaining its purpose."

In describing the TOT procedure, Father McCarthy explains that the retrieval of the ova and the re-positioning of the ova (plus the husband's sperm) is accomplished "through laparoscopy within an hour's time under general anesthetic and the couple can return home within three hours."[82] This "hour's time" would justify the claim of a *moral union* between the couple's engaging in conjugal union just before leaving for the outpatient facility of the hospital and the actual assisting or facilitating factor as provided by the laparoscopic re-positioning of the gametes in the fallopian tube. Since some theologians might insist that the TOT procedure could be morally acceptable only if there is some possibility of a causal relationship between the preliminary conjugal union and a conception, it should suffice to point out that there is always the *possibility* that the husband's sperm as deposited in the wife's vagina during the preliminary act of conjugal union could account for the fertilization of the re-positioned ova. Due to that undeniable possibility, the inseparable bond between the unitive and the creative dimension of that particular preliminary act of conjugal union remains intact with regard both to intent and fact.

This defense of the TOT procedure as being in harmony with Catholic moral standards is presented with all due sentiments of fidelity to the magisterium of the Church in the event that the Holy See might express disapproval of the opinion.

The Gamete Intrafallopian Transfer Procedure (GIFT)

The November 3, 1984, issue of *Lancet* announced "the first pregnancy obtained after 'gamete intrafallopian transfer (GIFT).' " This report of Dr. Ricardo Asch of the Department of Obstetrics and Gynecology of the University of Texas (San Antonio) and three colleagues explained that a 35-year-old wife had repeatedly submitted to a wide variety of up-to-date medical treatments for infertility over a period of seven years, but without success. These treatments included "artificial insemination and intrauterine insemination

---

[82]Article in the *National Catholic Register,* "Overcoming Infertility," Jan. 19, 1986, p. 9.

with washed semen." She then submitted to the GIFT procedure, conceived twins, and carried them to a safe delivery.

In this successful procedure (which is very similar to the TOT procedure described above), semen from the 37-year old husband (obtained 2¹/₂ hours before laparoscopy) were treated and centrifuged to a high degree of concentration and motility, and then transferred in separate applications to the fimbriated ends of each fallopian tube at a precisely-calculated period in the wife's menstrual cycle, along with two oocytes (ova) from his wife (one oocyte was preovulatory and the other was of doubtful maturity in each application). The oocytes had been obtained by laparoscopy just 15 minutes before the transfer (by injection) of the sperm and oocytes into the fallopian tubes. The transfer was accomplished by laparoscopy (entry into the abdomen through a small surgical incision) through a 16-gauge catheter attached to a syringe. In the loaded catheter, the sperm and oocytes were separated by a special medium and by airspaces so that fertilization could not take place until the two gametes (sperm and ova) had been deposited in the fallopian tubes. On the 25th day after the transfer, an ultrasound scan revealed that the wife indeed was gestating twins.[83]

The similarity between the TOT procedure and the GIFT procedure (above) is apparent. Provided that the GIFT procedure is restricted to two individuals who are husband and wife, and that the husband's sperm are obtained by legitimate means (NOT by masturbation), and that there is no other reasonable, available and legitimate method of promoting fertility, there is no apparent reason why the procedure could not be adapted to the TOT procedure practice of requiring the couple to engage in conjugal union immediately before they present themselves at the outpatient facility of the hospital. It appears that the time element between that preliminary act of conjugal union and re-positioning of the gametes could be somewhat less than one hour. The *Lancet* report on the GIFT procedure states that "the time elapsed from follicular aspiration to gamete transfer into the oviducts was about 15 minutes."[84] This factor would provide increased validity of the claim of a moral union between that particular act of conjugal union and the re-positioning of the gametes. These observations lead to the conclusion that the GIFT procedure (like the TOT procedure) could be managed so as not to be in violation of Catholic moral principles. It should also be mentioned that the availability of the TOT and GIFT procedures would dissuade Catholic cou-

---

[83]"Pregnancy After Translaparoscopic Gamete Intrafallopian Transfer," in *The Lancet*, Nov. 3, 1984, by Dr. Ricardo H. Asch and colleagues, pp. 1034, 1035.

[84]*Ibid.*, p. 1034.

ples from the temptation to submit to the morally objectionable (and more expensive) "in vitro" fertilization procedure.

It is interesting to note that studies on the possibility of re-positioning the gametes not by laparotomy and laparoscopy but by delivery through the vagina and the uterus (by transhysteroscopy) are being pursued. This could be the proper approach in cases of the occlusion of the distal portion of the fallopian tubes.[85] If that approach could be made as effective as the re-positioning of the gametes by laparoscopy, however (in both the TOT and the GIFT procedure), it would be somewhat less artificial, and more in keeping with the physiological route and sequence of human fertilization. It would enhance the symbolism of the procedure as assisting and facilitating with regard to the natural teleology of the process of human conception.

The Sperm Intrafallopian Transfer Procedure (SIFT)

Over sixty years ago (1922), a belgian Jesuit, Father Joseph Salsmans (nephew of a distinguished theologian, Father Edouard Genicot, S.J.) tested the theological atmosphere by suggesting that in situations where couples cannot have children due to the hyperacidity of the wife's vagina, the husband might use a condom in conjugal intercourse so as to collect enough sperm for later injection closer to the cervix. The opinion was rejected by many theologians. Father Salsmans eventually withdrew his suggestion.[86] There was no indication that he envisioned the injection of the collected sperm within the context of conjugal union. The opposition to his suggestion, therefore, could have been based on the suspicion that he was advocating artificial insemination. It is also possible that the opposition was based on the apprehension that the sperm might be obtained in some cases by masturbation or by the use of a closed condom.

The procedure which this writer has presumed to call "SIFT" (for Sperm Intrafallopian Transfer) involves transfer of the husband's sperm only. Human sperm can be immobilized by the inhospitable atmosphere of the cervical tract. One contemporary author lists four conditions under the heading of

---

[85]*Ibid.*

[86]Wakefield, John, *Artful Childmaking* (cf. note 72), p. 42, and note 76, p. 168. The advantage of treating the semen or sperm before injection into the cervical canal is realized more effectively by contemporary obstetricians. Such treatment is described as a process which ". . . involves the elimination of sperm-agglutinating and sperm-immobilizing antibodies by washing the sperm and then suspending them in a normal acellular seminal plasma. Filtration of whole semen with millipore filters (pore size 0.45 m) removes all spermatozoa and yields sperm-free seminal plasma." Cf. *Male Infertility,* by Richard D. Amelar, MD, Lawrence Dubin, MD, Patrick C. Walsh, MD (Philadelphia, Pa.: W.B. Saunders Co., 1977), p. 210.

"Hostile cervical mucus," namely: increased viscosity, increased infection, acid mucus and presence of sperm antibodies. These conditions may be found also in combination. Two of them are described as follows.

> The viscosity of cervical mucus is the greatest barrier in sperm penetration. There is no resistance to sperm penetration in thin mucus, but viscous mucus—such as that observed in the luteal phase, during pregnancy, and in the progestogen-treated woman—forms an impenetrable barrier. . . . Kremer and colleagues have shown that when sperm antibodies are found in the cervical mucus or on the surface of the sperm, the ability of sperm to penetrate cervical mucus is impaired and sperm lose their progressive movements, showing a local "shaking motion."[87]

Although such conditions often can respond to hormonal treatments or other substitute procedures (including morally-objectionable measures such as "in vitro" fertilization or surrogate embryo transfer), there could be situations where the only reasonable and available treatment would be to use a catheter to by-pass the inhospitable atmosphere of the cervical canal so as to deposit the husband's sperm closer to the fallopian tubes. The husband's sperm, obtained by morally-acceptable means, could be washed, centrifuged and treated as required before delivery by catheter through the vagina and uterus. Presuming that the procedure is restricted to husband and wife, with the requirement of conjugal union immediately before appearing at the hospital for the procedure (hence, within the context of conjugal union), the procedure would be in harmony with Catholic moral standards as observed in the foregoing discussions of the TOT and GIFT procedures. Although this writer has been unable to find any published articles with regard to this SIFT procedure, the fact that it is being promoted in basic outline has come to his attention through a consultation addressed to the Pope John Center.

Only time and clinical experience will tell whether or not the three procedures discussed above (TOT, GIFT and SIFT) may have unfavorable side-effects for pregnant mothers and/or infants thus conceived. With regard to the GIFT procedure in particular, apprehension has been expressed with regard to the added risk of ectopic pregnancies.[88] If adverse complications are encountered, however, there are solid reasons for anticipating that contempo-

---

[87]Moghissi, Kamran, S., MD, in *Infertility,* Mary G. Hammond, MD, and Luther M. Talbert, MD, editors (Oradell, N.J.: Medical Economics Books, 1985), pp. 93–95.

[88]"First Attempt With GIFT Yields Twins," in *Medical World News for Obstetricians, Gynecologists, Urologists,* Jan. 17, 1985, pp. 13, 14.

rary medical science will be equal to the challenge.

2) Lawful Means of Obtaining Human Sperm for Analysis

As mentioned previously, the analysis of the sperm of the husband often is the first item of investigation in infertility cases. Some authors have doubts about the morality of one or the other of the seven methods listed below. It is safe to say, however, that all of them are morally acceptable in practice if used for the purpose of overcoming human infertility. Most physicians probably would agree with an expert in pastoral medicine, Albert Niedermeyer, MD, Ph.D. in saying that "none of these methods fully satisfies the designated requirements [that is, in obtaining adequate specimens for analysis].[89] The one exception to such a statement might be the use of the plastic condom-type seminal pouch (cf.n.5) (below). Other experts insist that the entire semen specimen be delivered to the laboratory in its entirety: "Since the distribution of sperm cells is not uniform throughout the entire ejaculate, loss of the first or last portion may give entirely erroneous results."[90] Catholic moral principles rule out masturbation or withdrawal during the act of intercourse as methods of obtaining adequate samples of human sperm for analysis. The Church relies on the good will of physicians in their respectful understanding of the overriding importance of peace of conscience for the patient. It is with this confidence in mind that the following list is presented.[91]

---

[89]Niedermeyer, Albert, MD, Ph.D. translation by Fulgence Buonanno, O.F.M., *Compendium of Pastoral Medicine* (New York, N.Y.: Joseph F. Wagner, Inc., 1961), pp. 100, 101.

[90]Amelar, Richard, MD et al., *Male Infertility* (cf. note 86), pp. 107, 108.

[91]Of the seven methods listed, there should be no moral objection to methods (1), (2) and (7). As to the other 4 methods, they are listed as licit in the works of Jesuit authors Thomas O'Donnell (*Medicine and Christian Morality*, pp. 257–263) and Edwin Healy (*Medical Ethics*, pp. 147–149); presuming that Father Healy's reference to massaging the seminal vesicles is similar to the aspiration of the epididymis as proposed by Father Vermeersch—that is, similar in principle. Father Kelly (*Medico-Moral Problems*, pp. 221–225) approves of the use of the cervical spoon and lists the other 3 methods as "probably licit." With regard to the use of a perforated condom, Father Kelly mentions (*Ibid.*, pp. 222, 223) that it was considered licit by Father J. McCarthy of Maynooth College, Ireland, and by Father John Clifford, S.J. of the seminary at Mundelein, Ill. Father Healy's comments on the liceity of the use of the perforated condom include the following statement: "The perforation must be large enough to permit the greater part of the ejaculation to reach the female genital tract, for otherwise the coitus would be substantially contraceptive and unnatural" (*Ibid.*, p. 149). It should be noted, however, that distinguished theologians such as Father Henry Merkelbach, O.P., Father Francis Connell, C.SS.R., and Father Arthur Vermeersch, S.J., considered the use of the perforated condom to be immoral. In Father Vermeersch's opinion, such a means of collecting human sperm would involve "the direct will to deposit some of the ejaculate outside of the vagina—something which makes it a 'partial onanism' " (cf. Kelly, *Ibid.*, p. 222).

1) *Retaining the ejaculate from an involuntary emission:* This preferred method, often referred to as a "wet dream," is more likely to occur after a period of abstinence from intercourse corresponding to the couple's usual coital frequency.

2) *Removing the semen adhering to the male organ after intercourse:* This would be practical only if the analysis required only a minimal sample of semen.

3) *Retrieving semen from the vagina after intercourse:* This would require the presence of a cooperative physician or nurse at the time of intercourse. A sterile syringe could be used to retrieve the ejaculate and then spray or propel it closer to the opening to the fallopian tubes—or to retrieve a substantial portion of the ejaculate to serve as a sample for sperm analysis. The word "substantial" is of some importance. Theologians in the past were disposed to disapprove of retrieving a substantial portion or sample of sperm insofar as it might decrease considerably the likelihood of conception. They had no way of knowing in their day, however, that the median sperm-count of fertile men in the act of intercourse is over 80 million per milliliter of ejaculate. Hence even if a substantial amount of the ejaculate is retrieved for analysis purposes, the procreative significance and potential of the act of intercourse is not affected to any appreciable degree.

4) *Employing the "Cervical Spoon" or the "Vaginal Cup:"* The former, a concave lucite spoon, is inserted into the wife's vagina immediately *before* intercourse, so that it is positioned directly below the opening to the uterus. As she lies quietly for about an hour after intercourse, the spoon catches that portion of the ejaculate which drains from the opening to the uterus. The vaginal cup is inserted in the opening to the vagina immediately *after* intercourse so as to catch that portion of the ejaculate which drains from the vagina.

5) *Employing a perforated "condom" during intercourse:* Rubber or rubberized condoms are not recommended because "the sperm-immobilizing properties of the materials used in its manufacture will interfere with any evaluation of sperm motility."[92] The word "condom" is in quotation marks above because the recommended item is a plastic *condom-type seminal pouch;* but not the standard condom. A seminal pouch of this type can be obtained from Milex Products (Chicago, Ill., 60631). An improved version of the Milex product was developed in cooperation with the Dow Corning Co. of Midland, Mich. It is known as the *Silastic Seminal Fluid Collection Device.* It is said to have all of the advantages of a latex condom with none of its

---

[92]Amelar, Richard, MD et al., *Male Infertility* (cf. note 86), pp. 107, 108.

spermicidal qualities.[93]

It would be immoral, however, to use such a device for semen-analysis purposes unless a small perforation is made at the tip of the sheath so that a substantial amount of the ejaculate is allowed to be projected into the wife's vagina in the course of marital union. The word "substantial" does not have to mean the major portion or any quantitative percentage, but rather a *significant* portion: enough to "signify" that this is an act of normal conjugal union wherein the husband's ejaculation into the vagina of the wife is an essential component, and enough to satisfy the requirements for a potential fertilization. In view of nature's profuse abundance in providing the husband's ejaculate with millions of sperm, a perforation about the size of the writing tip of a lead pencil should suffice to meet both the demands of theology and the demands of technology.

6) *Aspiration of the Genital Organs:* One of the most influential theologians of the 20th century, Father Arthur Vermeersch, S.J. (1858–1936), did not approve of the use of a condom as a means of collecting human sperm (cf. footnote 91). In his cooperative efforts to work with physicians in finding a licit method of obtaining semen for analysis, he suggested that it would not be immoral to aspirate seminal fluid from the testicles or from the epididymides by using a needle or syringe. The argument was that such methods would not involve stimulation of the generative faculty. Several authors have compared such methods to the process of removing other body fluids (blood, bile, etc.) without causing any physical harm. Another suggested method, the stripping of the seminal vesicle by massage, is regarded as useless on the grounds that the seminal vesicles do not contain sperm.[94]

7) *Testicular biopsy:* This procedure, which requires a general anesthetic, is sometimes indicated for diagnostic purposes in determining why spermatogenesis is not taking place. It tells nothing about motility, which is critical in male infertility.[95]

---

[93]"Evaluation of a New Silastic Seminal Fluid Collection Device," by Cy Schoenfeld et al. in *Fertility and Sterility,* Sept., 1978, p. 319. The device is made of a silicone compound. If used properly, there is no spillage of the ejaculate.

[94]"Clinical Treatment of the Infertile Couple," by Thomas Nabors, MD in *Technological Powers and the Person* (St. Louis, MO.: The Pope John Center, 1983), p. 386. He lists most of the methods of obtaining sperm specimens as listed above, but prefaces his list with the following comment: ". . . moral theologians in the past have recommended other indirect, clumsy and downright meaningless methods" (pp. 386–388).

[95]*Ibid.,* pp. 387, 388. Dr. Nabors and others insist on "fractionation" of the ejaculate into several portions, for proper analysis: "The first part of the fluid portion of the ejaculate comes from the prostrate and the remainder from the seminal vesicles" (p. 388). Fractionation makes it possible to identify the area of malfunction.

One author referred to a technique, published in 1966, of using a simple hand electric vibrator as a means of obtaining semen for analysis. The contention was that this was accompanied by an erection "at times," but "at other times ejaculation occurs without erection."[96] Further research on this technique justifies the conclusion that the procedure would amount to mechanical masturbation. The procedure is described as follows: ". . . a simple electrovibrator . . . is fitted with a collection cup and applied to the glans penis before the apartus [sic] is turned on. The pulsatile vibrations are applied directly to the glans."[97] Such a procedure would be immoral.

The unfortunate fact that semen samples may have been obtained by masturbation should not put Catholic lab technicians or physicians under the obligation to inquire each time about the method employed to obtain the sample. If the patient's physician is a Catholic, both justice and charity should rule out the presumption that the physician would advise the patient to stoop to an immoral practice such as masturbation. Father Gerald Kelly, S.J. has prudent advice in this regard: inform that particular physician of the hospital directives in that regard, and state very clearly to a physician who may have submitted samples obtained by masturbation in the past that he may not submit any more samples which have been obtained in a morally-objectionable manner (masturbation, electric vibrator, etc.). He concludes: "If doctors who had been thus warned would later send more specimens, we should usually presume that these specimens had been licitly obtained unless there were some sound reason for questioning the good faith of the doctor."[98]

If any physician challenges the Catholic stand on masturbation and states that all of his or her patients will be advised to resort to masturbation, some person in authority at the Catholic hospital would have to inform that physician that semen samples from his or her patients would not be accepted at the Catholic hospital or clinic unless the patient can assure them, in each case, that the sample had not been obtained by masturbation. In this manner, the Catholic health facility could not be accused of illicit material cooperation in evil, and any basis of scandal would be obviated.

---

[96]*Ibid.*, p. 388.

[97]Amelar et al., *Male Infertility* (cf. note 86), pp. 208–209. Another immoral method would be the application of some type of electric prod to the genitals. Cf. Niedermeyer, Albert, *Compendium of Pastoral Medicine* (cf. note 89), pp. 100, 101. Such a method is said to be successful in "cattle-breeding."

[98]*Medico-Moral Problems* (cf. note 22), pp. 226, 227.

3) Fertility Procedures Which Must be Regarded as Immoral

All of the methods listed below come under Pope Pius XII's general condemnation of artificial insemination.[99] They all amount to an unfortunate but effective separation of the procreative element from the unitive element in conjugal love.

(a) *Artificial Insemination by the Husband* (AIH): If a husband had some professional expertise so as to be capable of taking the sperm which had been collected by one of the morally acceptable means mentioned above, placing it in a syringe or blow-type instrument (catheter, for example), and then injecting it close to or even beyond the cervix of his wife's uterus *but* outside of the context of conjugal union, his action would appear to be an illustration of what Pope Pius XII condemned as *artificial insemination* ("fecondazione" in the Italian original). After speaking of the propriety of conjugal union, Pius XII said, "This is much more than the union of two life-germs, which can be brought about even artificially, that is, without the cooperation of the husband and wife."[100] In other words, such a procedure could not pass as a *substitute* for proper conjugal union as a means of realizing the blessing of procreation.

As mentioned previously (pp.40 ff.) however, the procedure would not be a *substitute* for the conjugal act, but rather an element of *facilitating and assisting* "the natural act, placed normally, in attaining its purpose" *if the husband and wife engaged in conjugal union either soon before or soon after the injection of the collected sperm.* This would then be "within the context of" or "as an added part of" the conjugal act. As to the actual injection of the collected sperm within the context of a particular act of conjugal union, however, the more practical (and less risky) alternative would be to enlist the cooperation of a physician or trained nurse to accomplish the injection process. The condemnation of artificial insemination would apply, however, if the wife simply brought the collected sperm to a physician who was willing to perform the injection process and actually did so.

(b) *Artificial Insemination with Sperm from a Donor (AID):* In cases of male infertility, the wife can be inseminated with the sperm of an anonymous donor.

---

[99]Cf. his address to Catholic doctors, Dept. 29, 1949, and his address to the Italian midwives, Oct. 29, 1951, as found in the *Canon Law Digest,* vol. III (cf. note 43), pp. 432–434 respectively. Cf. also Paul VI's encyclical letter *Humanae Vitae* of July 25, 1968, n. 12, as found in *Love and Sexuality* (cf. note 61), pp. 336, 337.

[100]*Canon Law Digest,* III (cf. note 43), p. 434. For an extensive study of the background of the artificial insemination controversy, cf. Wakefield, John C., *Artful Childmaking* (cf. note 72), pp. 69–147.

It is estimated that 20,000 children are conceived in this manner each year.[101] In addition to obvious legal complications inherent in such "arrangements," there are also potential sorrows. Due to inadequate screening in selecting the semen-donor, some women have ended up with venereal disease, or with a genetically defective child. A survey in 1979 at the University of Wisconsin revealed that 70% of the physicians had kept no records of the identity of the sperm donor.[102] Pope Pius XII condemned this practice (AID) as detrimental both to the husband and wife (their conjugal right is "exclusive, non-transferrable, inalienable"), and to the child born of the procedure ("there is no link of origin, no moral and juridical bond of procreation" between such a child and the lawful husband).[103] Furthermore, there are overtones of infidelity on the part of the wife who allows herself to be inseminated by donor sperm, and of adultery on the part of the donor. There is also reliable evidence that the sperm usually is obtained by masturbation—and usually for profit.

(c) *"In Vitro" Fertilization (IVF):* If the wife has blocked or diseased fallopian tubes, or if the husband's sperm count is so low or of such poor quality that fertilization is unlikely, standard artificial insemination is not the answer. Medical technology offers them the hope of having a child by means of the "test tube baby" or "in vitro" (literally "in glass") technique. Thanks to ultrasound, fiberoptics and laparoscopy, the physician can "aspirate" or remove an ovum or several ova from the wife surgically a few hours before the calculated time of ovulation. The ovum (oocyte) is put into a shallow glass or plastic "petri" dish along with a suitable nutrient. Some of the husband's sperm is added, and the egg and sperm are allowed to interact. If fertilization occurs (detectable by the presence of the two pronuclei in the ovum), it usually occurs some 18 to 22 hours "after the mixing of the washed sperm with the oocytes." About 50 to 60 hours later, the embryo (or "embryos" if more than one ovum is involved) is transferred very carefully to the uterine cavity of the wife. At this time of transfer, the embryo generally has advanced to the 8 to 16 cell stage.[104]

[101]Andrews, Lori B., "The Stork Market: The Law of the New Reproductive Technologies," in the *American Bar Association Journal,* August, 1984, p. 50.

[102]*Ibid.,* p. 56.

[103]Address to Catholic doctors, Sept. 29, 1949. *Canon Law Digest,* III (cf. note 43), p. 433.

[104]Behrman, Dr. S.J., "Establishing an In Vitro Fertilization Program," in *Hospital Practice,* July, 1984, pp. 102, 103.

Third persons can be brought into the procedure. If the wife has ovarian failure, or does not want to risk passing on a genetic defect, another woman's ovum can be fertilized in the petri dish. If the husband is infertile or subfertile, a donor's sperm can be a substitute for, or even an additive to his sperm in the dish. The claim is made that all steps except implantation (transfer to the uterine cavity) have an 80% to 90% success rating. Unfortunately, most of the tiny embryos are lost, as indicated in the statement that "implantation is achieved 20% to 30% of the time."[105] It is estimated that about 1000 babies have been born worldwide (as of 1986) as a result of the "in vitro" procedure. The cost before a pregnancy is achieved (several attempts often required) can be up to $15,000.[106] If the couple plans on having a child "not now, but later," the embryo or embryos can be frozen between fertilization and implantation.

The immoral aspects of "in vitro" insemination are multiple. A report on the guidelines for this procedure as issued by the American Fertility Society includes assurances that all *ethical* concerns have been addressed, including "(the) destruction or disposition of extra zygotes, scientific examination of such zygotes, and cyro-preservation of extra concepti . . ."[107] So much for the evidence of disregard for human life. To a considerable extent, experimentation is the name of the game. In addition to most of the immoral aspects of artificial insemination by donor (AID), the following additional immoral features should be noted: a variety of ways of "playing God" through experimentation; the fact that surplus zygotes and embryos will be discarded, traded, abandoned, or simply consigned to the risk of death through cyro-preservation; the exposure of the embryos to the risk of death in the very delicate technique of transfer and implantation.

As of this writing, the prospect of injecting a Christian set of values into any state or federal regulations for "in vitro" procedures is not bright. Pope Pius XII's very brief pronouncement on the morality of this procedure in 1956 emphasized especially the experimental aspects of the procedure: "On the subject of experiments in artificial fecundation 'in

---

[105]*Ibid.*, p. 95.

[106]"Encouraging News for Childless Couples" by Earl Ubell in *St. Louis Post-Dispatch* (*Parade Magazine* Section), May 6, 1984, p. 12.

[107]"Fertility Society Issues Guidelines for IVF" in *Medical World News*, March 12, 1984, p. 41 (no author indicated). The article indicates that the prestigious American College of Obstetricians and Gynecologists is inclined to model their forthcoming guidelines on those of the American Fertility Society.

vitro,' let it suffice for Us to observe that they must be rejected as immoral and absolutely illicit."[108]

(d) *Surrogate Embryo Transfer (SET):* This technique might be called "temporary womb rental" so as to distinguish it from *surrogate motherhood* which might be identified with "full-term womb rental." Surrogate embryo transfer (SET) is designed for "A," the *infertile wife* of husband "B". Another woman, "C," who is known as the "donor," is inseminated by the sperm of husband "B" ("A" is the intended "recipient"). About five days after fertilization, "C's" uterus is subjected to a "lavage" or washing-out procedure. This may have to be done several times in order to find the tiny embryo. This is called "scanning time," and can go on for as long as 2 1/2 hours (as in one case). After the embryo has been recovered from the lavage fluid, it is transferred to the uterus of "A," the infertile wife or "recipient." The success of the transfer from donor "C" to recipient "A" depends on a very careful synchronization of the ovulation period of "A" the recipient, and of the ovulation period of "C", the donor.

On February 3rd, 1984, after considerable "preliminary experience" throughout 1983, researchers at the University of California (UCLA) announced the birth of the first child by embryo transfer. The procedure as described above was followed. The report of the preliminary experience of this group, headed by Dr. John E. Buster, MD, indicates not only possible legal complications, but also additional immoral aspects of the delicate procedure. As to legal problems, in one case the "recipient" had an ectopic pregnancy; in another case, the "donor" decided to retain the pregnancy. The moral dangers involve the loss of embryos: of 29 attempts to apply the procedure, only 12 embryos were recovered from the lavage fluid, and most of the attempts to transfer the embryo to the recipient were unsuccessful.[109]

There are indications that the legal climate for embryo transfer is not favorable for the spread of this procedure. The lavage technique could come under the prohibition of abortion in many cases (perhaps as many

---

[108]*The Human Body* (cf. note 61), p. 389. Ethicist Paul Ramsey also speaks of the experimentation aspects of IVF in an article entitled "Shall We Reproduce?" in the *Journal of the American Medical Association,* June 5, 1972, as follows: "*In Vitro* fertilization constitutes unethical medical experimentation on possible future human beings, and therefore . . . is subject to absolute moral prohibition" (p. 1347).

[109]Annas, George J., "Surrogate Embryo Transfer: The Perils of Patenting," in *The Hastings Center Report,* June, 1984, p. 25. Cf. also Buster, Dr. John et al., "Nonsurgical Ovum Transfer as a Treatment in Infertile Women: Preliminary Experience," in the *Journal of the American Medical Association,* March 2, 1984, pp. 1171–1173.

as 16 states) which have laws restricting fetal research. This and other potential restrictions are discussed in a recent article in the *American Bar Association Journal.* [110] Lawyers can circumvent the law, however, by arranging to have the procedure take place in states where restrictions do not apply.

4) The Morality of Surrogate Motherhood

Surrogate Motherhood or "full-term womb rental," is the converse or opposite of artificial insemination by donor (AID). Whereas the AID technique applies to a *male-infertile* couple, surrogate motherhood is an alternative for adoption for a *female-infertile* couple. In AID, the male-infertile couple achieves conception by using a donor's sperm; in surrogate motherhood, conception is achieved by using the husband's sperm to *impregnate a donor* (surrogate mother) who agrees to carry the embryo to full term.

An infertile couple may be attracted to the surrogate-motherhood concept for one or more of the following reasons: it is less cumbersome and a more immediate solution than legal adoption (no long wait, no legal adoption formalities, etc.); the wife may be a carrier of a genetic disease; the wife is a career-woman who cannot be tied down by the inconvenience of carrying and begetting a child; the wife has a history of several miscarriages; a single male or female may wish to have a child without the burden of having to support a spouse, etc. The technique could not be contemplated by a poor couple. The couple or individual must be willing and able to spend from $20,000 to $25,000, depending on the lawyer's fee and the supply and demand for surrogate mothers. [111]

It is misleading to compare surrogate mothers to Old Testament examples of solutions to the problem of infertility. It is true that Abraham's son, Ishmael, was the offspring of the patriarch and his wife Sarah's maidservant, Hagar (Genesis,16:1–16); likewise Jacob's sons, Dan and Naphtali, were the offspring of Jacob and his wife Rachel's maidservant, and his sons Gad and Asher were the offspring of Jacob and his wife Leah's maidservant (Genesis,30:1–13). These maidservants were not surrogate mothers. They were accepted as wives of the patriarchs Abraham and Jacob and as members of the patriarchal families (Genesis,30:4 and 9.; also 16:3). The same is true of the so-called "levirate law" ("levir" means "brother-in-law") whereby brothers who lived together were expected to take a sister-in-law as wife if one

---

[110]Andrews, Lori B. (cf. note 101), pp. 50–56.
[111]Robertson, John A., "Surrogate Mothers: Not So Novel After All," in *The Hastings Center Report*, October, 1983, p. 29.

of the brothers died childless (Deut.,25:5–6). As Jesus himself indicated, the Mosaic law tolerated certain practices "because of the hardness of their hearts, but it was not like this from the beginning" (Matthew,19:8).

Again, the Church must repeat the words of Pope Pius XII to all couples who regretfully must face the fact that they cannot have children of their own: namely that the marriage contract does not confer the right to have children, but rather the right to acts suitable of themselves for the procreation of off-spring. In surrogate motherhood, there is not only a separation of the *procreative* element of marriage from the *unitive* element in marriage, but also a separation of the *educational* element from the *procreative* (cf. Can.1055,1). This could be one of the reasons why there are statutes in many states which brand any adoption release as invalid if it is executed by the natural mother before the birth of the child.[112] Finally, there is the disturbing premonition of a scandalous "babies for sale" market if the donor-woman is allowed to demand a fee substantially in excess of the expenses actually incurred in gestating the child and giving birth (including, of course, her support and a fitting remuneration for her loss-of-other-employment income during the gestation and delivery period).

It is evident that the welfare of the child is not paramount in a surrogate-motherhood agreement. There have been situations where the baby was born with defects suggesting retardation, and neither the surrogate mother nor the presumptive parent or parents wanted the child. There have been situations where the surrogate mother decided to keep the baby as her own, or where a surrogate mother decided to have an abortion. In some locales, courts and civil authorities have declared the surrogate-mother contract or agreement to be in violation of public policy or of the state adoption laws.[113] There could be situations, however, where a generous woman, inspired by the *Principle of the Common Good,* would volunteer her services as a surrogate mother, in order to vindicate the right to life of an embryo which otherwise, of a moral certainty, would be destroyed, discarded or abandoned. Objectively considered, therefore, and divorced from the immoral aspects associated with artificial insemination (in which she was not involved), this rare aspect of surrogate motherhood could not be condemned as immoral.

---

[112]Holder, Angela R., "Surrogate Motherhood: Babies for Fun and Profit," in *Law, Medicine and Health Care,* June, 1984, p. 115.

[113]Gersz, Steven R., JD, "The Contract in Surrogate Motherhood: A Review of the Issues," in *Law, Medicine and Health Care,* June, 1984, pp. 111, 112. Cf. also *Technological Powers and the Person* (cf. note 94), for an address on the legal aspects of surrogate motherhood by Judge Carol Los Mansmann, pp. 406–420.

> *Directive 21:* Because the ultimate personal expression of con-
> jugal love in the marital act is viewed as the only fitting
> context for the human sharing of the divine act of creation,
> donor insemination and insemination that is totally artificial
> are morally objectionable. However, help may be given to a
> normally performed conjugal act to attain its purpose. The
> use of the sex faculty outside the legitimate use by married
> partners is never permitted even for medical or other laud-
> able purpose, e.g., masturbation as a means of obtaining
> seminal specimens.

5) Possible and Pending Genetic Techniques

In the realm of the *possible,* "cloning" must be mentioned. Frogs were
cloned from the intestine cells of tadpoles in 1966. By this alarming procedure, "carbon copy" babies could be produced asexually. Articles have been
published in bioethic circles which even suggest that human beings might be
cloned "to serve as an inventory of parts for human transplants."[114] It is
possible that cloning could be followed by attempts to produce half-man/half-
animal hybrids. If such efforts were to succeed, mythology could become
reality. It would be impossible to foresee the extent of the cataclysmic denigra-
tion of human dignity.

In the realm of the *pending,* it is only a question of time before a feasible
artificial placenta is developed—that is, a reliable life-support system for a
pregnancy outside of the original host womb. There is also serious speculation about a non-injurious method of removing an embryo from the womb of
a seriously ill or unwilling mother for transfer to a host mother. This would
involve embryos more advanced than the 5-day embryos which are "washed
out" of the uterus in the surrogate embryo-transfer technique (SET). In his
remarkable book entitled *Aborting America,* Dr. Bernard N. Nathanson speaks
of such a discovery (safe embryo-transfer method) as a solution both for infertile couples and for the abortion problem. It would simply be a matter of
detecting the embryo in its early stages, removing it from the ill or unwilling
mother, and transferring it "either to a life-support system, or re-

---

[114]Krimmel, Herbert T., "The Case Against Surrogate Parenting," in *The Hastings Center Report,* October, 1983. He speaks of "articles that foresee the use of comatose human beings as self-
replenishing blood banks and manufacturing plants for human hormones" (p. 36).

implantation into a willing and eager recipient." He adds: "There would then remain only the creation of a new word to replace abortion."[115]

Faith in human decency and in human dignity must prevail. This represents not only a moral medical problem of major proportions, but also an ethnic, social and political challenge to preserve the dignity and integrity of the human race. Medical experts and geneticists must be inspired to sort out and discard the possibilities of evil from the immense possibilities of good which are inherent in the pursuit of their profession. Reason and respect for human dignity will prevail if the medical world is faithful to the recently-revised American Medical Association's "Code of Medical Ethics" which begins (following the preamble) with the following statement:

> The principle objective of the medical profession is to render service to humanity with full respect for the dignity of man. Physicians should merit the confidence of patients entrusted to their care, rendering to each a full measure of service and devotion.[116]

2.4 PSYCHOLOGICAL AND SOCIAL NEEDS

Just being in a health-care facility can affect a person's sense of independence, self-confidence, self-worth, etc., in a gradual downward curve. In varying degrees, patients forfeit control over what to wear, what to eat, when to retire, etc. Personal privacy is invaded; highly personal facts become a part of the official and not-so-confidential record; trust must be placed in hurrying and scurrying service personnel who remain, for the most part, strangers to the lonely and fearsome individual. There is the tedium and inconvenience of the mechanics of diagnosis and the haunting fear of the perils of prognosis. The seriously ill and terminal patients often are overcome with anxieties. Considering that three-fourths of the deaths in the U.S.A. occur in hospitals or in long-term care facilities, the sense of alienation in such an atmosphere of "benign captivity" must often bring to mind sentiments similar to those expressed in psalm 137: "How could we sing a song of the Lord in a foreign land?" (v.4). How many yearn to die at home, surrounded by familiar faces and places!

Many of the psychological needs associated with the atmosphere of alienation in health-care facilities are being addressed today through enlightened

---

[115]*Aborting America* (New York, N.Y.: Pinnacle Books, 1981), p. 287.
[116]Reiser, Stanley J., MD, Ph.D., "Codes of Medical Ethics," in *Health Matrix,* summer, 1984, p. 43.

chaplain and pastoral care programs; and also by the "at home" orientation as sponsored by the Hospice Movement. Other problems, especially those associated with the pangs of decision-making and self-determination will be discussed in the chapter on the *Principle of Informed Consent*. As to the social needs of patients, the phrase "ready access to all that is necessary for living a genuinely human life" has little meaning without a basic understanding of the role of government, and the role of charity.

The Role of Government in "Ready Access" to Medical Care

Almost as certain as death and taxes are the two realities which must be faced in health-care planning: 1) "The poor you will always have with you . . ." (Matthew, 26:11), and 2) more and more, the U.S. Government will be less and less able to meet the medical needs of all of the citizens without outside-government help to take up the slack. The government cannot do it alone. The report of the *President's Commission For the Study of Ethical Problems in Medicine and Biomedical and Behavioral Research* (to be referred to hereafter as *The President's Commission*) tells it "as it is." The report develops the conclusion that it would be fiscally impossible in practical terms for the U.S. Government to provide fair or equitable access to health-care dollars either on the basis of *EQUALITY* (since some would use private funds to exceed the set standard), or on the basis of *WHATEVER CARE MIGHT BE NEEDED OR BENEFICIAL* (which would mean "whatever a person wants") without neglecting other very important societal needs.[117]

The President's Commission proposes that the concept of equitable access be based not on the two levels mentioned above (*equality* and *beneficial*) but rather "that everyone have access to *some* level of care: *enough care* to achieve sufficient welfare, opportunity, information, and evidence of interpersonal concern to facilitate a reasonably full and satisfying life."[118] With a price tag for the procurement and transplanting of body organs which ranges from $30,000 for a kidney, to $100,000 for a heart, and to $230,000 for a liver at current rates (subject to change), any *reasonable* person should appreciate the objective of a *"reasonably* full and satisfying life" as a goal which must be subject to some variation. Expending exorbitant sums for the *special* needs of a few could spell the neglect of the *ordinary* needs of so many others. There would be variations in that *adequate level of care*.

---

[117]*Securing Access to Health Care* (Washington, D.C.: U.S. Government Printing Office, 1983), I, pp. 18–22. This is a publication of *The President's Commission*.
[118]*Ibid.*, p. 20.

The President's Commission must be commended for stressing an aspect of an *adequate level of health care* which can easily be overlooked: namely, the *burdens* many must bear in order to *obtain* that health care (for example, painful waiting, travel time, cost and availability of transportation, financial cost of the care itself). No one should have to forego food, shelter, or educational advancement in order to obtain adequate care. In order to illustrate what burdens might be involved, one might imagine the sacrifices required of a family where one member is a victim of renal failure, and must be taken to a distant city several times per week for expensive renal-dialysis treatments (estimated cost: $35,000 per year). The full criterion, therefore, should be: society has a moral obligation (within its capabilities) to ensure that *everyone has access to adequate care without being subjected to excessive burdens.*[119]

What agencies might be expected to "take up the slack" to the extent possible? The report mentions the purchase of insurance, reliance on acts of charity in which "individuals such as relatives and care givers and institutions assume responsibility for absorbing some or all of the person's health care expenses," and also state and local agencies. To the extent that the market place (insurance, for example), private charity, and lower levels of government are insufficient in achieving equity in the matter, "the responsibility rests with the federal government."[120] There is no tendency in this report to gloss over sensitive and thorny issues.

The Role of Charity in the Mission of Healing

The report of *The President's Commission* pays tribute to the "strong tradition of private charity in the United States including free services by health professionals as well as the role of charitable organizations."[121] It must be admitted, regretfully, that this practice has declined with the expansion of *Medicare* and *Medicaid* ("let the government pay!") The decline in such deeds of charity in Catholic hospitals, however, is something that has developed beyond the control of the dedicated Religious Sisters who came to America to establish Catholic hospitals so as to help the poor and the indigent. In the 1880's, however, a change took place which explained the decrease in charity to the poor: the income from paying patients simply became insufficient to continue the charity role on a significant scale. Gradually, the prime focus of Catholic hospital care changed from concern for the poor and indigent to general service to all who were sick and injured regardless of their ability to

---

[119]*Ibid.*, p. 22.
[120]*Ibid.*, p. 25, 26.
[121]*Ibid.*, p. 29.

pay. The charity role had to be "spread out" to the many, instead of to the poor and indigent in particular.

During the 19th century and up to the present day, the private pay-patient became the "overpay-patient," in the sense that he or she had to be billed for more than the actual cost for that patient (but not for operating the hospital) so as to supplement the hospital fund for other purposes. Whereas those "other purposes" at first were primarily to cover concern for the poor, the trend today is to earmark most of the overpay for needed construction and modernization.[122] Most of the factors which contributed to this decreased concern for the poor and indigent (increased patient income, higher wages for hospital personnel, improved and expensive medical technologies, growth of health insurance, effects of Medicare and Medicaid, etc.) were simply beyond the control of the dedicated Religious Sisters and others who witnessed for Christ in the mission of healing throughout the years.

The shining glory of the mission of healing—concern for "the least of my brethren,"—currently is threatened with at least a partial eclipse. A series of surveys conducted by a task force of the Catholic Health Association in 1982 has delineated the challenge of the present and the future. Those requested to participate in the surveys included the following:

–Religious congregations who sponsor Catholic hospitals in the U.S.A.;

–422 CEO's, or Chief Executive Officers (over 50% of Catholic hospitals currently are headed by lay executives);

–35 leaders of multi-institutional systems (system leaders);

–33 major superiors of religious congregations which sponsor Catholic hospitals in the U.S.A.;

–151 Catholic bishops from throughout the U.S.A.

The overall commentary on the issue of service to the poor was: "[It] emerges as a problematic issue. It is perceived as important for the Catholic hospital's purpose, and yet it is currently difficult to provide charity and maintain fiscal solvency."[123] . . . The general commentary in the responses of all but the first group (sponsoring religious congregations) was that the ministry of hospitals "is being challenged to advance new methods, systems and structures for the service of the needy."[124]

Without doubt, the shortage of vocations to the religious life is one of the weak links in the Catholic tradition of service to the poor. Over 50% of the

---

[122]Collins, Thomas M., JD, "The For-Profit/Not-For-Profit Debate: Issues and Responses," *Religious Congregations and Health Care Facilities: Commitment and Collaboration, Colloquium II* (St. Louis, Mo.: Catholic Health Association, 1982), pp. 16–18.

[123]Callahan, Thomas E. and Sister Margaret John Kelly, D.C., Ph.D., "CHA Task Force on Stewardship Survey Report, Part IV," in *Hospital Progress*, April, 1983, p. 68.

[124]*Ibid.*, p. 73.

religious superiors who were interviewed in the survey "identified the poor as their main target population for service." It could be inferred that the continued presence of the Religious Sisters in the hospital apostolate would enhance the possibility of service to the poor. The respondents to the survey seem to harbor such sentiments. Although 85% of them rated the laity's ability to administer Catholic hospitals at an above-average level, "only 50% expressed the same confidence in lay sponsorship if religious sponsorship were not available."[125] Another source explains the lack of the presence of Religious Sisters in the hospital (besides the decrease in vocations) as follows: "We are seeing a diminishing number of sisters, the effects of renewal, and the recently won independence of religious to determine their own destinies."[126]

A possible solution must involve prayer and action on two fronts: the vocation front, and the "access to health care" front. Young men and women today seem to gravitate to volunteer work which involves the indigent and the elderly. The once-rewarding and fulfilling apostolate to the sick and needy may yet be re-discovered. As to prayer and "access to health care," it should be directed to a fervent plea that *common sense* may prevail, and not the "impossible dream" that government can and must do it all. *Adequate* health care for all is possible; enough to *facilitate* (not guarantee) a *reasonably* full and satisfying life. To this end, the following final paragraph of a popular book of the early 70's is presented as seasoned and sensible food for thought:

> We all have to die sometime and we shall all be grateful to scientific medicine when it is our turn to have our deaths postponed (unless they strive too officiously to keep us alive), . . . in the meantime we have to live, and it may be that the quality of our lives should carry more weight. Perhaps medicine should help us live more fully and spend less in averting our deaths. Medicine in crisis cannot do both to the full. In the end this is the biggest choice we have to make.[127]

---

[125]*Ibid.*, p. 73.
[126]Collins, Thomas M. (cf. note 122), p. 19.
[127]Leach, Gerald, *The Biocrats: Ethics and the New Medicine* (cf. note 59), p. 356.

CHAPTER III

The Principle of the Right to Life

For God, the Lord of Life, has conferred on men the surpassing ministry of safeguarding life—a ministry which must be fulfilled in a manner which is worthy of man. Therefore from the moment of its conception life must be guarded with the greatest care, while abortion and infanticide are unspeakable crimes . . . Furthermore, whatever is opposed to life itself, . . . whatever violates the integrity of the human person, . . . whatever insults human dignity . . . all these things . . . are infamies indeed (*The Church Today,* nn.51 and 27).

PRINCIPLE: PROCEEDING FROM THE WILL AND PLAN OF THE CREATOR, AND PRIOR TO THE VERY EXISTENCE OF HUMAN SOCIETY, THE FIRST RIGHT OF EVERY HUMAN INDIVIDUAL, AND THE FOUNDATION AND CONDITION FOR THE EXERCISE OF ALL OTHER RIGHTS, IS THE RIGHT TO LIFE—WHICH MUST BE RESPECTED AND GUARDED FROM THE MOMENT WHEN THE PROCESS OF HUMAN GENERATION BEGINS. ANY DISCRIMINATION AGAINST HUMAN INDIVIDUALS ON ANY GROUNDS OR IN ANY STAGES OF HUMAN GROWTH OR DECLINE, IS IMMORAL AND A GLARING INJUSTICE IN THE STRICT SENSE OF THE WORD (Adapted from The *Declaration on Abortion,* Nov. 18, 1974, nn.11,12).

John J. Noonan, Jr. begins his book *Private Choice: Abortion in America in the Seventies* by saying: "Once or twice in a century an issue arises so divisive in its nature, so far-reaching in its consequences, and so deep in its foundations that it calls for every person to take a stand."[128] This last quarter of the century is such a time, and abortion is such an issue. "Standing up for life" is not enough; enlightened leadership is also of the essence. Vatican II's document, *The Church Today* (n.15) emphasizes the need of wisdom in that leadership:

> Our era needs such wisdom more than bygone ages if the discoveries made by man are to be further humanized. For the future of the world stands in peril unless wiser men are forthcoming.[129]

The Pro-Life Movement has become something of a crusade in America as if in response to the words of *The Church Today* (quoted above) that the "ministry of safeguarding life" is a "surpassing" concern for all mankind—surpassing all other human concerns. The movement is no longer looked upon as merely a "Catholic" campaign, and truly has caught fire as a "catholic" one (small "c" for "widespread, universal"). The Heavenly Father has blessed this campaign with enlightened leadership to the extent that the President of the most influential nation on earth personally has championed this crucial campaign of "safeguarding life." No one can deny, however, that the opposition to this campaign is determined, influential and well-financed.

3.1 OUR HEAVENLY FATHER, THE LORD OF LIFE

Those who are ignorant or forgetful of man's divine origin, and would re-fashion man and woman to become caricatures of the divine image, might be likened to the maker of clay idols in the Old Testament as described in the Book of Wisdom (15:10 and 11).

> Ashes his heart is! More worthless than earth is his hope, and more ignoble than clay his life; because he knew not the one who fashioned him and breathed into him a quickening soul, and infused a vital spirit.

---

[128](New York, N.Y.: The Free Press, 1979), p. 1.
[129]The observation that "mankind today . . . is in danger of being ruined from within, by his own moral decay," is referred to by His Eminence Joseph cardinal Ratzinger in his opening address at the Bishops' Workshop as sponsored by the Pope John Center in Dallas, Texas, Feb. 6–10, 1984. Cf. *Moral Technology Today* (St. Louis, Mo.: Pope John Center, 1984), pp. 3, 4.

The Book of Genesis portrays the Creator as a Divine Potter: "The Lord formed man out of the clay of the ground and blew into his nostrils the breath of life, and so man became a living being" (literally, "a living soul"). The name "Adam" is a play on the word "ground" (in Hebrew, "adamah"). What heights from such humble origins: "God created man in His image" (Gen.1,27)! And what a reminder of the insignificance of the "shell" (for St. Paul, the "tent") when death signals the liberation of the soul from the body: "For you are dirt, and to dirt you shall return" (Genesis,3:19). Until that time, however, the origin of human life and conservation of life is in the hand of God: "For the spirit of God has made me, the breath of the Almighty keeps me alive" (Job,33:4).

The great minds of antiquity such as Plato and Aristotle considered the civil state to be the source of all rights. Plato recommended abortion as well as infanticide "when necessary,"—Aristotle wrote: "Let there be a law that no deformed child shall be reared . . ."[130] Throughout the early centuries and the Middle Ages, the Church vindicated the creative dominion of God, and insisted on the worth and dignity of every human individual as based on the will and plan of the Creator. Influential voices of the 17th century such as René Descartes (1596–1650), Baruch Spinoza (1632–1677) and Gottfried Leibnitz (1646–1716) prepared the way for the wave of resentment and eventual rejection of the biblical accounts of the creation and of any transcendent source of authority or guidance. The storm broke in Catholic France—at just about the time when George Washington was inaugurated as the first President of the United States of America (April 30, 1789). The French revolutionary campaign to nationalize church property was launched in May, 1789. Beginning in May, 1792, the focus was on "dechristianization." Prohibition of worship applied to all Christian churches; churches were closed or used for secular purposes; executions of those who opposed the new order spread from city to city; the "Goddess of Reason" was enthroned in the Cathedral of Notre Dame in Paris in November, 1793.[131] Rationalism triumphed, and became the basis for insisting that all human rights, including the right to life, are subject to the recognition and regulation of civil authority.

The challenging task of reinstating and renewing the faith in the dominion of God as the source of the right to life and of respect for life—of giving evidence of the "saving presence of Christ and His Church in the mission of healing"—is such a prime objective for Catholic health facilities, that the

---

[130]Gorman, Michael, *Abortion and the Early Church* (New York, N.Y.: Paulist Press, 1982), pp. 21, 22.

[131]LaTreille, A., article on the French Revolution, in *New Catholic Encyclopedia* (New York, N.Y.: McGraw Hill, 1967), pp. 187–191.

Ethical and Religious Directives for such facilities begin with a dedication to that challenge:

> Catholic health facilities witness to the saving presence of Christ and His Church in a variety of ways: by testifying to transcendent spiritual beliefs concerning life, suffering, and death; by humble service to humanity and especially to the poor; by medical competence and leadership; and by fidelity to the Church's teachings while ministering to the good of the whole person.
>
> (Preamble, paragraph one)

3.2 ALLOWING LIFE TO BEGIN

Most people would agree with author William Henry Hudson (1841–1922) who spoke of his long periods of sickness, poverty and loneliness, and added: "I could yet always feel that it was infinitely better to be than not to be."[132] Whether, in Shakespeare's words, it is "To be or not to be" depends on whether or not fertile married couples allow the blessing of offspring to flower from their conjugal love.

Pope Pius XII pointed out that marriage does not grant a right to have children. Children are gifts from above which may or may not result from the right couples do have, namely, the right over each other, as persons, to the acts suitable of themselves for the procreation of offspring (Can.1061,1). The phrase "over each other as persons" is significant. As Pope John Paul II said in his *Apostolic Exhortation on the Family* ("Familiaris Consortio") on Nov. 22, 1981: ". . . sexuality by means of which man and woman give themselves to one another through the acts which are proper and exclusive to spouses, is by no means something purely biological, but concerns the innermost being of the human person as such" (n.11).[133]

Do married couples have an obligation to beget offspring? That God wills "fertility and increase" is apparent in the account of the very act of creation: "God blessed them saying: 'Be fertile and multiply; fill the earth and subdue it' . ." (Genesis,1,28). That procreation is an essential human good should be

---

[132]*Familiar Quotations,* John Bartlett, ed., 13th edition (Boston, Ma.: Little, Brown and Co., 1955), p. 711.

[133]*The Pope Speaks,* Vol. 27, n. 1 (1982), p. 9.

clear not only from the Word of the Creator, but from right reason. God is the Author of Life, and retains His dominion over those joined in marriage who would cooperate with Him in the transmission of life. As Pope Paul VI wrote in his encyclical letter *Humanae Vitae* (n.10):

> In the task of transmitting life, therefore, (husband and wife) are not free to proceed completely at will, as if they could determine in a wholly autonomous way the honest path to follow; but they must conform their activity to the creative intention of God, expressed in the very nature of marriage and of its acts, and manifested by the constant teaching of the Church.[134]

This obligation to bring forth new life is not incumbent upon all married couples. Many couples are not blessed with fertility. Furthermore, there have been cases of "virginal marriage" where both parties have been inspired from spiritual motives to agree mutually before marriage to forego the use of the marriage right (that is, the *proximate* right to marital acts) over each other's person, leaving intact the *fundamental* right to that aspect of the conjugal relationship. Thus the marriage of the Blessed Virgin Mary and St. Joseph was a true marriage. Each knew of the others's vow NOT to request the use of the marriage right.[135] Other fertile couples may have serious reasons for not realizing the blessing of parenthood temporarily or even permanently, and restrict their use of the marriage right to periods of infertility. The extent of their obligation to realize parenthood would depend upon the serious nature and permanency of their reasons. The brunt of the obligation to "increase and multiply" devolves upon fertile married couples who have no serious reasons for not having children. This aspect of NOT excluding life from conjugal love in a positive manner is so essential, that if a couple agrees before marriage to prevent the conception of children absolutely and permanently, there is a very strong presumption that the marriage right itself was excluded. This would make the marriage invalid. In a matrimonial tribunal case, of course, the presumption would yield to definite proof to the contrary.[136]

---

[134]*Love and Sexuality* (cf. note 61), p. 336.

[135]The noted Jesuit theologian, Father John C. Ford, wrote his doctoral dissertation on the subject of *The Validity of Virginal Marriage* (Worchester, Ma.: Harrigan Press, 1938), with special application to the marriage of the Blessed Mother of Jesus and St. Joseph.

[136]Griese, Orville, doctoral dissertation entitled *The Marriage contract and the Procreation of Offspring* (Washington, D.C.: Catholic University of America Press, 1946), pp. 61–66. Cf. also the review of actual cases, *ibid.*, pp. 127–133. Pius XII refers expressly to such an exclusion of children as grounds for the invalidity of marriage in his address to the Italian midwives. Cf. *The Human Body* (cf. note 61), p. 163.

The Case Against Contraception

To say that contraception is wrong because it is a perversion of the generative faculty to use it while frustrating its natural orientation to bring about new life, is not a convincing or proper argument. This "scholastic natural law" argument infers that it is always wrong to pervert a natural faculty (eating, hearing, seeing, etc.) Author Germain Grisez points to the fallacy of this argumentation by saying: "People reasonably note that perverting faculties in this sense cannot always be wrong—no one objects to the use of earplugs or chewing sugarless gum."[137] The roots of the evil of contraception are to be sought on a level which is far more profound than the surface manifestations of the physiology of marital union. Those roots are to be sought on the level of the profound meaning of truth and dignity in the personal communion of marriage: a communion of persons.

This concept of the real truth and dignity of personal communion in marriage was introduced by Pope Paul VI in his encyclical letter, "Humanae Vitae" (n.12), where he insisted upon "the inseparable connection, willed by God and unable to be broken by man on his own initiative, between the two meanings of the conjugal act: the unitive meaning and the procreative meaning." In commenting upon this passage, Pope John Paul II explained this "inseparability" by saying: ". . . because both the one and the other pertain to the intimate truth of the conjugal act: the one is activated together with the other and in a certain sense the one by means of the other . . . in such a case [that is the separation of the unitive aspect from the procreative aspect] the conjugal act, deprived of its interior truth, because artificially deprived of its procreative capacity, ceases also to be an act of love." Pope John Paul II then completed his analysis of the evil of contraception as follows:

> It can be said that in the case of an artificial separation of these two aspects, there is carried out in the conjugal act a real bodily union, but it does not correspond to the dignity of personal communion: communion of persons. This communion demands in fact that the "language of the body" be expressed reciprocally in the integral truth of its meaning. If this truth is lacking, one cannot speak of the truth of self-mastery, or of the truth of the reciprocal gift and of the reciprocal acceptance of self on the part of the

---

[137] *The Way of the Lord Jesus,* Vol. I (Chicago, Ill.: Franciscan Herald Pres, 1983), pp. 105 f. Cf. also *Contemporary Moral Theology* by John C. Ford, S.J., and Gerald Kelly, S.J., Vol. II (cf. note 65), pp. 366, 367.

person. Such a violation of the interior order of conjugal union, which is rooted in the very order of the person, constitutes the essential evil of the contraceptive act.[138]

Coming now to a definition of contraception, the following is proposed as incorporating on the practical level the concepts developed by Pope Paul VI and Pope John Paul II as presented above:

Contraception, then, is a directly willed intervention of any positive kind to prevent the realization of the procreative good when it otherwise might follow from an act of sexual intercourse in which one has chosen to engage.[139]

The phrase "chosen to engage" is to be understood in the sense of *freedom* of choice. Thus it would not be immoral, for example, for a woman who is in danger of being raped to have recourse to some protective, contraceptive device.[140]

3.3 THE CHURCH'S CONCERN FOR COUPLES WITH A FERTILITY PROBLEM

The Church's concern for couples with an *infertility problem* was discussed in the previous chapter (2.3). Since this involved extended references to methods which are more popular in the effort to *regulate fertility* than in the effort to *promote fertility,* however, the discussion included basic descriptions of landmark discoveries such as the "Rhythm Method," the Billings Ovulation Method and the Sympto-thermal Method. When it comes to using such methods to regulate fertility, however, the following question must be antici-

---

[138]*Reflections on Humanae Vitae* (Boston, Ma.: St. Paul Editions, 1984), pp. 33, 34. Taken from his address at a general audience, August 22, 1984.

[139]Grisez, Germain, *Contraception and the Natural Law* (Milwaukee, Wis.: Bruce Publishing Co., 1964), p. 91. In the same vein, a distinguished Catholic physician of Chicago, Ill., Eugene F. Diamond, MD, and his wife Rosemary, state in *The Positive Values of Chastity* (Chicago, Ill.: Franciscan Herald Press, 1983), p. 18: "If there is no inseparable relationship between sexuality and reproduction, then what used to be called illicit—homosexual and extramarital heterosexual liaisons—are as valid and deserving of respect as conventional marriage."

[140]In the early 1960's, the Holy See tacitly accepted a solution to the danger of rape which faced the Religious Sisters in the Belgian Congo due to the unsettled civil status of that country. The Sisters were allowed to resort to the use of contraceptive pills as protection against the danger of rape. Cf. *Rape Within Marriage: A Moral Analysis Delayed,* by Father Edward J. Bayer, STD (Lanham, Md.: University Press of America, Inc., 1985), pp. 82, 83.

pated: "How can Catholics use such methods in effect to avoid conception (and with a good conscience) when the couples who use them with all of their good reasons nevertheless have a *positive* will to exclude the essential human good of procreation?"

Before attempting a response to that logical question, it is important to point out that, strictly speaking, the word "contraception" should be reserved for "a *directly willed* intervention of any positive kind" to prevent conception (cf.definition,p.73). The use of the "Rhythm Method" or of Natural Family Planning, on the other hand, is best described *not* as contraception, but as the *natural regulation of fertility*. Although both modes of action, based on reaction to the fertility problem, involve the avoidance of conception, they are intrinsically different from an ethical viewpoint. Pope Paul VI states in "Humanae Vitae" that, in having recourse to contraception, the couples "impede the development of natural processes," whereas in restricting the use of the conjugal right to sterile periods only, "the married couple make legitimate use of a natural disposition" (n.16). In commenting upon this passage, Pope John Paul II made the following helpful observation:

> From this there derive two actions that are ethically different, indeed, even opposed: the natural regulation of fertility is morally correct; contraception is not morally correct. This essential difference between the two actions (or modes of acting) concerns their intrinsic ethical character . . . . It might be observed at this point that married couples who have recourse to the natural regulation of fertility, might do so without the valid reasons spoken of above. This, however, is a separate ethical problem, when one treats of the moral sense of "responsible parenthood."[141]

An effective response to the question posed above requires a second preliminary observation: a distinction must be made between avoiding conception *directly* (contraception properly so-called) and *indirectly* through recourse to natural fertility regulation (often called indirect contraception). When couples have recourse to Natural Family Planning, which involves the avoidance of conception, it is a question of material cooperation in something which, objectively considered, would be morally wrong if directly intended—that is, positive opposition to a definite obligation which belongs to the very state of marriage. Objectively considered, the deliberate pursuit of sterility in marriage is contrary to the very concept of marriage as grounded on the

---

[141]*Reflections on Humanae Vitae* (cf. note 138), pp. 26 and 27. Taken from his address at a general audience on Aug. 8, 1984.

natural law as well as on the divine positive law. The difficulty is solved by the application of the *Principle of the Double Effect*. The *direct* and prevailing intention on the part of the couple in restricting the exercise of their conjugal rights to sterile periods only is the fostering of some good or the avoidance of some evil as indicated by the serious and proportionate reasons which obtain in their particular situation. The avoidance of conception is a concomitant side effect which is not intended but merely permitted. This distinction must be kept in mind whenever the natural regulation of fertility (as often is the case) is referred to as *indirect* contraception.

With a proper understanding of these two preliminaries, the following response to the question posed above is both revealing and adequate. It is taken from Pope Pius XII's address to the Italian midwives in 1951:

> . . . marriage binds to a state of life which, while conferring certain rights, at the same time imposes the accomplishment of a positive work which belongs to the very state of wedlock. This being so, the general principle can now be stated that the fulfillment of a positive duty may be withheld should grave reasons, independent of the good will of those obliged to it, show that such fulfillment is untimely, or make it evident that it cannot equitably be demanded by that which requires the fulfillment—in this case, the human race.[142]

Thus if it is morally certain that a woman has an irremedial condition whereby she can give birth only to dead infants, or only to infants with gross congenital defects, that couple is justified in using Natural Family Planning so as to regulate the wife's fertility. If medical science cannot later furnish a remedy for their unfortunate situation, this mode of solving their fertility problem can be justified for the entire duration of their married life.

It is not, therefore, the intention or purpose of regulating fertility in married life which constitutes the evil of contraception properly so-called, but the choice of *means to that end* which are *directly* designed and intended to "render procreation impossible" (*Directive 19:* a direct quotation from "Humanae Vitae," n.14). If such means are used not with the intention of *avoiding* conception, but as a medically-recommended means of enhancing the possibility of having children (for example, the temporary use of steroid pills to regularize the woman's cycles) as the only available and reasonable means of

---

[142] *The Human Body* (cf. note 61), p. 164. Pius XII repeated this principle in his address to the Hematological Congress on Sept. 12, 1958, cf. *The Pope Speaks* Vol. I (1959–1960), pp. 396 and 397.

fostering conception, the couple is acting not *against* nature but with nature. The side effect of temporary sterility (in the application of the *Principle of the Double Effect*) is not intended but merely permitted.

In having recourse to Natural Family Planning with sufficient reasons so as to regulate the fertility of their marital union, the husband and wife (in the words of Pope Paul VI) are making "legitimate use of a natural disposition of nature" (the succession of sterile and fertile days); they also submit to a certain degree of self-denial, and yet protect one another from temptations to infidelity: ". . . they are able to renounce the use of marriage in the fecund periods . . . while making use of it during infecund periods to manifest their affection and to safeguard their mutual fidelity."[143]

This is NOT to say, however, that the Catholic Church has "canonized" methods such as Natural Family Planning, or that the Church is promoting her own brand of "Catholic birth control." The question of appropriate reasons for regulating fertility will be discussed presently. To follow such a regime in married life without appropriate reasons—seeking always and deliberately to evade the procreative duty—"would be a sin against the very meaning of married life."[144] The mere fact that such couples (with no serious reasons for seeking the sterility route in marriage) are willing to accept and bring up a child or children who may be conceived and born notwithstanding their Natural Family Planning precautions, "would not in itself alone be a sufficient guarantee of a right intention and of the unquestionable morality of the motives themselves." In fact (as previously noted), there could even be reasons for questioning the validity of such a marriage.[145]

It must be stressed, however, that this "infertility route" is not for every couple with a list of sufficient reasons. Both parties must be *"willing"* and *"able."* Why *willing*? Because if one party is unwilling, and makes reasonable requests for conjugal union during the fertile periods, each refusal of intercourse by the other party would be a violation both of charity and of justice. Why *able*? Because the program of "periodic continence" involved in the practice of these methods could put one or both of the parties in proximate occasions of sin; for example, the use of artificial contraceptive devices during the fertile periods, infidelity, seeking satisfaction through masturbation, etc. In some cases, the real danger of a critical cooling in supportive love (considering the voluntary abstinence required) could militate against taking the infertility route. In other words, "God be with you" is required in view of the spirit of sacrifice and self-denial which is inherent in the method.

---

[143] *Love and Sexuality* (cf. note 61); n. 16 of "Humanae Vitae," p. 339.
[144] Address to Italian midwives, cf. *The Human Body* (cf. note 61), p. 164.
[145] *Ibid.*, pp. 163, 164.

There is much practical wisdom in the saying: "You don't know what you can do until you have to do it." Pius XII invoked the memory of both St. Augustine and the Council of Trent when he said: "God does not command what is impossible, but when He commands He warns you to do what you can and ask His aid for what is beyond your powers, and He gives His help to make that possible for you."[146] Drawing on sources of spiritual strength can confirm their *willingness,* and their *ability* to handle the challenge, and in the process, they may well find themselves coming closer to God and to one another.

Sufficient Reasons for Regulating Fertility

As indicated above, Paul VI refers to serious motives for spacing out births "which derive from the physical or psychological conditions of husband and wife, or from external conditions." Pius XII (17 years earlier) had mentioned serious reasons "often advanced on medical, eugenic, economic and social grounds" which can exempt a couple from having children "even for a considerable period of time, even for the entire duration of marriage."[147] That phrase "even for the entire duration of the marriage" is best interpreted in Paul VI's reference to "even for an indeterminate period" as found in *Humanae Vitae* (n.10); for the Church does encourage couples with even the most serious marital problems (e.g., serious danger to the health of the wife if conception occurs) to resort to prayer and to technological/medical progress in an effort to solve the problem. More than a few wives have become jubilant mothers despite the warnings of their family physicians regarding the threatening dangers of conception and childbirth. Surely "Don't lose hope" is more Christian than "Nothing can be done."

If "willing and able" couples with fertility problems who are inclined to take the Rhythm or NFP route have any doubts about the sufficiency of their reasons, they should have a confidential visit with their parish priest or confessor. There are no stock or taxative lists of "sufficient reasons"—the ultimate, prudential judgment must come from the couple themselves after prayerful pondering and consultation. The "social" grounds or conditions mentioned by Pius XII and Paul VI would stem from many contemporary factors such as the preponderance of working wives, the increased mobility of families, the rapid turnover in employment (layoffs, etc.), and even certain valid claims of the "womens' liberation movement" (wife not "tied down" to

---

[146]*Ibid.,* p. 167.
[147]*Ibid.,* p. 165.

the home, etc.). The following listing of possible reasons are offered as examples.

Examples of Sufficient Reasons for the Temporary Practice of Fertility-Regulation (mostly for the "spacing" of children): The wife is of frail health; she is unable to give birth except by cesarean section (expensive); she is unusually fecund (fertile, fruitful); she is in a highly nervous state of mind and cannot "even think of another child" now; the several tots in the home already temporarily require all of the wife's time and attention (especially if she is a working wife), etc. Similar reasons could justify the "caboose syndrome" (this is the last one) if the couple already has a fair-sized family.

Generally Insufficient reasons: The wife's unfounded and unreasonable fear of the ordinary inconveniences and pain of pregnancy and childbirth ("too delicate"); the desire of husband or wife or both to "enjoy life while they are young;" the couple plans on just one or two children to "keep the wealth in the family;" one or both of the spouses "just cannot stand children."

Doubtfully Sufficient Reasons: couple determined to have just one or two children so as to offer them exceptional educational advantages; the wife is determined to continue her professional career (entertainer, business venture); couple determined to have no children until the house and furniture are all paid for.

Examples of Sufficient Reasons for the LONG-RANGE Practice of Fertility-Regulation: Conception will very probably result in death or a permanent state of bad health for the mother; it is almost certain that the wife cannot bring forth living children or bring them to term (history of miscarriages); it is practically certain that the children will be born with serious and incurable hereditary defects which would render them unfit for the exercise of normal, social functions;[148] the financial condition of the couple is such that it would be morally impossible to support another child even if the wife is working; the wife has a proven incapacity, either physically or morally, to fulfill her maternal duties with regard to the children already born; one of the parties is absolutely opposed to having another child (threatening the stability of the marriage). Two "sinful situation" reasons might be added: one of the parties is determined to adopt contraceptive practices (condom, diaphragm) or continue such practices—OR one of the parties would be very likely to fall into sins of incontinence (masturbation, infidelity) *UNLESS the NFP Program is*

---

[148]In her book entitled *Fighting for Life* (Ann Arbor, Mich.: Servant Books, 1984), pp. 54–60, Melinda Delahoyde states that some individuals with Down syndrome "have even written books . . . They are capable of loving and learning and functioning in society just like every other citizen of our country."

adopted so that abstinence will apply to fertile periods only.[149] It is doubtful that an obstinate spouse would give up his or her evil ways in exchange for a diet of restricted-intercourse; but tender love for a delicate-conscience spouse could bring about that change.

3.4   CONTRACEPTIVE PROCEDURES, TECHNIQUES, DEVICES

Contraceptive (direct) sterilization includes recourse to any procedure, technique, or device "which of itself, that is, of its own nature and condition, has the sole immediate effect of rendering the generative faculty incapable of procreation." That statement from the Holy See's reply of 1975 on the subject of sterilization (2nd paragraph) points to the importance of the following three documents which will be found in the *Appendix* of this book with each line numbered for easy reference:

(1) *Reply of the Sacred Congregation for the Doctrine of the Faith on Sterilization* (to be referred to as *Reply of SCDF, 1975*).

(2) *Commentary on the Reply of the SCDF to the National Conference of Catholic Bishops on Sterilization in Catholic Hospitals* (to be referred to as *NCCB Commentary, 1977*).

(3) *Statement of the National Conference of Catholic Bishops on Tubal Ligation, July 3, 1980* (to be referred to as *NCCB Statement, 1980*).

The distinction between contraceptive (*direct*) sterilization and *indirect* sterilization must be kept in mind. The latter refers to procedures that induce sterility and are not always forbidden,—that is, procedures where contraception is not the purpose (*NCCB Commentary, 1977*, lines 85–94).

1) "Humanae Vitae" and the Morality of Contraception

There seems to be a prevailing attitude in some quarters that certain unpopular teachings of the Church are not obligatory if they are disputed by some theologians and/or are generally disregarded by the faithful. The implication is that matters of right and wrong could depend on a show of hands, or on reports or surveys with regard to the observance of laws and regulations. If this attitude had any basis for validity, the Church would have to temper her teachings on many fronts: for example, the scandalous manner in which the

---

[149]This listing of reasons for regulating human fertility by legitimate means is adapted from this writer's doctoral dissertation which later was published under the title of *The "Rhythm" in Marriage and Christian Morality* (Westminster, Md.: The Newman Press, 1948), pp. 75–79. Several other "lesser of two evils" cases are presented on pp. 107–109.

indissolubility of marriage is disregarded; or the repeated violations of justice in trades and professions whereby a patron or customer is charged for a small fraction of an hour of service as if it were for a full hour; or the obligation of the faithful to "assist with the needs of the Church" according to their ability (Can.222,1, and Vatican II's *Decree on the Ministry and Life of Priests,* n.20); or the almost flippant attitude of many of the faithful on the subject of pre-marital sex, etc. The Lord Jesus came to save sinners. With all of their rights and prerogatives, the glorious "People of God" is made up of sinners, and exists for sinners. The simple truth is that there is no one who does not have to pray with the psalmist (Ps.51:4): "Thoroughly wash me from my guilt and of my sin cleanse me." The fact is that "what is right is right even if nobody does it, and what is wrong is wrong even if everybody does it."

The three documents on the subject of sterilization as listed above provide ample evidence that the full subject of the documents includes both sterilization and contraception (temporary sterilization), and that, evidence of the dissent of "many theologians" to the teaching of the Church on this subject notwithstanding, the faithful may not invoke those expressions of dissent as a theological basis for rejecting the authentic magisterial teachings as emphasized and explained in those documents (cf. Appendix, lines 32 to 38; reference to Vatican II's *Dogmatic Constitution on the Church,* n.25). Another quotation from the same Vatican II document (*Dogmatic Const. on the Church,* n.37) touches on the core of the problem for many members of the faithful who are content to continue their contraceptive life-style, when it mentions the word "obedience:" "With ready Christian obedience, laymen as well as all disciples of Christ should accept whatever their sacred pastors, as representatives of Christ, decree in their role as teachers and rulers in the Church." These words are now enshrined in Canon 212,1, of the Code of Canon Law. The phrase "sacred pastors" refers to the Holy Father and to bishops in their role as representatives of Christ. It can be called "an obedience of faith" because the Church is a community of faith.[150]

It would be unfair to say, however, that all Catholic couples or individuals who claim to proceed with a good conscience in practicing contraception are *subjectively* violating the moral law. Even though such Catholics may have arrived at their judgment of conscience on the basis of sufficient information, and after serious reflection before God, they often can be free of moral guilt on the basis of invincible ignorance. In a true sense of the phrase "through no fault of their own," they may labor under an *erroneous* conscience and be absolutely convinced of the rectitude of their contraceptive behavior because

---

[150]*CLSA Commentary,* (cf. note 45), p. 145.

of circumstances beyond their immediate control. Examples of such circumstances could be a *family* background wherein marital and domestic strife abounded along with twisted and confused concepts of right and wrong; or an *educational* background from grade school and beyond which featured almost exclusively the liberal moral views of the proponents of dissent; or a *social* status which required close association with the critical and liberated members of the higher-income class, etc. Long-standing background obstacles such as these can blind individuals to the merits of any system of morality which requires obedience and can restrict human behavior. Such *invincibly* ignorant individuals must not be confused, however, with the legions of lax Catholics throughout the land who are little concerned about the loose moral code they follow, and the bad company they keep. Such individuals are *vincibly* ignorant.

The word "conscience," which is the proximate or "here and now" norm of moral conduct, is defined as "a judgment of the practical reason on the moral goodness or sinfulness of an action which is to be done or omitted here and now, or has been done or omitted in the past." It must be a right or true conscience; that is, a judgment or verdict of reason which agrees with objective truth. If it is a *certain* conscience—that is, it has been arrived at without reasonable fear of error—it must be obeyed. Yet, even an absolutely certain conscience can be erroneous (or false) because it is based on *invincible* error due to circumstances as mentioned in the above paragraph.[151] Vatican II's document, *The Church Today,* provides a practical guideline as follows:

> Conscience frequently errs from invincible ignorance without losing its dignity. The same cannot be said of a man who cares but little for truth and goodness, or of a conscience which by degrees grows practically sightless as a result of habitual sin (n. 16).

Those who err through *invincible* ignorance (and also *vincible* ignorance) are commended to the pastoral zeal of a dedicated confessor or spiritual guide. It should be clear from Holy Scripture that the Church should never "give up" on sinners. If Catholics who practice contraception truly are seeking truth

---

[151]Cf. standard authors in moral theology such as Prümmer, Dominic M., O.P., *Handbook of Moral Theology* (New York, N.Y.: P.J. Kenedy and Sons, 1957), pp. 58 ff.; Jone, Heribert, O.F.M. Cap., *Moral Theology,* 1st ed. (Westminster, Md.: Newman Bookshop, 1945), pp. 41 ff.; Merkelbach, Benedict H., O.P., *Summa Theologiae Moralis* 3 vols., I (Paris: Desclée de Brouwer, 1935), pp. 185 ff.

and moral goodness, they should conform to the expectations enunciated in Vatican II's *Declaration on Religious Freedom:*

> Hence every man has the duty, and therefore the right, to seek the truth in matters religious, in order that he may with prudence form for himself right and true judgments of conscience, with the use of all suitable means (n.3).

Those who "care but little for truth and goodness" (quotation above) such as those with a lax conscience, and those who are determined not to be enlightened by any instruction or persuasion on the morality of contraception, cannot hide behind the screen of invincible ignorance.[152] They are violating the moral law and constitute a challenge for a zealous confessor in his efforts to "open their eyes" to the evil of habitual sin.

In counseling married persons, either inside or outside of the confessional, who may be ignorant, in doubt, or simply confused on the subject of contraception, the following doctrinal principles must be kept in mind:

(1) One person's conscience in a particular matter cannot become the norm of morality for another person. Conscience is a "personal, practical dictate" for the individual, and not a "teacher of doctrine" for others. Hence those who insist that they are convinced "in good conscience" of the rectitude of their contraceptive behavior and *subjectively* free of moral guilt must be made to understand that they cannot presume to deny the *objective* evil of the practice of contraception.[153]

(2) Although circumstances surrounding an objectively evil human act such as contraception cannot make it *objectively* acceptable from a

---

[152]This is not to deny the "lawful freedom of inquiry and of prudently expressing their opinions on matters in which they have expertise" as enjoyed by both clerics and members of the laity who are engaged in graduate studies in seminaries and universities, professors of sacred studies, etc. Cf. Can. 218, and *The Church Today* of Vatican II, n. 62. Can. 218 insists, however, on "observing a due respect for the magisterium of the Church." As stated in the *CLSA Commentary,* p. 152: "A theologian should not express opinions that differ from the position of the magisterium in such a way as to lead to disrespect for the magisterium on the part of others." At times, qualified and respectful experts in theology, canon law, scripture studies, etc., have a duty to "speak up" respectfully, but with due regard for the common good. Cf. Canons 212,3, and 223, and the *CLSA Commentary* (cf. note 45), pp. 146, 147, and 158, 159.

[153]Statement of the American Bishops on "Human Life in Our Day," Nov. 15, 1968, as printed in *Pastoral Letters of the United States Catholic Bishops,* Vol. III, 1962-1974 (Washington D.C.: United States Catholic Conference, 1983), pp. 170-172, nn. 37-45.

moral viewpoint, they can make it, in varying degrees, *subjectively* inculpable, diminished in guilt, or even defensible.[154]

(3) Every person has the obligation (and the right) to be guided by *objective* moral norms of conduct, including the authentic Church teachings as advanced by both the infallible and the non-infallible declarations of the Church (*The Church Today,* n.50).

(4) In the case of a person who is honestly trying to lead a good Christian life, the confessor or counselor should not be too quick either to presume complete innocence, or to presume a deliberate rejection of God's loving commands. The fact that a penitent mentions contraception as a matter or confession or of spiritual concern means that he or she has the need (and the right) to receive instruction and prudent persuasion with regard to the authentic teachings of the Church (as in (3) above). This need (and right) is even more pressing if ignorance (either vincible or invincible) makes the person subject to an erroneous conscience.

(5) Especially in cases of an erroneous conscience which is based on *invincible* ignorance, there will be situations when the best spiritual interests of the penitent will require that he or she be left in good faith (if indeed the person is in good faith) at least for the time being. This is in accord with traditional principles of sacramental and pastoral theology. If the invincible ignorance, in due time, becomes vincible ignorance, the penitent can become fully reconciled with God with a *true* (or *right*) conscience due to prayer, instruction and prudent persuasion.

(6) In the final analysis, no one is to be forced to act in a manner contrary to his or her personal conscience. This does not mean, however, that the confessor is to abandon his prudent efforts to provide the penitent with the basis for a true and informed conscience. The following chapter in this book on the *Principle of Religious Freedom* will emphasize how easily the phrase "freedom of conscience" can be subject to a false interpretation.[155]

(7) It should be apparent to all experienced spiritual guides that habits of sin are not eradicated in one or two sessions with the priest in the confessional. Prayer and patience—and acts of self-denial—are of the

---

[154]*Ibid.*, p. 169, n. 30. Cf. also standard authors on the obstacles to the full imputability of human acts, e.g., Jone, Heribert, O.F.M. Cap. (cf. note 151), pp. 7 ff.

[155]*Ibid.* (Bishops' pastoral letters), p. 144, n. 222, and pp. 356, 357, nn. 98–101.

essence (Matthew,21:22) In the words of Pope Paul VI in "Humanae Vitae" (n.25):

> . . . let [married couples] implore divine assistance by persevering prayer, above all, let them draw from the source of grace and charity in the Eucharist. And if sin should still keep its hold over them, let them not be discouraged, but rather have recourse with humble perseverance to the mercy of God, which is poured forth in the sacrament of Penance.[156]

(8) Far more consideration than in the past must be given to the propriety and the effectiveness of Natural Family Planning as a means of providing peace of conscience to Catholic couples who have a fertility problem (cf. pp.37 and 89).

One can only speculate as to the immense number of contraception situations in which one of the partners in marriage is not a sinner, but rather sinned against. These are situations in which one of the partners is opposed to contraception, but forced into cooperation in the practice of contraception because the other partner is determined to use contraceptive devices during the fertile periods or throughout the entire span of the wife's capability to conceive a child. Often the alternative to compliance with a contraceptive regime in marriage is so damaging to marital harmony, that non-compliance could mean infidelity in the marriage, or the real threat of an abortion in the event of a pregnancy, or constant badgering and bickering in the home to the detriment of the children, or recourse to alcohol or other drugs on the part of husband or wife, or the complete break down of the marriage with recourse to the divorce courts, etc. The zealous confessor will be guided by traditional

---

[156]*Love and Sexuality* (cf. note 61), p. 345. The Latin original of the last three lines of this quotation, reads as follows: "Si autem peccatis adhuc retineantur, ne concidant animo, sed humiles et constantes ad Dei misericordiam confugiant, quam abunde Paenitentiae Sacramentum dilargitur." Cf. *Enchiridion Vaticanum, vol. 3, Documenti Ufficiali Della Santa Dede 1968–1970* (Bologna: Edizioni Dehoniane, 1977), p. 312. *Cassell's Latin Dictionary* (New York, N.Y.: Funk & Wagnalls Co.) lists two verbs "concidere" (both of the 3rd conjugation), and the first of these would seem to apply in the phrase "ne concidant animo" insofar as the meaning, as applying to persons, is "to be ruined, overthrown, fail." Hence the word "discouraged" above is a good translation. The word "animo" in the phrase, however ("animus" being the spiritual principal of life), would favor a meaning of "with God's help you can find a way out, and overcome the sin;" rather than "Keep on as you are, God understands." The latter meaning would be spiritual defeatism! In many, if not most situations, where couples are having recourse to contraceptive practices, the solution could well be the practice of Natural Family Planning (NFP).

principles of sacramental and pastoral theology in dealing sympathetically with those who are "sinned against rather then sinning" in their search for peace of conscience in marital life.

2) The Sterilization "of the Faculty Itself"

One of the most controversial procedures involving the sterilization "of the faculty itself" (that is, the generative faculty) is tubal ligation (Appendix, lines 16–18). The American bishops resorted to a prudential understatement when they spoke of a "certain confusion" with regard to this procedure (Appendix, lines 181–186). The Holy See spoke of an awareness of "the dissent against this teaching" (on direct contraceptive sterilization) on the part of "many theologians," but denied any doctrinal significance to such dissent. To be guided by such dissent would be tantamount to rejecting the authentic magisterium in favor of "opinions of private theologians" (Appendix, lines 32–38).

Sterilization procedures such as tubal ligation (fallopian tubes tied or cut), its masculine counterpart, vasectomy ("vasa deferentia" tied or cut), hysterectomy (surgical removal of the uterus), oophorectomy (surgical removal of the ovaries), salphingectomy (surgical removal of the fallopian tubes), radiation of the generative organs with X-ray, etc., come under the heading of contraceptive (direct) sterilization if they are done solely for the purpose of rendering the person sterile. The argument of the "opposition" is that such procedures should be allowed when a woman's kidney, heart, lungs, etc., are in such a weakened or diseased condition, that another pregnancy would constitute a serious danger to her physical or mental health (*Reply of SCDF, 1975,* lines 11–15). Some have tried to justify such procedures on the basis of the *Principle of Totality.* The *Reply of the SCDF, 1975,* makes it very clear that such a principle will not justify the efforts of married couples to obviate their obligation to realize the essential human good of procreation:

> Likewise, neither can one invoke the principle of totality in this case [that is, direct sterilization], in virtue of which principal interference with organs is justified for the greater good of the person; sterility intended in itself is not oriented to the integral good of the person as rightly pursued, "the proper order of goods being preserved," [reference to *Humanae Vitae,* n.16] inasmuch as it damages the ethical good of the person, which is the highest good, since it deliberately deprives foreseen and freely chosen sexual activity of an essential element (lines 22–31).

Pius XII was even more specific in ruling out the *Principle of Totality* argument. The following is taken from his allocution to the delegates at the 26th Congress on Urology on Oct. 8th, 1953:

> The appeal to this principle [the Principle of Totality] here is unjustified, for in this case, the danger which threatens the mother does not derive at all—either directly or indirectly—from the presence or normal functioning of the oviducts, nor from the influence they exercise over the diseased organ—kidneys, heart, or lungs. The danger comes only when free sexual intercourse causes a conception which can menace the organs mentioned, because they are too weak or diseased. But the conditions which permit a part to be disposed of in favor of the whole, in virtue of the principle of totality, do not exist.[157]

Another prime focus of the three documents mentioned above, namely, the extent to which the authorities of Catholic hospitals might appeal to the *Principle of Material Cooperation* in tolerating some degree of material cooperation with the evil of direct sterilization, will be discussed under the chapter on material cooperation.

Directive n.18: Sterilization, whether permanent or temporary, for men or for women, may not be used as a means of contraception.
(Taken from *Humanae Vitae,* n.14)

---

3) Directly-Contraceptive Techniques and Devices

As mentioned in the previous chapter, the use of contraceptive steroids so as to enhance a woman's chances of conceiving a child could be justified if recommended by her physician as a *fertility* measure. This would not be contraception in the strict sense of the word; there is no purpose of "rendering contraception impossible." Two of the traditional *techniques* for avoiding conception are "withdrawal" whereby the husband withdraws the male organ from the wife's vagina just prior to ejaculation; and "copula dimidiata" which involves only half-way penetration in the act of intercourse. Both prac-

---

[157] *The Human Body* (cf. note 61), p. 279.

tices are morally objectionable; both are rather ineffective means of separating the creative from the unitive element in marriage.

There was a time when the more popular methods of contraception involved the use of either chemical or mechanical devices. As of December, 1984, however, a leading weekly magazine announced: "The pill has been superseded by male and female sterilization."[158] After surgical sterilization, therefore the "popularity" list must be changed to read: oral contraceptives (OC's) or "the pill," condoms, and in fourth place, intrauterine devices known as IUDs.[159] Two of these deserve a brief special commentary: the IUD (used by about 6.5% of married women in the U.S.A.), and the "morning after" pill. Both are abortifacients.

The "intrauterine devices" (IUD) category includes various types such as flexible metal and plastic loops and coils, as well as "T" and "7" shaped designs. The latter are wound with copper wire. IUDs are inserted into the womb by a physician and can stay "in situ" for a year or more. They require periodic checking by a physician. While their contraceptive effect is thought to be due to a "sterile tissue reaction in the endometrial cavity" (a foreign body reaction), they can also cause a toxicity not only to the sperm but also to the early stage of the embryo known as the blastocyst. In the theological sense of abortion as any effort to destroy life from the moment of conception, therefore, the IUD is an *abortifacient*. The same must be said of the "morning after" pill. This popular pill is a composite of the compound known as diethylstilbestrol (DES) and estrogen. If a woman has been exposed to the possibility of conception (by having intercourse around the middle of her menstrual cycle), she can reduce the probability of pregnancy by taking the "morning after pill" for five days or so after exposure. Consequently if conception had occurred and the zygote reached the uterus about one week later for implantation, it would face a fatally hostile environment due to the pill.[160]

Devices Used "in Anticipation of the Conjugal Act" (*Directive* 19): Although the *Physicians' Desk Reference* mentions reducing the likelihood of implantation as a possible side effect of *oral contraceptive pills,* it is clear that the primary effect is the "inhibition of ovulation" (cf. pp.39,40). They also could cause the endo-

---

[158]*Time* magazine, Dec. 7, 1984. The report was based on figures from the U.S. Center for Health Statistics. As reported in the Dec. 19, 1985, issue of the *Boston Globe* (p. 28), the discovery of a substance known as "inhibin" could lead to the production of a contraceptive pill for *both men and women*. This substance "apparently prevents the pituitary gland from secreting a hormone called FSH that stimulates the sex glands of men and women to produce sperm or eggs."

[159]These contraceptives and the ones to follow are listed and explained in *The Merck Manual* (cf. note 56), pp. 1699–1705.

[160]On the "morning after pill," a more complete description is found in *The Dignity of Life* by Father Charles McFadden, O.S.A. (cf. note 65), pp. 113, 114.

metrium of the uterus to become thin, and the cervical mucus to become thick and impervious to sperm. *Spermicidal Foams, Creams and Suppositories* not only immobilize or kill sperm on contact, but also provide a mechanical barrier to sperm. They must be placed in the vagina before each act of intercourse. The use of *Vaginal Spermicidal Sponges* is also very popular as a contraceptive device. A 1984 report on one brand of spermicidal sponge (known as "Today") from the Federal Centers for Disease Control reveals that the product presents a very low danger of getting the dreaded toxic shock syndrome if properly used.[161] The *Diaphragm*, made of soft rubber with a flexible spring around the cup, must be fitted by a physician. The woman must know how to insert it so that the cervix is covered. Usually spermicidal foam or jelly is used along with the device so as to prevent any live sperm from entering the opening to the uterus. The *IUD* (discussed above) also is in place in anticipation of intercourse.

Devices Used in the "Accomplishment of the Conjugal Act" (*Directive* 19): The *Condom* is widely used to prevent the ejaculate from entering the vagina of the woman. It is said to be more accurate in theory than in practice. It is a thin sheath made of rubber, latex or similar materials and is designed to fit over the erect male organ (the penis). The device does help to prevent the transmission of venereal disease. A special type of condom known as a "seminal pouch" was discussed in chapter II as a reliable device for collecting specimens of human semen for analysis.

Devices Used in the "Development of Natural Consequences" (*Directive* 19): It would be immoral for a woman to have recourse to a *douche* or "washing out" of the vagina soon after a freely-engaged act of intercourse with contraceptive intentions in mind. As a contraceptive technique, such a practice would be quite ineffective. Contraception takes place not in the vagina or womb but in the fallopian tubes. The time element in the passage of sperm to the fallopian tubes is a matter of minutes.[162] A douche often is recommended by the physician for hygienic reasons. A woman's vagina could be so badly infected or diseased as to require repeated douching. If the physician prescribes douching for a serious reason and insists that it be done (excluding contraceptive reasons or intent) within a reasonable interval after intercourse, the woman could follow his prescription in good conscience. This would be an application of the Principle of the Double Effect.

---

[161]*St. Louis Post-Dispatch,* Nov. 13, 1984, p. 8, a. For a brief contemporary review of other contraceptive devices which can be implanted or injected so as to prevent pregnancy for months or even years, cf. *Time,* "Birth Control: Vanishing Options," Sept. 1, 1986, p. 78. Some of these devices are not available in the U.S.A.

[162]*The Merck Manual* (cf. note 56), states that under experimental conditions, sperm have been seen to travel from the vagina to the fimbriated end of the uterine tube in five minutes, p. 1708.

As this book was in the process of publication, the communications media abounded with announcements and commentaries on the "contragestive" (v. "contraceptive") known as RU-486. Based on one study of 100 European women who sought abortions, this experimental abortion pill gives promise of an effectiveness rating of 85% in terminating pregnancies when the woman takes it within the first 10 days after a missed menstrual period. This progesterone-blocking pill may be approved for marketing in some European countries (but not in the U.S.A.) within the current year (1987). It is a sinful substitute for a criminal procedure (surgical abortion). Tragic experience with the damaging side effects of other once-acclaimed panaceas against fertility such as DES (diethylstilbestrol), the Dalkon shield, thalidomide, the IUD, etc., must put society and the medical world on guard against possible long-range side effects of a revolutionary drug such as RU-486. The word "revolutionary" is well chosen. Increasing recourse to such a pill would make abortion a private matter between the young girl or woman and her doctor.[163] What must be stressed on the subject of *fertility regulation* is that the *natural* means as provided by Natural Family Planning can mean peace of conscience to so many Catholic couples who are living in sin because they have chosen the directly-contraceptive solution to their fertility problem. In addition to peace of conscience, Catholic couples who have appropriate reasons for adopting the NFP method, and who are "willing and able" to abide by its moderate restrictions without spiritual harm, can be protected against the host of dangerous side effects (physiological, psychological, even psychiatric) which can be associated with the directly-contraceptive route. With a modicum of personal discipline and a pinch of self-sacrifice, they can be persuaded by a caring and zealous counselor or confessor to understand and appreciate the advantages of *natural family regulation*. A powerful "selling point" is provided by a pamphlet-publication of the U.S. Department of Health and Human Services entitled *Natural Family Planning*. As to NFP's reliability in regulating human fertility, all three methods as included under the heading of Natural Family Planning are given a *98% rating* for "method effectiveness" (that is, the "Basal Body Temperature Method," the "Ovulation Method," and the "Sympto-Thermal Method"). The publication states that the success of "natural methods" depends upon (a) the motivation of the couple, (b) the quality of instruction the couple receives, and (c) the follow-up by the instructor to insure that the couple properly understands the method.[164] Members of

---

[163]"Termination of Early Pregnancy By the Progesterone Antagonist RU 486 (Mifepristone)," by Beatrice Couzinet, MD et al., in *The New England Journal of Medicine*, December 18, 1986, pp. 1565–1569.

[164]*Natural Family Planning* (6 page pamphlet), published by the *U.S. Dept. of Health and Human Services,* public Health Service, Health Services Administration, Bureau of Community Health Services, DHHS Publication No. (HSA) 80-5621 (not dated).

the Catholic clergy should be on the forefront in promoting "peace through NFP."[165]

> *Directive 19:* Similarly excluded is every action which, either in anticipation of the conjugal act, or in its accomplishment, or in the development of its natural consequences, proposes, whether as an end or as a means, to render procreation impossible (taken from "Humanae Vitae," n.14).

4) Procedures that Induce Sterility—Indirect Sterilization

In the procedures, techniques and practices discussed above, contraception is the *end,* and sterilization is the *means* to that end. Not all sterilization is contraception in the moral sense of the word, but all contraception in the moral sense of the word is sterilization. There are cases when sterilization (indirect) can be allowed for non-contraceptive ends—for example, the surgical removal of a cancerous uterus. The procedure "brings with it" (hence "induces") necessarily the condition of sterility.

The campaign to widen the basis for allowing the direct pursuit of sterilization includes both the demand for the right to use contraceptive devices and practices and the claim that a woman has the right to seek medical/surgical protection against the danger or even against the inconvenience of having another child. The contraceptive mentality has found favor throughout the nation and throughout the world. To say that this campaign has been a bone of contention among Catholic authors in the past score of years would be something of an understatement. In the wake of Paul VI's encyclical letter "On the Regulation of Birth" (*Humanae Vitae*), the pressure on Church authorities to address more "realistically" the plight of women who would be put in a precarious health situation if they conceived another child, took on the proportions of a crusade. Good intentions were in evidence. Even more evident, however, was the trend to forget or to overlook basic principles of morality—to overlook, in the words of Paul VI, the "profound relationship (of responsible parenthood) to the objective moral order established by God"

---

[165]Two very helpful books are available: *Natural Family Planning* (Printed in Japan: Copyright by De Rance, Inc., 1980), distributed by The Human Life Center, St. John's University, Collegeville, Minn., 56321 (apparently available for postage only), 262 pages, and *The Art of Natural Family Planning* (Cincinnati, Ohio, 45211, 1977), 228 pages. Authors: John and Sheila Kippley. Fifth printing, 1977.

(n.10). The same pontiff alluded to the "too numerous . . . voices . . . contrary to the voice of the Church" as "amplified by the modern means of propaganda" (n.18).

The argument that a widened base for allowing contraception and sterilization could be based on the *Principle of Totality* was rejected definitely as noted earlier in this chapter. In "Humanae Vitae," Paul VI listed several other *unacceptable* arguments of the opposition: that deliberately making conjugal acts infecund "could be made honest and right by the ensemble of a fecund conjugal life" (n.14); that it is reasonable in many circumstances to have recourse to artificial birth control "if, thereby, we secure the harmony and peace of the family and better conditions for the education of the children already born" (n.16); that the Church's teaching on the regulation of births "will easily appear to many to be difficult and even impossible of actuation" (n.20).

Application of the Principle of the Double Effect

Some of the confusion referred to above could be traced to a faulty interpretation of *Hospital Directive n. 6* which normally would be applied on the basis of the *Principle of Totality*. That directive states: "ordinarily the proportionate good that justifies a medical or surgical procedure should be the total good of the patient himself." As Father O'Donnell, S.J. observes, however, the word "ordinarily" is used precisely to indicate that the *Principle of Totality* (in the interests of the whole body) cannot be used to justify direct sterilization. In other words, contraceptive sterilization is an exception to *Directive 6:*

> *If the procedure were taken precisely as a contraceptive measure, even in the interests of the whole body, this would be contrary to Catholic teaching on contraception.* This is so because the generative organ, precisely as generative, is not, to this extent, viewed as subordinated to the good of the individual.[166]

This is clearly understandable in the light of all that has been said about the essential good of procreation (subordinated to the good of society) and about mankind's limited dominion over the generative function.

Since sterilization cannot be willed *directly*, it can be justified only with the application of the *Principle of the Double Effect* whereby it becomes a foreseen but merely permitted side effect of a necessary surgical procedure. This prin-

---

[166]*Medicine and Christian Morality* (cf. note 31), pp. 115–118.

ciple will be discussed at length in a special chapter. It may be summarized for illustration purposes by considering the case of a woman who is being treated for cancer of the ovaries. The onset was silent and insidious; it is far too late to consider any alternatives. The physician decides that the ovaries must be removed as a life-saving procedure. In viewing this situation in the light of the *Principle of the Double Effect:*

(1) The proposed standard surgical procedure is morally good in itself;

(2) The intended good effect ("direct voluntary") is to save the woman's life; there is no reasonable alternative available which would not involve the danger of sterility;

(3) The "merely permitted" evil effect (sterility) is foreseen, but not directly willed or intended (indirect voluntary). As a causal effect, it cannot be avoided.

(4) The good effect (life of the mother) is not realized through the evil effect (sterility)—the latter is not the *means* of bringing about the good effect;

(5) There is a due proportion between the good effect that is intended and the evil effect which is permitted. The connection between (5) and (2) is important. If the same good effect could be obtained by another reasonable, equally effective and available means with less chances of causing sterility, there would be no proportionate reason for proceeding with the surgery.

To "Cure, Diminish, or Prevent a Serious Pathological Condition"
(*Directive* 20)

In the example above, the woman presumably was cured of cancer and became *permanently* sterile. Another case of a permanent cure might involve a woman with a fairly-large family who is in great pain, physical debility and constant distress because of lacerations and infections of the vaginal area and erosions of the cervix of the uterus. She has a history of several difficult deliveries, and her uterus has not returned to normal size since her last delivery. It has become heavy, boggy, enlarged and weakened to the extent that ordinary home and family duties became painful burdens. If a troublesome appendix or gall bladder caused similar misery which could not be diminished with medications, surgical removal of the organ would be the answer. If the physician decides that only surgery can remedy the condition of the woman with the lacerated and infective uterus, he would be justified in performing a hysterectomy.[167] In similar circumstances, there could be estab-

---

[167]Similar cases of indirect sterilization are found in *Medical Ethics*, by Edwin J. Healy, S.J. (cf. note 46), pp. 178–185. Cf. also Kelly, Gerald, S.J., *Medico-Moral Problems* (cf. note 22), pp. 208–215.

lished suspicions of a precancerous condition. In such a case, the surgical removal of the uterus would not only be a cure of the woman's present serious pathological condition, but also a diminishing or preventing of an even more serious pathological condition.

Directive 20 mentions several other procedures which might be used more as a "diminishing or preventing" measure than as an outright cure. Thus if a simpler treatment is not reasonably available, a woman with breast cancer could submit to surgical removal of her ovaries or to scheduled X-ray treatments of the ovaries *if* such measures are foreseen and calculated as effective in preventing the spread of breast cancer. The same would apply to the removal of a man's testicles in treating cancer of the prostate gland. Today, however, simpler treatments are available for many such cancerous conditions. Needless to say, if a woman has been rendered sterile by the removal of her ovaries, any possible diagnosis which might indicate the need of removing her uterus could be decided on the basis of the *Principle of Totality*—since her reproductive function has already been lost through the previous surgery.

Directive 20: Procedures that induce sterility, whether permanent or temporary, are permitted when: a. They are immediately directed to the cure, diminution, or prevention of a serious pathological condition and are not directly contraceptive (that is, contraception is not the purpose); and b. a simpler treatment is not reasonably available. Hence, for example, oophorectomy or irradiation of the ovaries may be allowed in treating carcinoma of the breast and metastasis therefrom; and orchidectomy is permitted in the treatment of carcinoma of the prostate.

3.5   SAFEGUARDING HUMAN LIFE

This chapter began with an argument for "Stand up for life—Together," and presented the scriptural basis for our belief that the "breath of life," which makes every human individual a "living being" (literally "a living soul"), comes from God. It is precisely the question of just when that principle of human life is communicated—known as the question of animation or ensoulment (hominization)—which dampens the zeal of many in standing up for the sanctity of human life from the moment of conception.

For well over 1000 years, Church scholars (including St. Augustine and St. Thomas Aquinas) were influenced by the view of the great Aristotle (384–322 B.C.) who held that life began at the moment of conception, but that it is not human life ("formed") until 40 days after conception for the male, and 90 days after conception for the female. St. Thomas wrote: "The answer therefore is that a soul pre-existed in the embryo, at first a nutritive soul, after that a sensitive soul and then an intellectual soul."[168] There is no evidence whatever that he would have permitted an abortion during the early period of gestation. It was not until the 14th century that the distinction between the formed and unformed (animated and unanimated) fetus was used in discussions about the general condemnation of abortion. These discussions, however, did not affect the Church's position on abortion. In his scholarly study of this subject, Father John Connery, S.J. concludes as follows:

> Whatever one would want to hold about the time of animation, or when the fetus became a human being in the strict sense of the term, abortion from the time of conception was considered wrong, and the time of animation was never looked on as a moral dividing line between permissible and immoral abortion. As long as what was aborted was destined to be a human being, it made no difference whether the abortion was induced before or after it became so. The final result was the same: a child was not born.[169]

No Longer Any Reasonable Doubt About When Life Begins

Aristotle and his host of followers must be excused for their misunderstandings in the field of human embryology. It was almost 2000 years later before the discovery of magnifying devices made it possible to advance the study of embryology by building on facts instead of on speculation. The cellular nature of spermatazoa was not established until 1841. The nuclei and cytoplasms of sperm cells were not demonstrated until 1869. The chromosomes were first described in the 1870's.[170] The past century of medical re-

---

[168]*Summa Theologiae* (Taurini-Romae: Marietti, 1952) pars I, Q.118, art. 2, ad 2: "Et ideo dicendum est quod anima praeexistet in embryone a principio quidem nutritiva, postmodum autem sensitiva, et tandem intellectiva . . . Sic igitur dicendum est quod anima intellectiva creatur a Deo in fine generationis humanae, quae simul est et sensitiva et nutritiva, corruptis formis praeexistentibus." p. 554.

[169]*Abortion: The Development of the Roman Catholic Perspective* (Chicago, Ill.: Loyola University Press, 1977), pp. 304 ff.

[170]Krumbhaar, E.B., M.D., Ph.D., *A History of Medicine* (New York, N.Y.: Alfred Knopf, 1941), p. 674.

search has led to a definite answer to "When does life begin?" The report of the *Subcommittee on Separation of Powers* to the *U.S. Senate Committee on the Judiciary* conducted extensive hearings on *Human Life Bill, S 158* in 1981. After considering the testimony of a total of 57 witnesses (geneticists, biologists, physicians), their report read as follows:

> The testimony of these witnesses and the voluminous submissions received by the subcommittee demonstrate that contemporary scientific evidence points to a clear conclusion: the life of a human being begins at conception, the time when the process of fertilization is complete.[171]

It should suffice (space being limited) to present one typical quotation from an expert in medical genetics. Dr. Hymie Gordon, Professor of Medical Genetics at the Mayo Clinic in Minnesota, made the following conclusive statement:

> I think we can now say that the question of the beginning of life—when life begins—is no longer a question for theological or philosophical dispute. It is an established scientific fact. Theologians and philosophers may go on to debate the meaning of life or the purpose of life, but it is an established fact that all life, including human life, begins at the moment of conception.[172]

This remarkable consensus on the part of experts in the biological sciences constitutes convincing evidence that the new life within the womb must be regarded as at least "incipiently human." It does not and cannot settle the vexing question of just when the spiritual soul is infused. The following quotation from the *Declaration on Abortion* as issued by the Sacred Congregation for the Doctrine of the Faith on Nov. 18, 1974, explains why the solution of the time-of-ensoulment question is not crucial to the Church's teaching on the criminal nature of direct abortion:

> The present declaration deliberately leaves untouched the question of the moment when the spiritual soul is infused . . . For two reasons the moral position taken here on abortion does not depend on the answer to the question: 1) even if it is assumed that

---

[171]Hall, Theodore, O.P., "Human Life Begins: Integrated Senate Report," in *Linacre Quarterly*, August, 1983, p. 254.
[172]*Ibid.*

animation comes at a later point, the life of the fetus is nonetheless incipiently *human* (as the biological sciences make clear): it prepares the way for and requires the infusion of the soul, which will complete the nature received from the parents; 2) if the infusion of the soul at the very first moment is at least *probable* (and the contrary will in fact never be established with certainty), then to take the life of the fetus is at least to run the *risk* of killing a human being who is not merely awaiting but is already in possession of a human soul. [173]

> *Directive 11:* From the moment of conception, life must be guarded with the greatest care. Any deliberate medical procedure, the *purpose* of which is to deprive a fetus or an embryo of its life, is immoral.

Abortion—"Directly Intended"

The crime of abortion applies to the "directly intended termination of pregnancy before viability" . . . including the "interval between conception and implantation of the embryo"(*Directive* 12). That critical ten-day interval is a succession of quiet (and often undetected) processes of budding-forth, expansion and protection.

Conception (fertilization) takes place usually near the fimbriated end of the fallopian tube when two *gametes* (germ cells), namely the ovum of the wife and the sperm of the husband, become united as one. Appropriately the resulting cell is called the *"zygote"* or the bonding stage, after the Greek word for "yoked." That tiny speck of new life contains all that the human individual inherits from his or her parents. It then takes from 3 to 5 days for the zygote to move from the site of conception down to the uterine cavity, and another 1 to 2 days to arrive at the site of *implantation*. It has been dividing as it moves along. At the time of implantation, it has formed a single layer of cells surrounding a central cavity. This is called the *"blastocyst"* stage (from the Greek word for "sprout"). By the 9th or 10th day after conception, the process of burrowing into the center layer of the three-layer lining of the uterus (implantation) is complete. Soon thereafter, when the outer layer of the blastocyst forms the amniotic sac, the newly-conceived becomes recognizable

---

[173] *The Pope Speaks*, Vol. 19 (1974, 1975), p. 256, note 19. All living embryos, even the smallest, are to be baptized *absolutely* (NOT conditionally).

as an *"embryo"* (from the Greek word meaning "to swell inside"). The sac fills with fluid and expands to cover the embryo.[174]

At the end of the 8th week, this unique individual, programmed by a genetic code which will never be repeated, is called a *"fetus"* (Latin for "off-spring"). If this 56-day-old wonder could be seen alive outside the womb—less than 2 inches in length in its egg-shaped amniotic sac with transparent "shell,"—it would appear to be a boy or girl in miniature complete with a primitive skeletal system, with a functionally complete cardiac system, with an ability to respond to touch and to make slight changes in position, and with features definitely recognizable as human even to the extent of thumb-sucking. One could well imagine these future citizens of our planet singing the praises of the Creator.

> I give you my thanks that I am fearfully, wonderfully made; Wonderful are your works. My soul also you knew full well; nor was my frame unknown to you when I was made in secret . . . (Psalm 139,14 f.).

All that they need in order to know the light of day and the joy of life in the world seven months later is divine love, and loving human care and protection. Strange to say, at this amazing juncture in embryonic human life, many women do not even realize that they are pregnant.

Quite naturally, the Church's prohibition of abortion extends to every procedure whose sole immediate effect is the separation of a non-viable *living* fetus from the uterus,—that is, a *direct* attack on the *life* of a non-viable fetus. The prohibition does not include *indirect* abortion, that is, when the termination of pregnancy is not intended, although it is foreseen and tolerated as a side effect of a procedure which is designed to cure a serious pathological condition of the mother. The procedure simply cannot safely be postponed until the fetus is viable. When such an urgent medical procedure and the intention behind it is viewed in the light of the *Principle of the Double Effect,* it is only reasonable to conclude that those who are involved in the procedure are not guilty of immorality. A special chapter will be reserved for a discussion of that important principle as well as cases of indirect abortion which are classic applications of that principle.

The accusation that recourse to the "double effect" principle is the Church's back-door justification for sacrificing the life of the fetus for the health or life of the mother must be regarded as a *grave distortion of fact and of*

---

[174]For an inspiring commentary on human embryology, cf. *Abortion, the Myths, the Realities, and the Arguments* (New York, N.Y.: Corpus Books, 1970), by Germain Grisez, pp. 11–23.

intent. It is a *distortion of fact* because the mother-or-child dilemma (so-called) is a relic of the early days of obstetrics. Obstetrics research and practice has improved to the point where the "mother and child" dilemma is scarcely ever encountered. Father Thomas J. O'Donnell, S.J. has a likely explanation as to why the dilemma-scare is kept alive:

> As obstetric research and improved technique reduced the medical indications for abortion to near zero, the discouraging fact remained that many pregnant mothers simply did not want to give birth to their babies. Thus there was a long period in which obsolete medical indications became medical excuses rather than reasons for aborting . . . Finally, while the civil law still required a medical indication if abortion was to be done, there was a shift to nebulous and unproven psychiatric indications and to the unusual concept of abortion in the interest of the unborn baby under the questionable presupposition of "better dead than deaf" (the rubella rubric) or "better dead than disdained" (the unwanted baby warranty).[175]

The accusation is a *distortion of intent* because the Church has always looked upon the life of the mother and the life of the unborn child as of equal value. In the words of Pius XII: "Never and in no case has the Church taught that the life of the child must be preferred to that of the mother . . . In the one case as in the other, there can be but one obligation: to make every effort to save the lives of both, of the mother and of the child."[176]

Abortion—"Before Viability"

It is for the physician who is handling the case to decide whether or not the fetus should be considered as viable. In medical technology, a delivery after the 20th week is called a *premature delivery;* presuming that the fetus would not be viable at 20 weeks, the Church calls such a termination of pregnancy an abortion.

The word "viable" is a relative term. The former dividing line of 26 to 28 weeks in determining viability is bound to be pushed downward with the rapid progress in medical technology. Even apart from such progress, however, viability depends on more than the number of weeks or days within the

---

[175]*Medicine and Christian Morality* (cf. note 31), p. 152. Cf. also Healy, Edwin, S.J., *Medical Ethics* (cf. note 46), p. 196.

[176]Address to large families, Nov. 26, 1951. Cf. *The Human Body* (cf. note 61), pp. 180, 181.

womb. Other important considerations include the anatomical and functional development of the fetus, the weight and length of the fetus, the race of the parents, etc. Furthermore, it is only a question of time before hospitals acquire not only improved incubators, but also artificial *"placentas"* which will surround and nourish fetuses well below the 26–28 week of uterine life.[177] Naturally, the determination of "viability" in a given case would depend upon the availability of such equipment and adequate professional personnel in the area in question.

The author of *Aborting America,* Dr. Bernard Nathanson, mentions that up to the 70's, obstetricians used 1000 grams (a little over 2 pounds, and around 27 weeks) as the point "where they should exert every effort to salvage the life by such techniques as Caesarean section and the respirator." At the time of the publication of his book (1981), the usual rule of thumb was 750 grams (1 pound , 10½ ounces, and around 25 weeks). In the New York hospital where he was practicing (as of 1981) 6 of 9 infants admitted to the Special Care Nursery in the 751–1,000 gram category did survive (a 66.7% survival rate), whereas only one infant of the 501–750 gram category survived. These were 1977 statistics. He describes viability realistically as "the current reflection of medical achievement," and urges consideration of non-medical factors by adding: "An infant could be "viable" in New York City but not in a rural U.S. town, or in the rural town, but not in Bangladesh."[178] The question of viability is of special importance in determining whether or not a person guilty of the *sin* of abortion has incurred the canonical penalty for abortion known as excommunication.

The Extent and Effects of Excommunication for Abortion

Canon 1398 states: "A person who procures a successful abortion incurs an automatic (latae sententiae) excommunication." The penalty applies to all involved in the deliberate and successful effort to eject a non-viable fetus from the mother's womb.[179] The word "successful" as a translation of "effectu secuto" of canon 1398 is appropriate: it means that the abortive effect really must have followed or resulted from the means or procedure used. Since this law of the Church is one that establishes a penalty, it is subject to a strict interpretation (Can. 18). Remembering that this refers to a *living* non-viable fetus, it should be clear that if the fetus actually was dead at the time of the

---

[177]Noonan, John T., Jr., ed., *The Morality of Abortion, Legal and Historical Perspectives* (Cambridge, Ma.: Harvard University Press, 1970), p. 87.
[178]*Aborting America* (cf. note 115), pp. 215–217.
[179]*CLSA Commentary* (cf. note 45), p. 930. Cf. also their commentary on canon 1329, pp. 905, 906.

abortive effort, those involved in the criminal deed would be guilty of the *sin* of abortion (presuming that they thought that the fetus was living), but would not incur the penalty of excommunication. The same would be true (regarding the sin and penalty of abortion) if the action or procedure employed resulted in the ejection of a *viable* fetus. Undoubtedly the hardy infant would be badly scarred and weakened due to the abortive efforts, but the perpetrators would not incur excommunication. They would, however, be guilty of serious sin, and liable to substantial deprivations and prohibitions for "mutilating or seriously wounding" another human being (for example, loss of office, faculty or function, dismissal from the clerical state, etc., cf. Cann.1328,1336,1397).

The restrictive nature of the penalty of excommunication for abortion also explains why procedures such as *criminal* craniotomy (compression of the skull of the fetus after the contents have been removed) and *criminal* embryotomy (any unnecessary mutilating operation on the fetus) would not involve excommunication. As noted above, however, such crimes would be punishable in other ways.[180]

There are only two automatic or "latae sententiae" excommunications listed in the present Code of Canon Law which are not reserved to the Holy See. One applies to Catholics who fall away from the faith and become apostates, heretics or schismatics (Can.1364,1). The other applies to those who are involved in a "successful abortion" (Can.1398). This includes not only the woman who consents to an abortion but also to all the principal or necessary collaborators provided that the abortion would not have been committed without their efforts" (Can. 1329, 2). Examples of such accomplices would be those involved in the abortion process either *physically* (physician and his assistants in the medical or surgical procedure, physical violence by husband or boyfriend, etc.) or *morally* (husband or boyfriend who "talked her into it," etc.), provided that the abortion would not have been committed without their efforts.

The average priest will encounter few cases of abortion in his pastoral life. The new Code of Canon Law has simplified the entire subject of penalties such as excommunication. The procedure to be followed canonically, however, still remains somewhat complicated. The following observations will not address the extremely rare situation when the penalty of excommunication has been made public by a formal intervention of Church authority. In

---

[180]Craniotomy is never allowed, of course, if the fetus is living. Embryotomy refers to the necessity of removing an arm or a leg of the infant in the delivery process when no other solution is possible. Cf. Healy, Edwin, S.J., *Medical Ethics* (cf. note 46), pp. 250 ff. (many case studies presented).

such very rare cases, the individuals are included among those who "obstinately persist in manifest sin" (Can.915), and the reconciliation process is more complicated. If a confessor should encounter such an unusual situation, he will find an explanation of that rare type of penal action in the following chapter on the *Principle of Religious Freedom*.

It is important to remember that excommunication is called a "medicinal" or "correctional" penalty which is intended for the spiritual welfare of the penitent. It could be compared to a penalty imposed by a parent upon a misbehaving child "for your own good." An excommunicated person does not cease to be a Catholic and is not cut off entirely from the source of spiritual benefits. Temporarily the individual is outside ("ex") the community ("communio") of the faithful. For their interior peace, such individuals can regain grace by making an act of perfect contrition. In *external* affairs, however, their spiritual rights and privileges are restrained until they have been absolved of the excommunication (Can.1331,1). Since they are excluded from receiving the sacraments, they cannot be absolved of the *sin* of abortion until the penalty of excommunication has been remitted.

The confessor's role in handling an abortion case is limited to the *internal* forum. Usually the case will come to his attention through sacramental confession. If it comes to his attention through non-sacramental confession (often called the "forum of conscience") he can persuade the person to make it a matter of sacramental confession. The following procedural steps are presented in an effort to simplify the confessor's role. It is safe to say that in most situations, the penalty of excommunication will not apply. In such cases, he will have to deal only with the *sin* of abortion.

(1) Whatever excuses the penitent from a *serious sin* excuses him from the penalty of excommunication (Can.1321,1). Even if there is evidence of a serious sin, however, the penitent may be excused from excommunication on the basis of Canon 18 which states that laws which establish penalties are to be strictly interpreted. Hence, in keeping with the canonical axiom that "a doubtful censure is no censure," the penitent may be given the benefit of any positive doubt, for example: was abortion actually achieved?—could the abortive effect have resulted from some other cause than the action placed by the attempt at abortion? was the termination of pregnancy of a non-viable fetus or embryo directly intended?

(2) If it looks like a valid case of excommunication due to a directly-intended, procured abortion, the confessor must recall the circumstances which can excuse a sinner from excommunication (Can.1323) especially with regard to automatic or "latae sententiae" penalties (Can.1324, note especially section 3). In summary, it can be said that the penitent incurred the excommunication only if he or she was over 18 years of age (no longer a

minor), and had (a) full *knowledge,* and (b) full *deliberation,* and (c) full *freedom,* and (d) *full responsibility.* [181]

A brief commentary on each of these four factors may be helpful:

(a) Full *knowledge* would be lacking if the penitent did not know that abortion was a serious sin, or that it was subject to a special penalty (for example, excommunication).

(b) Full *deliberation* would be lacking if the person had been "in the serious heat of passion" at the time (provided it had not been voluntarily stirred up or fostered) (Can.1324,1,n.3).

(c) Full *freedom* would be lacking if the person had been compelled by fear or physical force, or under the influence of a chance happening which could not have been foreseen, or if foreseen, could not have been avoided. This would be applicable even if the person erroneously and culpably thought he was under even relatively grave fear, or under necessity or grave inconvenience; or thought he was acting in self-defense or in defense of another (Can.1324,1,n.8, and Can.1323,nn.4 and 5).

(d) Full *responsibility* would be lacking if the penitent had only the imperfect use of reason, or lacked the use of reason at the time (even if due to drunkenness or a similar culpable mental disturbance).

One author summarizes the above circumstances by saying:

". . . any of the above lists of excuses will exempt from the penalty. Or to look at it the other way, there will be a penalty present only in the case of very full deliberation and knowledge." [182]

(3) If there is no doubt but that the excommunication has been incurred, the hospital chaplain has the faculty to absolve from the excommunication in the *internal* forum (Can.566,2). If the confessor is not a duly-appointed hospital chaplain, the procedure is simplified in the following situations:

(a) If the penitent is in danger of death, any priest can licitly and validly absolve the penitent both from the penalty of excommunication and from the sin of abortion. (Can.976). It is left up to the prudential judgment of that priest to determine whether or not the case is one which would require special admonitions or an appropriate penance (Canons 1358,2, and 1348). The law of the Church no longer requires the penitent to have recourse to the

---

[181]Stenson, Alex, "Penalties in the New Code, the Role of the confessor," in *The Jurist,* vol. 43 (1983), n. 2, pp. 412–414. Cf. also *CLSA Commentary* (cf. note 45), pp. 902–904 (Canons 1323 and 1324).

[182]*Ibid.* (Stenson), p. 414.

diocesan bishop or others after the danger of death has passed.[183] If the excommunication has been *imposed* or *declared* (rare indeed), consult the following chapter (4.1).

(b) If the penitent is not in danger of death, but "it would be hard on the penitent to remain in the state of serious sin" during the time it would take to have recourse to the diocesan bishop or to his representative (Can.508), any confessor can remit the excommunication in the *internal* forum. The rest of the canon is self-explanatory:

> In granting a remission, the confessor is to impose on the penitent the burden of having recourse within a month to a superior or to a priest endowed with faculties and obeying his mandates under pain of reincidence of the penalty; in the meantime he should impose an appropriate penance and the reparation of any scandal or damage to the extent that it is imperative; recourse can be made by the confessor without mentioning any names (Can.1357,2).

The "superior" in this case would be the bishop. The "priest endowed with faculties" would be the priest designated by the diocesan bishop for that purpose (if Can.508 has been activated in the diocese). It is highly recommended that the confessor volunteer his good services in making recourse for the penitent, without mentioning any names. The purpose of the recourse is not to have the penalty of excommunication remitted (which already has been done) but to obtain the "mandata" or instructions and/or admonitions of that superior which are designed to reform the penitent and repair damages which may have resulted from the sin and crime of abortion. The confessor is encouraged to use his powers of persuasion to "make it hard to remain in the state of serious sin" and thus motivate him or her to proper sentiments of

---

[183]*CLSA Commentary* (cf. note 45), commentary on Canon 976, p. 688. The phrase "danger of death" does not mean that the danger must be certain. A well-founded probability of death suffices (impending major operation, serious sickness, victims of war or natural catastrophies, presence in an area where life is in danger due to war, tornadoes, earthquakes, etc., passenger in a seriously malfunctioning ship or airplane, etc.) Cf. Healy, Edwin, S.J., *Medical Ethics* (cf. note 46), p. 368; Bouscaren, T. Lincoln, S.J., and Ellis, Adam C., S.J., *Canon Law, A Text and Commentary* (Milwaukee, Wis.: Bruce Publishing Co., 1946), p. 821.

The prohibition against receiving the sacraments is suspended for the duration of the danger of death (Can. 1352,1) if the patient is properly disposed. The patient will have greater peace of mind, however, if the "danger of death" situation or the "spiritual hardship of remaining in serious sin" (Can. 1357) is used to absolve the patient of both the excommunication and the sin of abortion.

repentance and spiritual need. Father Felix M. Cappello, S.J., states that the period of time (in serious sin) should be considered subjectively. For some penitents the full course of one day might suffice; for others (such as a penitent who is a cleric, a priest, a religious, etc.) it could be merely the space of a few hours.[184]

(4) If the possibilities above do not apply (penitent not in danger of death, and not the type of person who "finds it hard to remain in serious sin"), the confessor may either direct the penitent to approach the hospital chaplain (who can absolve from the penalty in the *internal* forum), or to the diocesan bishop or his representative (Can. 508), or to any bishop (who also can absolve from the penalty in the *internal* forum). If these choices are not available, the confessor should obtain the penitent's permission to apply for him or her to the diocesan bishop or his representative to have the excommunication remitted. The confessor would then have to arrange for the penitent to return to him in the setting of sacramental confession in order to receive the "mandata" or instructions with regard to spiritual reformation and repair of damages caused by the crime of abortion.[185] In the event that the penitent is directed to see the hospital chaplain or a bishop other than the diocesan bishop, however, that person (as confessor) would have to attend to the matter of recourse in order to receive and communicate the "mandata." The formula for absolving from the penalty of excommunication is:

By the power granted to me, I absolve you from the bond of excommunication. In the name of the Father, and of the Son, and of the Holy Spirit. Amen.

Authors speculate regarding the possible situation when there is a space of time between the abortive action or procedure and the effect, and the pregnant woman (or others who are involved) sincerely repents of her role in the process. Since there is doubt as to responsibility in such a situation, it is safe to say that the excommunication was not incurred.[186]

---

[184]Cappello, Felix, S.J., *Tractatus Canomico-Moralis De Censuris,* 3rd ed. (Rome: Marietti, 1933), n. 124, 4.

[185]Stenson, Alex (cf. note 181), p. 418.

[186]Ayrinhac, H.A., S.S., and Lydon, P.J., *Penal Legislation in the New Code of Canon Law* (New York, N.Y.: Benziger Brothers, 1936), p. 242; Genicot, Edward, S.J. and Salsmans, I., S.J., *Institutiones Theologiae Moralis,* 2 vols, II, 14th ed. (Buenos Aires: Ediciones Declée de Brouwer, 1939), n. 572; O'Donnell, Thomas, S.J., *Medicine and Christian Morality* (cf. note 31), p. 147. It is to be noted that Canon 1328 of the present code of canon law projects a sense of leniency in the matter.

> *Directive 12:* Abortion, that is, the directly intended termination of pregnancy before viability, is never permitted nor is the directly intended destruction of a viable fetus. Every procedure whose sole immediate effect is the termination of pregnancy before viability is an abortion, which, in its moral context, includes the interval between conception and implantation of the embryo. Catholic hospitals are not to provide abortion services based upon the principle of material cooperation.

3.6 DISCRIMINATION AGAINST HUMAN LIFE

The directly-intended termination of the life of the infant after birth is called infanticide. Both crimes, that of abortion and of infanticide, are forms of euthanasia or "easy death" (from the Greek "eu" and "thanatos"). The Holy See's *Declaration on Euthanasia* (May 5, 1980) defines "euthanasia" as "any action or omission that by its nature or intention causes death with the purpose of putting an end to all suffering. Euthanasia is, therefore, a matter of intention and method."[187] The word often is cloaked in the concept of "mercy killing." The defenseless victim of euthanasia can be an embryo or fetus, an infant, or an adult who is advanced in age, incurably ill, or in a moribund state.

Prenatal Euthanasia

Genetic screening techniques today have made it possible to gain a fairly reliable preview of the child-to-be, and to provide diagnostic guidelines in the management of pregnancy and of obstetric procedures and treatments. Some of these techniques can be used only at certain stages of embryonic or fetal development, and their use implies certain risks which must be balanced against the anticipated benefits; but considered as a whole, these techniques constitute a singular blessing in the contemporary practice of obstetrics.

Many of the technological procedures which are used commonly in the practice of medicine can serve the obstetrician in the management of pregnancy. Fetal heartbeat, for example, can be monitored through electrocardi-

---

[187] *The Pope Speaks,* 1980, p. 292. The declaration was released by the Sacred Congregation for the Doctrine of the Faith on June 27, 1980.

ography (EKG). Through the use of a transcervical catheter, a continuous monitoring of electrocardiographic data and of uterine contractions can be provided. Contemporary techniques in fetal screening and in the monitoring of pregnancy increase the possibilities of measuring alpha fetoprotein levels (AFP) in the amniotic fluid and in the blood serum of pregnant mothers so as to detect neural tube defects (NTD's) such as anencephaly and spina bifida.[188] A brief review of these techniques is both enlightening and encouraging.

Amniocentesis is a procedure whereby a needle is inserted through the abdominal wall into the amniotic sac which surrounds the fetus. A small amount of the amniotic fluid can be withdrawn and used to grow a culture for diagnostic analysis of cells that have flaked off the body of the fetus into the fluid. The procedure has been used routinely since 1956 when it was demonstrated as a reliable aid in the management of an Rh-immunized pregnancy.[189] When used for genetic-screening purposes (to detect chromosome abnormalities, metabolic disorders, neural tube defects, etc.) the ideal time is 15 to 17 weeks of gestation when the amniotic fluid volume increases rapidly. Preliminary to the insertion of the needle, ultrasound scanning is used to document and evaluate fetal life and formation, and to avoid the placenta and the fetus in the search for pockets of amniotic fluid. During the second half of pregnancy, it is rarely used for genetic reasons, but it is useful (during that period) for determining fetal condition in Rh disease or other blood group immunizations, and also to determine fetal maturity and to check for infection and maturity in the setting of premature rupture of the membranes.[190]

Dr. John T. Queenan states that this procedure, once considered to be daring, risky, "and even reckless," is now routine in approximately 15% of pregnancies. He emphasizes the importance of adequate training in this procedure in residency training programs. He does not deny the risks involved, but adds: "With careful consideration of the indications, the benefits of amniocentesis far outweigh the risks. Amniocentesis is safe when careful judgment and skill are used."[191]

Ultrasonography for medical diagnostic purposes can be traced to the development of radar and sonar (and the flaw detector for materials testing) during

---

[188]For a review of these techniques, cf. *Genetic Medicine and Engineering* (St. Louis, Mo.: Catholic Health Assoc. and Pope John Center, 1983), Albert S. Moraczewski, O.P., ed., pp. 16–26; *Genetic Counseling, the Church and the Law* (St. Louis, Mo.: The Pope John Center, 1980), Albert S. Moraczewski, O.P., and Gary M. Atkinson, eds., pp. 12–24; Nathanson, Bernard, *Aborting America* (cf. note 115), pp. 200 f.

[189]Queenan, John T., MD, "Amniocentesis," in *Management of High-Risk Pregnancy*, 2nd ed., John T. Queenan, MD, ed. (Oradell, N.J.: Medical Economics Books, 1985), p. 201.

[190]*Ibid.*, pp. 201, 202, 213

[191]*Ibid.*, p. 213.

World War II. It is described as "The use of pulse-echo imaging technics to detect tissue density differences within the body and thus display pathologic processes that are not adequately seen by other diagnostic procedures."[192] Although it is safe to say that, as of 1985, "there have been no reports in the literature of harmful effects due to diagnostic imaging with commercially available instruments," it must be admitted that the effect on future generations or in ways still untested remains an open question. Hence, "the prudent physician should not 'guarantee' the safety of ultrasound."[193] Since ultrasonography does not involve x-radiation, it is the diagnostic method of choice in obstetrical practice.

In standard ultrasonic diagnostic equipment, a transducer (usually a crystal of barium titanate), designed to oscillate at high-cycle levels, is pulsed at a rate between 300 and 1000 times per second, producing bursts of ultrasonic energy that are directed into the tissue as a collimated or focused beam. When the ultrasound strikes a tissue or fluid interface of different density, sonic echoes are reflected back to the transducer face, converted into electrical impulses, amplified, and displayed on an oscilloscope as pips or dots. A major advance in ultrasonography known as *real-time scanning* employs a *multiple* transducer array *interphased* successively to display motion of the heart, the fetus, and the larger blood vessels without use of contrast media at up to 40 frames per second.[194] This version, in which the transducers operate in a planned pattern instead of successively, is the favored type of ultrasonography in obstetrical practice. As a unit of equipment, it can be moved easily from the physician's office to the hospital bed or to the delivery room. The importance and many uses of real-time ultrasonography are described as follows:

> The impact of diagnostic ultrasound in perinatal management has been monumental. Within the past decade we have seen two-dimensional imaging move from the research laboratory into the clinician's office. Ultrasound has become an integral part of perinatal medicine. Included among its many uses are determining gestational age and presentation, detecting multiple gestations, establishing early fetal life by the detection of fetal heartbeat and movement, diagnosing fetal congenital abnormalities, locating the placenta, monitoring fetal growth and determining well-being by

---

[192]*The Merck Manual* (cf. note 56), p. 2157.

[193]Queenan, John T., MD, and Warsof, Steven L., MD, "Ultrasonography," in *Management of High-Risk Pregnancy* (cf. note 189), pp. 229, 230.

[194]*The Merck Manual* (cf. note 56), pp. 2158, 2159.

the biophysical profile, confirming fetal maturity, and enhancing parental bonding.[195]

Fetoscopy involves the use of a solid optical endoscope known as a "Needlescope" or "Dyonics Fetoscope" (roughly equivalent in size to a 16-gauge needle) to sample blood and tissues as a means of diagnosing some fetal hemoglobinopathies, hemophilia, immunodeficient diseases and chromosomal abnormalities in the face of equivocal amniotic fluid findings, and various serious fetal skin defects. Although this technique is used for the diagnosis of conditions which are beyond the reach of amniotic fluid cell studies or ultrasonography, it is employed in combination with ultrasound (to determine the position of the fetus, placenta, cord, and uterine wall before and during the procedure). The patient is mildly sedated. The time required to obtain fetal blood varies from 3 to 45 minutes.[196]

Since fetoscopy is a more invasive procedure than amniocentesis, efforts are being made today to diminish the need for fetoscopy in diagnosing cases of β-thalassemia (a type of hereditary hemolytic anemia) and sickle cell disease by the DNA analysis of cells found in amniotic fluid through amniocentesis.[197] Due to the consequences and complications of the fetoscopy procedure itself, the recommendation is that it should never be done routinely by the practicing obstetrician. Furthermore, it is a procedure that should be done only in medical centers.[198]

Chorionic villus sampling (CVS) has the advantage of being a first trimester procedure for detecting fetal abnormalities. The cellular, outermost extraembryonic membrane known as the *chorion* develops threadlike projections growing in tufts on its external surface about two weeks after fertilization. This is known as the "shaggy" surface of the chorion (*chorion frondosum*) which eventually becomes the *placenta*.[199] Samples of such villi have been obtained by direct vision with the help of a hysteroscope or fetoscope, but better results are obtained by ultrasound-guided aspiration through a soft tube (cannula) at about 8—10 weeks gestation. The difficulties in chorionic villus aspiration are listed as: failure to negotiate the cervical canal; problems in placing the cannula at the suitable site; inadvertent rupture of the amniotic sac.[200]

---

[195]Queenan-Warsof (cf. note 189), p. 215.

[196]Hobbins, John C., MD, "Fetoscopy," in *Management of High-Risk Pregnancy* (cf. note 189), pp. 231, 232.

[197]*Ibid.*, p. 233.

[198]*Ibid.*, p. 238.

[199]*Dorband's Illustrated Medical Dictionary*, 26th ed. (Philadelphia, Pa.: W.B. Saunders Co., 1981), p. 264 (chorion) and p. 1456 (villus).

[200]Ward, Humphry, MD, "Chorionic Villus Sampling," in *Management of High-Risk Pregnancy* (cf. note 189), pp. 242–245.

Chorionic villus sampling (CVS) still is in the research stage. The risks involved would indicate that the procedure be restricted to medical centers. As stated above, the need for fetoscopy can be diminished due to rapid advances today in the DNA analysis of cells obtained through amniocentesis. These same advances can decrease dependance on the CVS procedure. The DNA methods may soon be available not only to detect such disorders as cycstic fibrosis and phenylketonuria (a metabolic abnormality), but also for conventional chromosomal and biochemical studies.[201] The following analysis of the CVS procedure should be kept in mind:

> It is still difficult to assess the true risk of chorionic villus sampling. It must be compared with the risk of patients of the same age group who have a sonographically normal fetus at 8—12 weeks, and who do not undergo CVS. The risk of fetal loss in that group is approximately 3%. In some of the larger series of CVS, fetal loss ranges from 1.8% to 5.5%. The risk in CVS appears to be several times that of genetic amniocentesis. Still to be determined are the effects of bleeding and cramping over a prolonged period following the procedure; the effect, if any, on birth weight; and the long-term effects of CVS. Nonetheless, the procedure appears to be safe in skilled hands.[202]

From an ethical viewpoint, it should be emphasized that any woman who requests or agrees to undergo any of these tests (including amniocentesis, ultrasonography or fetoscopy) with the intention of aborting her pregnancy if the test results are unfavorable, is guilty of a serious sin. Of the four procedures discussed above, such a sinful intention is more likely to be found in requesting or submitting to the chorionic villus sampling procedure—precisely because it is a first-trimester procedure. An abortion at this early stage of pregnancy would present lower physical risks and less psychological trauma than an abortion late in the second trimester when the infant is approaching viability . . . a time when "maternal-fetal bonding may well be accelerated."[203] This also explains why CVS is used in population-control countries such as in China and in the Soviet Union.[204]

With regard to all four procedures, however, the obvious positive benefits must be stressed, regardless of the possible abuses which cloud the glory of so

---

[201] *Ibid.*, p. 240.
[202] *Ibid.*, Editor's comment, pp. 245, 246.
[203] *Ibid.*, p. 240.
[204] *Ibid.*, p. 242.

many achievements of human creativity (drug therapy, laser technology, nuclear science, etc.). The danger of abuse undoubtedly is more likely in a first-trimester procedure such as chorionic villus sampling. There is a sense, however, in which appropriate pro-life counseling and favorable test results can save infants who would otherwise be aborted. In discussing fetoscopy, for example, one obstetrician presents the following clinical observation:

> I'm often asked about the ethics of what we're doing. We diagnose conditions we cannot satisfactorily treat at present. We are diagnosing early, and the usual option is termination of the pregnancy if the fetus is afflicted with untreatable disease. Most of our patients, especially those who have already had a thalassemic child or who have someone in the family with this disease, say that if we can't give them any information about the fetus's condition, they will terminate the pregnancy. Theoretically, we are saving 75% of the fetuses that would ordinarily be aborted . . . As of February 1984, we had performed 301 fetoscopies, and 222 patients continued their pregnancies; 77 elected to terminate their pregnancies based on information we gave them.[205]

Father Richard McCormick, S.J. presents valid reasons why amniocentesis should be provided in a Catholic hospital (with "counseling and support for continuing the pregnancy") rather than in non-Catholic hospitals where the administrators have no qualms of conscience about abortion. He states: ". . by providing amniocentesis as a regular service, the Catholic facility will potentially and probably be involved in a service that will save fetal lives that would otherwise be lost." As if in confirmation of his statement, he mentions that about six-hundred fifty amniocentesis procedures are performed at the Georgetown University Medical Center in Washington, D.C., annually, and adds: "About ten of these will reveal problem pregnancies. Five of them will end in abortion (not performed at Georgetown)."[206] Based on studies done at several major obstetrical centers throughout the U.S.A., Father Charles McFadden, O.S.A. expresses the opinion that most amniocentesis procedures are done to ascertain the precise degree of fetal maturity, and that at least 90% are done for therapeutic purposes (helpful in prenatal and postnatal therapy for the infant).[207]

---

[205]Hobbins, John C., MD (cf. note 189), pp. 234, 235.
[206]*Health and Medicine in the Catholic Tradition* (New York, N.Y.: Crossroad Publishing Co., 1984), pp. 140, 141.
[207]*Challenge to Morality* (Huntington, Ind.: Our Sunday Visitor, 1977), p. 72–74.

The anticipated benefits of the use of these diagnostic procedures might be summarized as follows: (1) In advancing scientific research in genetic diseases. The field is vast. Not only do infants and children with birth defects constitute about one-third of all pediatric admissions to hospitals, but "patients with genetic diseases enter hospitals and stay longer, at least five times as frequently as patients with non-genetic diseases;"[208] (2) In promoting responsible parenthood in keeping with Catholic moral standards. The role of couples in begetting children is conditioned by their capability to provide for them. (3) In facilitating the prompt treatment of infants with birth defects. Physicians can obtain blood and tissue samples directly from the fetus at 18 to 20 weeks of gestation, and can give blood transfusion to the fetus within the womb from 22 weeks on. Intrauterine surgery, already attempted "only a few dozen times," may yet become feasible.[209]

Due to the risks involved in these various procedures, the anticipated benefits must be balanced with the dangers in each particular case. This is in keeping with the *Principle of the Double Effect;* it would be morally objectionable to submit to a risky and dangerous procedure if the same anticipated benefit can be obtained through a reasonable and available alternative procedure which presents a lesser danger. As mentioned above, future medical advances in the DNA analysis of cells obtained through amniocentesis and ultrasonography should decrease dependence on fetoscopy and chorionic villus sampling as procedures of choice. To submit to any risky procedure without a proportionate reason (for example, merely a routine measure) would be morally objectionable. This would apply to amniocentesis, and even to ultrasonography if the management of the pregnancy is proceeding normally. The cost factor of such specialized procedures must also be given due consideration in the evaluation of a proportionate reason.

Postnatal Euthanasia

The April, 1984, issue of the *Hasting Center Report* included three articles on the subject of "Care of Imperiled Newborns." One of them contains the following realistic but chilling statement: "Ethical ambiguity pervades the issue. Most seriously impaired children should be treated, some should be allowed to die. Substantive principles are available, but their application is

---

[208]*Genetic Medicine and Engineering,* Albert S. Moraczewski, O.P., Ph.D., ed. (cf. note 188), presentation on "Genetic Disorders" by Kutay Taysi, MD, p. 4.
[209]Lyon, Jeff, *Playing God in the Nursery* (New York, N.Y.: W.W. Norton and Co., 1985), p. 323. For an excellent presentation of the issue in "Genetic Screening and Counseling," cf. Ashley-O-Rourke, *Health Care Ethics* (cf. note 80), pp. 316–323.

fraught with difficulty and danger."[210] The author refers to both medical and non-medical aspects contributing to this ambiguity such as medical and prognostic uncertainty, parental neglect, etc. Unless something is done to dissipate this ethical ambiguity, "quality of life" considerations will prevail in determining whether a defective infant should be treated and allowed to live, or neglected and allowed to die. Some physicians admit that in making decisions for such infants they are influenced by the following "handy guide" for perplexed physicians: "QL = NE X (H & S)." Translation: the estimated quality of life (QL) for the infant equals his natural endowment, physical and intellectual (NE), multiplied by the amount of support he is likely to get from his home (H) and from society (S).[211] The problem is compounded by the wide variety of congenital malformations—in reality, in excess of several thousand.

The Sources of Congenital Malformations

As of 1983, statistics revealed that 33% of infant mortality was related to genetic factors. Developmental disorders in newborns can be traced to one or more of four factors: 1) *Single-gene Disorders* caused by abnormal (mutant) genes, which run in families, follow certain predictable types of inheritance, and express themselves by conditions such as retardation (both physical and mental), cysts in the kidneys, spastic paralysis of the lower legs, some skeletal abnormalities, etc. 2) *Chromosomal Disorders;* due to either one chromosome too many or one too few in each body cell (for example, the Down Syndrome, trisomy 21); 3) *Polygenic Diseases,* also called "multifactorial" because both genetic and non-genetic factors apparently are involved (congenital heart defects, cleft palate, open spine defects, etc.); 4) *Teratogenic Diseases,* so-called because they are caused by substances or factors which induce birth defects (exposure of the mother to the rubella virus or "German Measles" during pregnancy, X-ray radiation, chronic heavy alcohol intake by the mother, etc.).[212] Granted that the victims of many of these diseases will not live more than a few days or weeks or months, human dignity demands that they be allowed to live out their full span of life with due attention to their basic

---

[210]Arras, John D., "On the Care of Imperiled Newborns," in *The Hastings Center Report,* April, 1984, p. 33

[211]Hentoff, Nat., "Nursery Lottery Means Death for Many Handicapped Babies," in *NLR News* (Baltimore, Md.), May 3, 1984, p. 14.

[212]Dr. Kutay Taysi, director of the Medical Genetics Clinic at St. Louis Childrens' Hospital in St. Louis, Mo., who discusses these causes in *Genetic Medicine and Engineering* (cf. note 188), pp. 3–13, states that the number of different diseases in the single-gene-disorder group alone is approximately 3000 (p. 5).

medical and comfort needs (nutrition, hydration, etc.). They are the most defenseless of God's human family. Any efforts, or any willful omissions of ethically-obligatory procedures, which are designed to allow them to die, would amount to criminal euthanasia.

The presumption that parents are best qualified to make appropriate decisions with regard to their handicapped infants must yield to reliable evidence to the contrary. It cannot be denied that in some cases, parents have a significant conflict of interests which impairs their judgment negatively with regard to a handicapped infant. The *"Baby Doe" Case* in Bloomington, Ind. (1982) aroused public indignation when the media announced that the parents of this Down Syndrome infant had refused to authorize a simple and routine operation which would have repaired an internal blockage which prevented the infant from ingesting food. The medical personnel of the hospital allowed the infant to starve to death. In a very similar case in 1974, known as the *Baby Houle Case,* a Maine court appointed a guardian to give consent for corrective surgery contrary to the wishes of the parents. In the *Chad Green Case* in 1978, the Supreme Court of Massachusetts took custody of the 20-month-old leukemia victim whose parents had refused to allow appropriate treatment (chemotherapy). In the *Cicero Case* in 1979, a New York court ordered corrective surgery for an infant who had an open spine. The courts were saying that the state's interest in protecting the life of the infant outweighs the parents' right to determine the medical treatment of the infant.[213]

The Call for Help Through Ethics Committees

These cases and others throughout the nation have emphasized the need of going beyond the parents-physician-family triad in order to protect the best interests of defective newborns. Most observers of this sensitive problem would admit that referring the case to the courts should be an absolute last-resort procedure. The trend has been growing to have recourse in difficult cases to the consultative role of ethics or moral-medical committees in each health care facility. The beginning of this trend can be traced to the decision of the New Jersey Supreme Court (March 31, 1976) in the *Karen Quinlan Case* (lapsed into an irreversible coma in 1975). That decision reads as follows:

> Upon the concurrence of the guardian and family of Karen should the responsible attending physicians conclude there is no reason-able possibility of Karen's ever emerging from her present coma-

---

[213]Horan, Dennis J., and Grant, Edward R., "Prolonging Life and Withdrawing Treatment: Legal Issues," in *Linacre Quarterly,* May, 1983, pp. 159–160.

tose condition to a cognitive, sapient state, and that the life-support apparatus now being administered to Karen should be discontinued, they shall consult with the "Ethics Committee" or like body of the institution in which Karen is then hospitalized. If that consultative body agrees that there is no reasonable possibility of Karen's ever emerging from her present comatose condition to a cognitive, sapient state, the present life-support system may be withdrawn and said action shall be without any civil or criminal liability therefore on the part of any participant, whether guardian, physician, hospital or others.[214]

In the wake of the wide publicity given to the "Baby Doe" case (Bloomington, Ind., 1982), President Reagan issued a statement on April 30, 1982, in which he directed the Department of Health and Human Services (HHS) to notify health care providers that *Section 504 of the Rehabilitation Act of 1973* could be applied to the situation;—a claim which was contested strenuously throughout the turbulent history of the so-called "Baby Doe" regulations. It is important to quote from the first directive on the subject as issued from the office of the Director of Civil Rights on May 18, 1982:

This notice is intended to remind affected parties of the applicability of Section 504 of the Rehabilitation Act of 1973 . . . Section 504 provides that 'No otherwise qualified handicapped individual . . . shall, solely by reason of his handicap, be excluded from the participation in, be denied the benefits of, or be subjected to discrimination under any program or activity receiving Federal financial assistance.' . . . Under section 504 it is unlawful for a recipient of Federal financial assistance to withhold from a handicapped infant nutritional sustenance or medical or surgical treatment required to correct a life threatening condition, if:
1) the withholding is based on the fact that the infant is handicapped; and
2) the handicap does not render the treatment or nutritional sustenance medically contraindicated.[215]
It was not until March 7, 1983, however, that the HHS issued regulations dealing with the problem.

---

[214]Veatch, Robert M., "Hospital Ethics Committees: Is There a Role?," in *The Hastings Center Report*, June, 1977, p. 22. Quotation and commentary.

[215]These directives are found in the report entitled *Deciding to Forego Life-sustaining Treatment* (Washington D.C.: U.S. Government Printing Office, 1983), a publication of *The President's Commission*, pp. 467–474.

The regulations of March 7, 1983, issued as an "Interim Final Rule" from the Secretary of the HHS, met with opposition from many in the health care profession. The offending features included the following stipulations: the required posting of a notice in each hospital ward likely to treat disabled newborns to the effect that "discrimination is prohibited by federal law;" the clearance given to federal investigators to visit the hospital at any time so as to detect violations and enforce compliance with the regulations; the publication of a toll-free 24-hour hotline whereby suspected denials of "food or customary medical treatment" could be reported confidentially to the HHS Office or to the Office of Civil Rights.[216] These regulations were challenged by the District of Columbia federal district court, by the American Academy of Pediatrics and by other medical groups. On April 14, 1983, Judge Gerhard Gesell enjoined the regulations, calling them "arbitrary and capricious." In response, the HHS proposed a *second* version of the regulations which mollified some of the offending features of the first version. The American Academy of Pediatrics proposed a detailed alternative which would provide for *no applicability of Section 504 of the Rehabilitation Act of 1973.*[217]

The next turn of events introduced the subject of some type of ethics committee to deliberate contested cases of denial of food and treatment to handicapped infants. The proposal of the American Academy of Pediatrics (mentioned above) incorporated a recommendation of the *President's Commission* (report published, March, 1983) that an ethics committee "or similar body" be formed in hospitals that care for seriously ill newborns "to review the decisionmaking process."[218] The American Academy of Pediatrics proposal, dated July 5, 1983, approved of the creation of infant bioethical review committees as a "direct, effective, and appropriate means of addressing the existing education and information gaps."[219]

As of November, 1983, Surgeon General C. Everett Koop became involved in the effort to bring about an acceptable set of "Baby Doe" regulations. The *second* version (as above) actually received the support of 97.5% of the 16,331 comments received during the 60-day comment period. Not only

---

[216]*Ibid.*, appendix H. pp. 469–474.

[217]Horan, Dennis J., JD, and Balch, Burke J., JD, "Infant Doe and Baby Jane Doe: Medical Treatment of the Handicapped Newborn," in *Linacre Quarterly,* February, 1985, pp. 45–72. Reference on pp. 60, 61. Cf. also Bopp, James, Jr., JD, and Balch, Thomas J., JD, "The Child Abuse Amendments of 1984 and their Implementing Regulations: A Summary," in *Issues in Law and Medicine,* September, 1985, pp. 91–130 for another excellent survey of the Baby Doe regulations and legislation.

[218]*Deciding to Forego Life-Sustaining Treatment* (cf. note 215), p. 227.

[219]Fleischman, Alan R., and Murray, Thomas H., "Ethics Committees for Infants Doe?," in *The Hastings Center Report,* December .983, pp. 5–9. Reference on p. 5.

the American Academy of Pediatrics, but also hospital and physician groups, however, denounced that *second* version. In all probability, the proposal of the American Academy of Pediatrics, as well as his negotiations with medical groups, right to life organizations and others, had convinced Dr. Koop that the time was ripe for a *third* and final set of "Baby Doe" regulations. These compromise regulations (the *third* version), announced publicly on January 9, 1984, failed to please the opposition:

> These regulations were struck down on June 11, 1984, in a suit brought by the American Hospital Association. That federal district court ruling was affirmed by the Second Circuit Court of Appeals on December 27, 1984. Both courts regarded themselves as bound by an earlier Second Circuit ruling which had held that 'congress never contemplated that section 504 would apply to treatment decisions of this nature.' The United States Supreme Court granted certiorari [that is, a writ requesting a transcript of the proceedings of a case for review] to review the decision striking down the 504 Baby Doe Regulations on June 17, 1985.[220]

The last chapter in the perils of the "Baby Doe" regulations was written by the U.S. Supreme Court on June 9, 1986, by a 5–4 decision which struck down the "Baby Doe" regulations.[221] Since this decision ruled that the federal government cannot challenge life-or-death decisions that parents make for handicapped infants (by withholding sustenance or treatment), it will be discussed under the heading of the care of handicapped newborns in chapter V (Principle of Informed Consent).

While the executive branch of the U.S. Government was reacting to the public outcry over Baby Doe—with the unfavorable ending as mentioned above,—the U.S. Congress went into action to fashion its response to the problem. A bill introduced by Representative John Erlenborn on May 26, 1982 served as the beginning of a series of hearings followed by committee and floor action, which culminated in the *Child Abuse Amendments of 1984.*[222] Although it can be said that the route of *legislation* succeeded where the route of *regulations* failed, it is also valid to suspect that the legislators were willing to learn from the pitfalls of the "Baby Doe" regulations. The Child Abuse

---

[220]Bopp-Balch, "The Child Abuse Amendments of 1984 and Their Implementing Regulations: A Summary" (cf. note 217), pp. 98, 99.

[221]*Boston Globe,* June 10, 1986, pp. 1 and 8.

[222]Bopp-Balch, "The Child Abuse Amendments of 1984 and Their Implementing Regulations: A Summary" (cf. note 217), pp. 99, 100.

Amendments of 1984, which were signed into law by President Reagan on October 9, 1984 (to go into effect on October 9, 1985) stated that the statute under Sections 127(a) and (b) "shall not be construed" to affect any right or protection under *Section 504 of the Rehabilitation Act of 1973.*[223] The legislation also recommended Infant Care Review Committees (ICRC) which are quite similar to those published together with the Section 504 "Baby Doe" regulations.

This legislation expanded the definition of child abuse to include medical neglect in all cases of handicapped infants. The only exception is in the cases where, in the "physician's reasonable medical judgment," the infant is irretrievably comatose or would not survive even with treatment."[224] A full discussion and analysis of this legislation will be found in chapter V under the heading of the care of handicapped newborns.

Decreasing the Ethical Ambiguity

The high level of U.S. Government policies now in place with the passage of the *Child Abuse Amendments of 1984* provides a favorable atmosphere for Catholic health facilities to assume leadership in the campaign for respect for life. The ethical ambiguity is diminished considerably when U.S. government agencies champion principles as "Catholic" in tone and tradition such as the principle that medical care must be provided regardless of actual or anticipated handicaps; the principle that a person's disability must not be the basis for a decision to withhold treatment, etc. Furthermore, Catholic health facilities have had considerable experience with consultative discernment in difficult cases in the form of ethics committees. A 1983 survey of Catholic health facilities revealed that 41% of the responding hospitals in the U.S.A. have functioning ethics committees, whereas the figure for all other hospitals in the nation is only 1%.[225] Another superior advantage is that the principles and parameters for seeking guidance in perplexing cases (the "gray areas") are

---

[223]Rosenblum, Victor G., JD, and Grant, Edward R., JD, "The Legal Response to Babies Doe: An Analytical Prognosis," in *Issues in Law and Medicine,* March, 1986, pp. 391–404. Reference on pp. 398, 399.

[224]For an extended report on the *Child Abuse Amendments of 1984,* including the "Conference Report" of the House of Representatives, the "Joint Explanatory Statement of the Committee of Conference" (House and Senate), and the "Joint Explanatory Statement . . ." on the Amendments from the Appendix to the July 26, 1984, *Congressional Record* (44 pages in all), cf. *Report 98–1038* of the House of Representatives, 98th Congress, 2nd session. Available from the U.S. Gov. Printing Office, Washington, D.C.

[225]"Ethics Committees and Ethicists in Catholic Hospitals," by Sister Joan Kalchbrenner, R.H.S.J., Sister Margaret Kelly, D.C., and Father Donald McCarthy, in *Hospital Progress,* Sept., 1983, p. 47.

provided and spelled out in the *Ethical and Religious Directives for Catholic Health Facilities*. Catholic hospitals are singularly equipped to lead the campaign for respect for life.

In order that ethics committees may become effective as "the moral conscience of the hospital" (in the words of Father Thomas O'Donnell, S.J.) however, representation on the committee must be tailored to the variety of options contemplated; that is, the professional disciplines represented on an effective ethics committee should include, in addition to moral theology, the fields of medical practice, law, administration, social work and nursing. The subject of ethics committees will be discussed at length in the chapter VIII on the *Principle of the Common Good*. It may suffice to say for now that such committees can become the "conscience of the hospital" to a considerable extent if the members keep in mind that their role is not decision-making but rather educational and consultative or advisory. Success will attend their efforts if their priority of functions are understood and practiced as: 1) education, 2) recommending goals and policies, 3) availability for consultation.[226] The effectiveness of such committees can diminish considerably the possibilities of intervention by courts or by federal and state agencies.

Adult Euthanasia

The discussion of adult euthanasia can be presented more advantageously in chapter VIII on the *Principle of the Common Good*. At this juncture, it should suffice to state briefly what is NOT euthanasia. The *Declaration on Euthanasia* states:

> The pleas of the very seriously ill as they beg at times to be put to death are hardly to be understood as conveying a real desire for euthanasia. They are almost always anguished pleas for help and love.

The document goes on to say (quoting Pius XII) that the use of narcotics or painkillers even at the approach of death is allowed even though it is foreseen that the use of narcotics will shorten life, "provided that no other means exist and if, in the given circumstances, the action does not prevent the carrying out of other moral and religious duties."[227] The dying person is not to be

---

[226]*Ethics Committees: A Challenge for Catholic Health Care*, eds., Sister Margaret John Kelly, D.C., and Father Donald McCarthy (St. Louis, Mo.: Pope John Center and the Catholic Health Assoc., 1984), results of survey, p. 7.

[227]Declaration on Euthanasia, issued, May 5, 1980. Cf. *The Pope Speaks*, 1980, pp. 292, 293.

deprived of consciousness, however, unless there are serious reasons for doing so. The dying person may have unfulfilled moral or religious obligations such as making peace with God, becoming reconciled with estranged family members, settling important inheritance matters, etc. Furthermore, there is the importance of consciousness so that the dying persons can "dispose themselves with full awareness for their meeting with Christ."[228]

> *Directive 29:* It is not euthanasia to give a dying person sedatives and analgesics for the alleviation of pain, when such a measure is judged necessary, even though they may deprive the patient of the use of reason, or shorten his life.

---

[228]*Ibid.*, p. 294

CHAPTER IV

The Principle of Religious Freedom

It is in accordance with their dignity as persons—that is, beings endowed with reason and free will and therefore privileged to bear personal responsibility—that all men should be at once impelled by nature and also bound by a moral obligation to seek the truth, especially religious truth. They are also bound to adhere to the truth, once it is known, and to order their whole lives in accord with the demands of truth (Vatican II, *Declaration on Religious Freedom,* n.2).

THE HUMAN INDIVIDUAL HAS A RIGHT TO RELIGIOUS FREE-DOM, WHICH HAS ITS FOUNDATION IN THE VERY DIGNITY OF THE HUMAN PERSON . . . THIS FREEDOM MEANS THAT ALL MEN AND WOMEN ARE TO BE IMMUNE FROM COERCION ON THE PART OF . . . ANY HUMAN POWER, IN SUCH WISE THAT IN MATTERS RELIGIOUS, NO ONE IS TO BE FORCED TO ACT IN A MANNER CONTRARY TO HIS OR HER OWN BELIEFS. NOR IS ANYONE TO BE RESTRAINED FROM ACTING IN ACCORDANCE WITH HIS OR HER OWN BELIEFS WHETHER PRIVATELY OR PUBLICLY, WHETHER ALONE OR IN ASSOCIATION WITH OTHERS, WITHIN DUE LIMITS (Adapted from the *Declaration on Religious Freedom,* n.2).

The *obligation to seek and uphold the truth* and the *right to religious freedom* are not mutually exclusive. The right to religious freedom is not conditioned by the fact the many individuals, in seeking and in upholding the truth as they see it, may have a false or erroneous conscience. It is significant that Vatican II's *Declaration on Religious Freedom* does not base the right of religious freedom on "freedom of conscience." That phrase is not even mentioned. Due consideration must be given to the fact that many will say: "My decision does not bother me (abortion, living in an invalid marriage, having recourse to artificial insemination, etc.) because I am only doing what my conscience tells me to do." The right to religious freedom is based on our common human dignity, defined as personal responsibility. Every human individual must be free to follow, faithfully and without hindrance, the light of truth as he or she knows himself or herself to be *obliged* to act.[229] No judgment is leveled against those who may labor under a false or erroneous conscience. As Jesus said in narrating the parable of the wheat and the weeds: "Let them grow together until harvest time" (Matthew, 13:30). The *Declaration on Religious Freedom* continues:

> . . . the leaven of the Gospel has long been about its quiet work in the minds of men. To it is due in great measure the fact that in the course of time men have come more widely to recognize their dignity as persons, and the conviction has grown stronger that in religious matters the person in society is to be kept free from all manner of human coercion (n.12).

4.1 RESPECTING FREEDOM IN MINISTERING TO THE SPIRITUAL NEEDS OF CATHOLIC PATIENTS

One of the most vexing problems in a Catholic health facility is to encounter wayward and even belligerent Catholics who cannot be persuaded to make their peace with God. This writer has done parish work for several decades, and remembers the sense of frustration one evening when an embittered, dying Catholic gent summoned his last show of strength to raise himself up on his elbows and curse him out of the hospital room; or the many other occasions when efforts to mend an invalid marriage or bring a lapsed Catholic back into the fold was met with "Mind your own business!" Salvation cannot be force-fed. Such situations call for inspired diplomacy,

---

[229]*Commentary on the Documents of Vatican II*, 5 vols., IV, Herbert Vorgrimler, ed. (New York, N.Y.: Herder and Herder, 1969), pp. 64–68 and 80–83.

finesse, loving care, and, in many cases, a holy diet of prayer and fasting (Matthew,17:21).

The Catholic hospital chaplain is well fortified canonically to attend to the spiritual needs of patients by virtue of his appointment by the bishop. Since the *pastoral* care of the community within the hospital enclave is entrusted to his care "in a stable manner" (Can.564), that circumscribed area could be called, in a wide sense, his parish. Clerical courtesy requires that he maintain a proper relationship ("debitam conjunctionem") with the pastor of the area (Can.571), and by due implication, also with the pastors of Catholic patients in the hospital. Although he is admonished not to involve himself in the internal governance of the hospital, he is responsible for the celebration and regulation of liturgical functions (Can.567,2).

In addition to faculties which should be granted to him by particular law or special delegation from the bishop (566), the chaplain not only enjoys the faculties to hear confessions, preach the Word of God, administer Viaticum, anoint the sick and administer the sacrament of confirmation (the latter in danger-of-death cases only), but also the faculties to absolve from automatic ("latae sententiae") censures such as excommunication incurred by the sin of procuring an abortion (Can.1398) and also excommunication incurred by the sins of apostasy, heresy or schism (Can.1364). This grant of absolving penitents with an abortion problem or who have worries over having "left the Church" is rather significant. These are precisely the types of deep concerns which would trouble a conscientious Christian who faces the uncertainties of illness (perhaps serious) in a hospital setting: a now-repentant woman with a record of several abortions; or a now-serious adult with sentiments of apostasy ("Left the Church years ago in disgust"), and now feeling guilty about possible heresy (serious doubts about the Catholic faith approaching denial of basic Catholic doctrine), or schism ("shopping around" for another religious affiliation).

The present code of canon law provides a definition of apostasy, heresy and schism as follows:

> Heresy is the obstinate post-baptismal denial of some truth which must be believed with divine and catholic faith, or obstinate doubt concerning the same; apostasy is the total repudiation of the Christian faith; schism is the refusal of submission to the Roman Pontiff or of communion with the members of the Church subject to him (Can.751).

In fairness to individuals who may be guilty of such aberrations in good faith, these definitions should be interpreted in the sense that essential doctrines of the Church are denied or repudiated in rejection of the authority of God revealing or the Church teaching.[230] These essential doctrines which "must be believed with divine and Catholic faith" are elaborated clearly in Canon 750. The procedure to be followed when confronted with an authentic case of possible excommunication for the crime of abortion or for heresy, apostasy or schism, is outlined in chapter III on the *Principle of the Right to Life* (cf. pp.99ff.)

A point which was omitted in speaking of excommunication in chapter III must be introduced briefly at this time. Except in danger-of-death cases, when "any priest validly and licitly absolves from any kind of censures and sins" (Can.976), the hospital chaplain's faculty to absolve from excommunication in the situations mentioned above (abortion, etc.) does not apply if the excommunication has been imposed or declared (Can.566,2). This restriction applies to all priests who serve the needs of the faithful whether in the confessional or in a non-sacramental setting. The phrase "imposed or declared" puts an excommunicated person in very bad company; he or she joins the company of those who "obstinately persist in manifest grave sin" (Can.915). In extremely rare cases, when a penalized member of the faithful (excommunicated, for example) cannot be persuaded to reform and/or make up for scandal and injustice in any other way, the penalty can be imposed or declared by either a judicial or administrative procedure (Cann.1341,1342). The Church seeks the reconciliation of the sinner, and looks upon the rare process of declaration or imposition of the penalty as a last resort. The crime of the excommunicated person thus is made public in the hopes that such an unusual action may persuade the "obstinate sinner" to repent and to make reparation for scandal and injustice, or at least to promise seriously to do so. Once this has been done to the satisfaction of the superior who imposed or declared the excommunication (cf.Can.1341), remission of the censure "cannot be denied" (Can.1358,1).

These observations bring into relief the magnitude of the challenge to the chaplain and pastoral care personnel. The call to repentance and reconciliation comes through more effectively when bitter, lapsed or reluctant Catholics are lying flat on their backs, often tormented with anxiety over a forthcoming serious surgical procedure or an unfavorable prognosis. In many cases, it is a matter of "now or never" with regard to spiritual salvation. As St. Paul wrote

---

[230] *Vatican Council II,* Austin Flannery, O.P., ed. (cf. note 51), The Decree on Ecumenism, n. 3, p. 455. Cf. also *Directory Concerning Ecumenical Matters: Part I,* n. 19, *ibid.,* p. 490. which makes it clear from the *Decree on Ecumenism* of Vatican II (n. 3) that the penalty for heresy, apostasy or schism does not apply to baptized Christians of other denominations who are received into the Catholic faith. Cf. also *CLSA Commentary* (cf. note 45), pp. 547, 548; Bouscaren-Ellis, *Canon Law* (cf. note 183), p. 895.

to Timothy, after reminding him that the "servant of the Lord . . . must be kindly toward all:"

> He must be an apt teacher, patiently and gently correcting those who contradict him, in the hope always that God will enable them to repent and to know the truth (II Timothy, 2:24,25).

Some Catholics seem unwilling or unable to understand just why the Church should have to be concerned about penalties in any form. The following quotation is presented for serious consideration:

> To those questioning the need of penalties in a community of love, one might respond that the community can ill afford to be mute and inactive in the face of significant breaches of its faith or order; otherwise its identity as a sign of God's kingdom would be seriously jeopardized. While a certain type of diversity clearly enriches the Church, it simply cannot tolerate certain divergent patterns of thought or activity if it is to be fair to its own members who joined a reasonably well-defined community and have definite expectations from it.[231]

The general rule is that, except in danger-of-death situations, the sacraments of baptism, confirmation and marriage are not administered in a hospital setting (Cann.860,2;881;1118). This does not mean that the chaplain and pastoral care personnel should not, on occasion, seek the approval of the pastor of the patient in order to participate in some of the preparatory stages of the process of preparing a child or adult for baptism, initiating instructions in the faith for a non-Catholic who has expressed interest in becoming a Catholic, etc. As to regularizing a Catholic patient's marital status, "strike while the iron is hot" may apply in many cases. Many patients are more likely to agree to a convalidation or radical sanation of their marriage during their hospital tenure (even though not in danger of death) than after their discharge from the hospital.

With such practicality in view, the bishop may either extend full pastoral status to the chaplain within the hospital boundaries, or appoint him as an associate pastor of the local parish—or these needs might be covered by particular laws or by special delegation from the bishop. To quote Canon 566,1: "A chaplain should possess all the faculties required for proper pastoral care." The chaplain must remember, however, that such convalidation activities (except in danger-of-death situations) would entail all of the paperwork and

---

[231]*Ibid. (CLSA Commentary)*, p. 894.

legwork encountered in a convalidation, sanation, etc., in a parish setting. In many if not most cases, it might be more practical and prudential to put the patient in touch with his or her pastor, and offer to assist in any preliminary work while the patient is in the hospital. If there is evidence of a possible annulment of an existing marriage, the chaplain might offer to help the patient with the preliminary application questionnaire (used in many dioceses) while in the hospital. The initiation or restoration of a good pastor-chaplain relationship by deferring convalidation proposals to a parish setting could be a prime dividend of the patient's hospitalization. That feature should be taken into consideration.

If the chaplain does baptize an adult or receives one already baptized into full communion with the Catholic Church, he may also administer the sacrament of confirmation (Can.883,2).[232] This also applies to danger-of-death cases. He may baptize a child only "in case of necessity or some other compelling pastoral reason," unless otherwise permitted by the bishop (Can.860,2). The question of such infant baptisms in danger-of-death cases was discussed at length in the previous chapter. It remains to discuss sacramental ministrations to adults and to children beyond the infant category—and always with regard for the Principle of Religious Freedom.

1) Few Restrictions in "Special Need" Situations

The law of the Church is especially generous in facilitating the reconciliation of the patient with God. In the standard general hospital, many patients are not in danger of death. Hence the even-more-generous concessions for danger-of-death cases (to be discussed presently) would not apply to those patients. If a parish priest who is "making the rounds" of his parishioners in the hospital found out that one of them was under an excommunication (a women who had an abortion, for example), the general rule is that such a person may not receive the sacraments (Can.1331,1) without submitting to the canonical procedures for absolution from the crime of abortion as outlined in the previous chapter. The priest can justify the administration of the sacraments to such a patient, however, if he motivates that person to find it hard to "remain in a state of serious sin during the time necessary for the competent superior to provide" (that is, to complete the canonical requirements for absolution from abortion). Canon 1357 allows this consoling turn of events (but for the internal sacramental forum only) provided that the

---

[232]*Ibid.,* commentary on Canon 883, p. 636, explains why this faculty to administer confirmation cannot apply to a person "baptized Catholic who has simply never been catechized or admitted to the other sacraments."

excommunication has not been made public knowledge by a formal declaration (a rare situation).

In attending to the recourse procedure (Can.1357,2) in the course of sacramental confession, the excommunicated person might present valid reasons to explain just why it might be morally impossible for the penitent to return to that same confessor later in the confessional to receive the instructions ("mandata") of the recourse-person. If the reasons are considered valid on the basis of "no one is obligated to do the impossible," there would be no point in insisting on the need of recourse. In that event, the confessor's role in imposing "an appropriate penance and the reparation of any scandal or damage to the extent that it is imperative" (Can.1357,2) is of special importance. If the penitent were to manifest an unwillingness to accept such a penance and reparation measures with an attitude of obstinacy and contempt for authority (known as "contumacy"), it should be interpreted as an indication that the penitent would fall back into the censure of excommunication. A sincere manifestation of willingness to accept such a penance and reparation responsibilities is an absolute or "sine qua non" condition for the remission of the censure.[233] As noted previously, however (cf. pp.99ff.), the priest should be sure that the excommunication actually was incurred.

2) Even Less Restrictions in "Danger of Death" Situations

The following canon applies in *danger-of-death* cases (cf.footnote 183) for the full duration of the danger:

> Any priest, even though he lacks the faculty to hear confessions, can validly and licitly absolve penitents who are in danger of death, from any censures and sins, even if an approved priest is present (Can.976).

If, however, the penitent is under a censure (excommunication, for example) which has been "imposed or declared," or under a censure which is reserved to the Holy See, the penitent is still bound by the obligation to have recourse to the diocesan bishop or his representative after recovery from the illness.[234]

---

[233]*Ibid.*, commentary on canon 1357, p. 918.

[234]*Ibid. (CLSA Commentary)*, commentary on Canon 1357,3, pp. 917, 918. Besides the two excommunications previously discussed (for abortion and heresy, schism and apostasy), there are 4 censures as interdicts which are "latae sententiae" and could possibly be encountered in hospital ministrations: physical attack on a bishop (Can. 1370,2), pretended celebration of the Eucharist or absolution by one who is not a priest (Can. 1378,2), falsely accusing a confessor of solicitation (Can. 1390,1) and a religious (non-cleric) in perpetual vows who attempts a civil marriage (Can. 1394,2). If a cleric is the perpetrator in any of these situations, he is also suspended.

It seems appropriate to follow the opinions of pre-Vatican II authors, however, who would leave it up to the prudential judgment of the confessor to determine whether or not the danger-of-death patient (censure imposed or declared) should be reminded of the obligation. As one of the reasons for *not* reminding the penitent of that obligation, Father Felix Cappello, S.J. mentions "the very great indulgence of Mother Church towards the infirm." [235]

If the penitent is reminded of the obligation of recourse, the time element (30 days) should be given a benign interpretation. Some would extend this to a generous 30 days *after recovery.* [236] A caring confessor will offer his good services in making the recourse in the name of the penitent. Since the censure is, in a sense, public knowledge (imposed or declared), there would be no need to use fictitious names in making recourse. It is interesting to note that the reason why patients in danger of death may receive the sacraments is not because the prohibiting penalty is *remitted*—it is merely *suspended* (Can.1352,1). [237] The patient still must have the penalty remitted if he or she survives the life-threatening situation. Thanks to the Church's deep concern for all sinners who face the spectre of death in any way, however, the penalty can be remitted by virtue of Canon 976 above. Outside of danger-of-death situations, the "special need" canon can be used as noted above. The Church does tailor her laws to fit human needs.

Another indication of the Church's deep concern for the spiritual welfare of the sick and the infirm is found in making consoling "death bed" convalidations of marriage possible and convenient—as well as the marriages of careless Catholics who recover from their stay in the hospital and are challenged to "turn over a new leaf," giving witness to the sacramental beauty of marriage. The generous canon reads as follows:

> In danger of death, if other proofs are not available, it suffices, unless there are contrary indications, to have the assertion of the parties, sworn if need be, that they are baptized and free from any impediment (Can.1068).

Both parties must affirm that at least one of them was baptized, and both must affirm that they are free of impediments or other possible invalidating factors. Naturally this canon could not apply if it is known that the couple had been living together and that one of them was bound by a former and still existing marriage bond (both conditions required). Likewise, if despite the danger of death, there is time to obtain certificates of baptism and proof of

---

[235] *Tractatus Canonico-Moralis De Censuris* (cf. note 184), n. 116.
[236] Cappello, Felix, S.J., *Ibid.*, n. 115, 7.
[237] *CLSA Commentary* (cf. note 45), p. 915.

freedom to marry, those inquiries should be pursued as far as possible. If the diocesan bishop is not considered to be accessible (Can.1079,4), the pastor or attending priest can dispense "from the form to be observed in the celebration of marriage, and from each and every impediment of ecclesiastical law, whether public or occult, with the exception of the impediment arising from the sacred order of the priesthood "(Can.1079,1 and 2).

Naturally this canon is not operative beyond impediments of the ecclesiastical law. If the marriage is invalid because of an impediment of the *natural* law (for example, impotence) or because of an impediment of the divine positive law (for example, existing bond of a previous valid marriage), the marriage cannot be convalidated. Likewise, in the case of a mixed marriage, every effort must be made to secure the pledge of the Catholic party with regard to removing any dangers of falling away from the faith, and "to do all in his or her power to have all the children baptized and brought up in the Catholic Church" (Cann.1125,1126). Considering that one of the parties may be seriously ill or dying, it may happen in some cases that there is just no time to attend to this matter of protecting the faith of parent and offspring (in truth, "future offspring"). If this is overlooked in rare cases either because it is morally impossible (lack of time, patient terminal, etc.) or because it was simply forgotten, the dispensation nevertheless would be valid.[238]

If there are *occult* impediments (for example, the impediment of consanguinity based on unknown, illicit sexual union), the confessor can dispense from them in the *internal* forum (Can.1079,3). There is no need to inform the bishop of such *occult* dispensations. As to the *public* impediments (which can be proved in the external forum), the priest may also dispense from them if recourse to the bishop is impossible.[239] Soon thereafter, however, he is obligated to inform the bishop of such *external* forum dispensations (Can.1081). The bedside ceremony of convalidation can be very brief. Family members or hospital personnel (or other patients) can serve as witnesses. In the unlikely situation when witnesses simply are not available, and the ceremony could not be delayed due to pressing circumstances (death imminent, etc.), it is safe

---

[238]Bouscaren-Ellis, *Canon Law* (cf. note 183) state that if there is no time to attend to the "cautiones," the dispensation nevertheless would be valid "because no purely ecclesiastical law binds in such extreme necessity;" p. 440, n. 7. Cf. also A Coronata, P. Matthaeus Conte, O.F.M. Cap., *Institutiones Juris Canonici, De Sacramentis,* III (Rome, Italy: Marietti, 1946), p. 164 and note 8.

[239]Canon 1079,4. Even though contact with the chancery office is not required in such cases, it often is advisable to make contact by phone or personal visit in difficult and doubtful cases. In order to respect confidentiality, however, fictional names should be used.

to say that the exchange of consent would be valid without witnesses.[240] The priest is also required to attend to Canons 1121 to 1123 relative to the notification and registration of such convalidations.

4.2 MARITAL-STATUS PROCEDURES BEYOND SIMPLE CONVALIDATION (In Danger-of-Death Situations)

The procedure mentioned above refers to simple convalidation—when a marriage is invalid due to some impediment, or to defect of consent or defect of form. The justifying reason for the use of such a generous *danger-of-death* faculty was stated in the former code of canon law as "for peace of conscience and, if warranted, the legitimation of children." Such sentiments may be considered as expressive of the spirit of the present Code of Canon Law as well. For the same reasons, other canonical solutions are possible when a simple validation is out of the question. If the marriage cannot be convalidated (for example, the impediment of impotence or existence of a prior valid marriage bond), and the parties cannot separate for valid reasons (serious illness of one party, children need parental care, etc.), peace of conscience might be provided if both parties make a sincere promise to live as brother and sister.

The brother-and-sister solution is possible only if several conditions are verified: (1) It is the only practical solution available; (2) Continued cohabitation will not occasion grave scandal; (3) The age and motivation of the parties is such that effective means can be taken to change the danger of continued cohabitation into a *remote* occasion of sin (for example, use of separate bedrooms, daily prayer, presence of relatives in the home, etc.). If it is publicly known that the marriage is invalid and that it cannot be validated, the verification of condition No. (2) (absence of grave scandal) would be most difficult and doubtful. In such cases, the proper solution would be to refer the case to the diocesan bishop or his delegate and to motivate the couple to abide by the bishop's decision.[241]

Another possible solution in danger-of-death cases would be to consider a radical sanation of the invalid marriage (also known as "retroactive validation"). In the former code of canon law, only the Apostolic See could grant a

---

[240]*CLSA Commentary* (cf. note 45), p. 762 (Can. 1079).

[241]Mathis, Marcian J., O.F.M., and Meyer, Nicholas W., O.F.M., *The Pastoral Companion*, 12th ed. (Chicago, Ill.: Franciscan Herald Press, 1961), pp. 301–304.

radical sanation. The present code (Can.1165,2) reads as follows:

> [A radical sanation] can be granted by the diocesan bishop in individual cases, even if a number of reasons for nullity occur together in the same marriage, assuming that for the sanation of a mixed marriage, the conditions stated in canon 1125 will have been fulfilled; it cannot be granted, however, if there is an impediment whose dispensation is reserved to the Apostolic See in accordance with canon 1078,2, or if there is question of an impediment of the natural law or of the divine positive law which has now ceased.

Canon 1078,2, refers to the impediment arising from sacred orders or from a public perpetual vow of chastity in a religious institute of pontifical rite, and to the impediment of crime (Can.1090).

As an example, the patient may be in an invalid marriage because she is a Catholic but was married before a justice of the peace. The non-Catholic husband refuses to renew consent: "it will be an admission that I was never married in the first place. Once is enough." By granting a radical sanation, the bishop would be dispensing from the need of renewing consent. By a fiction of law, the marriage would be considered as having been valid from the beginning (Can.1161,1 and 2). It would also render legitimate the children born as of the date of their mutual consent before the justice of the peace, as well as children born before that date (Can.1139) provided that there was no impediment to the marriage at some time from the conception to the birth of such children.[242]

The conditions which must be verified before a radical sanation can be considered are the following: (1) There must be a serious reason such as the refusal of one party to renew consent (as above), or the invalidity is known to only one of the parties who is concerned about the serious inconvenience or harmful effects to telling the other party about the invalidity, or because the invalidity was due to the ignorance or neglect of others (for example, the pastor neglected to obtain a dispensation from disparity of cult);[243] (2) The case does not involve any of the impediments as excluded in Canon 1165,2, as stated above; (3) It must be probable that the parties intend to persevere in conjugal life (Can.1161,3). If consent was wanting on the part of either hus-

---

[242]A Coronata, P. Mattheus Conte, O.F.M. Cap., *Institutiones Juris Canonici, De Sacramentis,* III (cf. note 238), n. 609. Cf. also Mathis-Meyer, *Ibid.,* p. 297.

[243]As Canon 1164 indicates, a sanation can be granted even if both parties are unaware of the invalidity. Such would be the case if the pastor neglected to apply for an essential dispensation.

band or wife from the beginning (for example, at the time of the justice-of-peace ceremony as above) but was given later, validation can be granted from the moment when consent was given (Can.1162,2). In addition, if it is a mixed marriage or a disparity-of-cult marriage, the chaplain must seek assurances from the Catholic party that every effort will be made to have future children baptized and reared in the Catholic faith. If possible, the same assurance should be obtained with regard to children already born of the union.

The form for applying for a radical sanation is obtained from the chancery office. The convalidation takes place as of the moment when it is signed by the bishop (unless otherwise indicated, cf.Can.1161,2). The chaplain should inform the proper pastor of the convalidation so that proper notations can be made in the registers of marriage and of baptism (Can.1123).

4.3   ADMINISTRATION OF THE SACRAMENTS OF PENANCE AND OF THE EUCHARIST

The danger of encroaching upon a patient's religious freedom would appear to be more likely with regard to the sacraments of penance and Holy Communion. Two factors may explain a Catholic patient's reluctance to receive Holy Communion: the desire to "go to confession," and the failure to mention that desire because of the lack of privacy for hearing confessions. Screens and curtains provide visual privacy, but cannot allay the uneasy feeling of being heard by a roommate or by ward-mates. In such situations the patient can be advised to acknowledge his or her sinfulness in general and reserve the specific sins and significant details for a future confession. This affords slight comfort, however, to the devout souls who prefer to "tell all." Most patients can be transferred to a wheel chair and taken to a small alcove or conference room for private confession. In planning hospital and health-facility construction, the architect should be instructed to provide for such a small "sacramental-confession facility" on each floor. This significant need has been overlooked in the past.

Although other members of the pastoral care team such as deacons, sisters, brothers or laity, cannot give absolution, they can dispose a patient to want to see a priest, and thus become ministers of reconciliation in situations where anti-Church or anti-clerical sentiments do surface. Patients who are unwilling to confess to a priest may reveal some of their violations of the commandments spontaneously in the course of pastoral visits by pastoral care personnel. They can be assisted in making an act of contrition (preferably an act of perfect contrition) and other pleas for forgiveness such as the "Our Father." Such an act of recommending a patient to the mercy of God can be a source of internal peace.[244] It does not, however, substitute for sacramental confession.

> *Directive 40:* In wards and semi-private rooms, every effort should be made to provide sufficient privacy for confession.

---

1) Administration of the Sacrament of the Eucharist

The Sacrifice of the Mass, "the summit and source of all worship and Christian life," is a powerful means of bringing about the unity which is signified by the Eucharist. Unfortunately, hospital patients often are not able to attend Mass, and the reception of the Eucharist must be conducted as a separate ministration. Some Catholic hospitals have overcome this anomaly in part by broadcasting the Mass to the hospital rooms by closed circuit T.V., and by distributing the Eucharist to the patients in their rooms soon thereafter. If this cannot be done, the pastoral care team should establish a meaningful ritual which involves more than the hasty "in and out" practice of distributing the Eucharist. The Revised Roman Ritual (1983) entitled *Pastoral Care of the Sick, Rites of Anointing and Viaticum,* should be consulted. The comforting prayer "Deliver us, Lord, from every evil . . ." which follows the "Our Father" at Mass could be included. Another excellent suggestion is found in the 1982 publication entitled *Ministry to the Sick* which was written by a hospital chaplain and a registered nurse:

> Another custom is to distribute Communion in the evening after visiting hours are over. The chaplain assists the patients in their preparation with night prayers over the loudspeaker. In concluding the prayers the chaplain reminds the patients who plan to receive our Lord to make their own private preparation.[245]

Except for those who are in danger of death and receive Viaticum (Can.921), the general rule is that the Eucharist is to be received only once each day unless a patient participates in the Sacrifice of the Mass that same day (Can.917). Abstinence from all food and drink except water and medi-

---

[244]Ashley-O'Rourke, *Health Care Ethics* (cf. note 80), p. 406, emphasize the role of non-ordained personnel as ministers of reconciliation.

[245]Niklas, Gerald R. and Stefanics, Charlotte, R,N, *Ministry to the Sick* (New York, N.Y.: Alba House, 1982), p. 35.

cine (whether liquid or solid) is required for one hour before receiving the Eucharist. An exception is made for the elderly and for those who are suffering from some illness (Can.919,3). The words "elderly" and "illness" are to be interpreted broadly. Not only are such patients not bound by any Eucharistic fast and abstinence, but the concession applies also to those who care for the sick or elderly when they are actually caring for such individuals at the time they receive Holy Communion. This can include also visitors and family members (provided that they are Catholics, and properly disposed) who are present at Communion time inasmuch as they are providing moral and emotional support.[246]

As to the "properly disposed" requirement, it could happen that a newly-admitted patient who is in a state of serious sin insists upon receiving the Eucharist. If the chaplain is away and no other priest is available, and if there is a serious reason for such a request (for example, the patient is scheduled for serious surgery the next morning), he or she may receive the Eucharist after having made an act of perfect contrition, "which includes the resolve to go to confession as soon as possible" (Can.916). Children should not be given the Eucharist unless they have been adequately prepared (Can.913). As a general rule, this would exclude children who have not made their First Holy Communion. Children who are in danger of death, however, may receive the Eucharist provided that they can distinguish the Body of Christ from ordinary food and that they are disposed to receive the Eucharist reverently (Can.913,2).

2) Precautions Required to Avoid Irreverence

The proviso "that there be no danger of irreverence" must be added to all of the situations to be mentioned here and in the following paragraphs. The Eucharist should not be given to a mentally incompetent person who never had the use of reason, nor to a person who had become mentally incompetent after having received the use of reason. If such patients have intervals when they truly are lucid (conscious and able to understand what is being done for them), they may be given the Eucharist *at such times*. In the latter case (mentally incompetent who once had the use of reason), if there are indications that such individuals previously (when competent) had desired the Eucharist at least implicitly and had never revoked that desire, they may be given the Eucharist *when in danger of death* provided that they are, in all proba-

---

[246]*CLSA Commentary* (cf. note 45), p. 655.

bility, in the state of grace.[247] Those who are profoundly mentally retarded from birth, and those who have become mentally incompetent as a result of old age, may be given the Eucharist several times each year (especially during the Easter season and when in danger of death) provided that they are able to distinguish the Eucharist from ordinary food.[248]

A wise precaution in all situations when it is logical that a danger of irreverence might be present, is to give the patient a fragment of an unconsecrated wafer or a small piece of bread—explaining discreetly that this is "just a test." This is recommended especially in giving the Eucharist to patients who are victims of protracted coughing or vomiting spells. If their stomachs can tolerate the unconsecrated fragment, it should be safe to administer the Eucharist. In cases of *intermittent* coughing, once the Sacred Host has been swallowed, there is but little reason to fear that It will be expelled with the phlegm—which comes not from the stomach but from the trachea.[249] In all cases of coughing and vomiting, the physician is best qualified to assess the danger of expelling the Sacred Host.

Some authors infer that a Catholic patient who is unconscious could be given the Eucharist. This could apply if the patient has true lucid intervals or is in a semi-conscious state (but dimly realizes what is being done) and is otherwise properly disposed. If the person is completely unconscious, however, administering the Eucharist is not only unnecessary (can be deferred until later), but it could involve irreverence to the Blessed Eucharist.[250] The same should apply if the patient is delirious. What if an unconscious patient is brought to the hospital who had fallen into the unconscious state in the very act of committing a serious sin (robbery, rape, etc., and rendered unconscious by police action), or is known as a notorious sinner (professional prostitute, living in open concubinage, etc.). Such an individual may be given conditional absolution and conditional anointing of the sick based on even a slight or doubtful probability of repentance before becoming unconscious.

---

[247]Cappello, Felix M., S.J., *De Sacramentis,* I, 4th ed. (Rome, Italy: Marietti, 1945), n. 402. Cf. also Jone, Heribert, O.F.M. Cap., *Moral Theology* (cf. note 151), n. 501.

[248]Dr. Albert Niedermeyer, MD, Ph.D., *Compendium of Pastoral Medicine* (cf. note 89), describes this "mental weakness" category as follows: "In complete idiocy, there exists from birth an extreme mental inferiority. Speech is deficient or very imperfectly developed; . . . They neither learn to read nor write. Their vitality is often surprisingly intense: indomitable gluttony and sexual appetite (many times, excessive ipsation). In imbecility we encounter a mental weakness which is mostly congenital: deficient capacity of judgment and lack of the higher ethical ideas. Debility passes over little by little into common stupidity (weak intelligence);" p. 329.

[249]Davis, Henry, S.J., *Moral and Pastoral Theology,* 4 vols., III, 4th ed. (New York, N.Y.: Sheed and Ward, 1943), p. 205.

[250]Merkelbach, Benedict Henry, O.P., Summa Theologiae Moralis, 3 vols., III (Paris, France: Desclee de Brouwer, 1936), n. 277,1.

Even after regaining consciousness, such an individual could not be given the Eucharist unless he or she had given a fairly certain ("satis certum") sign of repentance.[251]

It bears repeating that the Eucharist is to be denied to those who are under an excommunication or interdict which has been imposed or declared. They are included among those who "obstinately persist in manifest grave sin" (Can.915). If such a person repents, however, and at least promises to make due reparation for damage and scandal (Can.1347,2), the Eucharist can be administered (Can.1358).

Patients who find it difficult to swallow should be given a small fragment of the consecrated Host and a sip or two of water to facilitate the process. Seriously ill patients who can take no food at all except through what is known as a Levine tube may be given a small fragment of the Host or even a small amount of the consecrated Wine. To avoid spilling the Sacred Species due to needless "manipulations," the wine should be consecrated in a special container which has a pointed spout; a purificator should be placed at the mouth of the tube as the Wine is poured carefully into the tube. A small amount of water should be given through the tube (ablution from the small container) so as to cleanse the tube of any vestiges of the Sacred Species.[252] A physician or nurse can best advise as to the opportune time to administer Communion via the tube.

Hospital regulations with regard to patients who are in isolation (mask precautions), or in an oxygen tent, or on a "nothing by mouth" regimen should be checked before making contact with the patients regarding the reception of the Eucharist. Since the divine presence remains as along as the appearance of bread has not disintegrated, this factor must be considered before giving the Eucharist to dying patients, victims of persistent coughing or vomiting, etc. Authors differ in their estimates of the dissolution rate— from non-existent (Host dissolved while in the mouth), to a minimum of one-half hour and a maximum of several hours or more (for victims of high fever illnesses).[253]

---

[251]Cappello, Felix M., S.J., *De Sacramentis,* I (cf. note 247), n. 407,2.

[252]On Dec. 12, 1959, in a private response, the Holy Office granted permission to a person who had a severe allergy to wheat, to receive Holy Communion in the oriental rite under the Species of Wine only. Cf. *Canon Law Digest,* V (Milwaukee, Wis.: Bruce Publishing Co., 1963), p. 434, and also *Canon Law Digest,* VI (Milwaukee, Wis.: Bruce Publishing Co., 1969), pp. 562–565 for several other private responses. Canon 925 of the present code of canon law states expressly that Holy Communion may be given "even under the form of wine alone in case of necessity." Cf. *CLA Commentary* (cf. note 45), pp. 658, 659.

[253]For a summary of such opinions, cf. Cappello, Felix M., S.J., *De Sacramentis,* I (cf. note 247), nn. 360, 361.

In a study published by a physician and a priest in 1955, the gastric juices of 50 fasting individuals (ages 26 to 81) were aspirated from the stomach by means of a Levine tube and then mixed with salivated fragments of unconsecrated communion wafers. In only 9 of the cases did the time required for the wafer to become unrecognizable ("corrupt" but not completely dissolved) exceed 10 minutes. The longest period was 21 minutes. The conclusions of the authors of this testing included the following: except in most unusual circumstances, there is no basis for undue concern about the desecration of the Host when an autopsy is performed on a recent communicant; the Eucharist should not be administered to victims of uncontrollable vomiting; a patient who requires nasogastric suction may receive the Eucharist if the suctioning can be interrupted for a period of 20 to 30 minutes after the reception of the Eucharist.[254]

If it should happen that the Sacred Host is ejected through vomiting or nasogastric suction, whatever remains of the Host should be picked up reverently, placed in a clean cloth, and given to the chaplain. Nurses and doctors should be instructed accordingly. The chaplain will put that Fragment (those Fragments) into an ablution cup. After complete dissolution, that water is to be poured down the sacrarium. In all cases, the freedom of the patient must be respected if he or she indicates an unwillingness or refusal to receive the Eucharist.

Directive 38: It is the mind of the Church that the sick should have the widest possible liberty to receive the sacraments frequently. The generous cooperation of the entire staff and personnel is requested for this purpose.

Directive 39: While providing the sick abundant opportunity to receive Holy Communion, there should be no interference with the freedom of the faithful to communicate or not to communicate.

---

3) Administration of the Eucharist as Viaticum

There are two situations when the reception of the Eucharist is emphasized as a definite and specific obligation: from First Communion Day

---

[254]"Medical Aspects of the Holy Eucharist," by Eugene G. LaForet, MD, and Rev. Thomas F. Casey, *Linacre Quarterly,* Feb., 1955, pp. 11–16.

onward, every Catholic is obligated to receive Holy Communion at least once a year, preferably during the Easter season (Can.920); and all baptized Christians who are able to receive Communion "are bound by reason of the precept to receive Communion when in danger of death from any cause."[255] The former (Easter duty) is critical in the passage through this life; the latter (Viaticum) is critical in the passage from this life. The *Revised Roman Ritual* recommends that Viaticum (which literally means "with you on the journey") be received within Mass "so that the sick person may receive Communion under both kinds." Another recommendation is that the profession of faith be included in the celebration of Viaticum.[256] Circumstances may limit the application of the first recommendation to rare cases; the second recommendation should be warranted frequently. A third recommendation, that Viaticum be administered while the patient is fully conscious, can be observed in most cases with proper planning and foresight (Can.922). The patient who is in danger of death may receive Viaticum even though he or she may have received Holy Communion that same day (Can.921,2).

The chaplain is the ordinary minister of Viaticum if he is available. In case of necessity, any other priest may substitute for him (with at least the presumed permission of the chaplain). If the proper pastor of the patient or his associate pastors are available, they also rate as ordinary ministers of Viaticum. The same applies to the superior of a clerical religious institute for members of his jurisdiction. If no priest is available, Viaticum may be administered by a deacon or by any member of the laity (man or woman) who has been duly appointed for the distribution of Holy Communion. The slight difference in the administration of Viaticum if done by a lay person is indicated in the *Revised Roman Ritual.*[257] The scenario thus far applies usually to a becalmed and treated patient lying in an assigned room. What about the emergency cases?

When patients are brought to the hospital in proximate danger of death as in cases of stroke, accident victims, etc., the emergency room, intensive care unit or coronary care unit are scenes of orderly confusion. If the patient is conscious, he or she usually is disoriented by sentiments of anxiety, helplessness, isolation, varying degrees of anger, etc. It is a debilitating challenge to body and soul to fall into the frenzied hands of physicians, nurses, technicians, etc. The imperative of the moment is to bring the patient to a semblance of physical and psychological equilibrium through medical

---

[255]*Pastoral Care of the Sick, Rites of Anointing and Viaticum,* Revised Roman Ritual (New York, N.Y.: Catholic Book Publishing Co., 1983), n. 27. Cf. also Canon 921.

[256]*Ibid.,* nn. 26 and 28.

[257]*Ibid.,* n. 29.

ministrations. This affords but slight entry for the chaplain except for sooth-
ing words of comfort and reassurance and, at the opportune moment, the
quick administration of conditional absolution, the conditional anointing of
the sick (forehead only) and the recitation of the apostolic blessing. Later,
when the patient has been calmed, treated, tidied and tucked in, the continuous rite of penance, anointing and the Eucharist as Viaticum can be administered as a single celebration.

If death is imminent, there may be time only for sacramental confession
(even if only in generic form), the administration of Viaticum and, if there is
time, also the anointing. If the patient is unable to receive Holy Communion,
the anointing of the sick should not be omitted. If the patient has not been
confirmed, and if time allows, the sacrament of confirmation should follow.
The chaplain is empowered to administer the sacrament of confirmation in
danger-of-death situations (Can.566). Pastors, associate pastors and assistant
priests are among those who also enjoy the faculty to confirm in these circumstances. The faculty definitely is denied to a priest who is under censure or
under a canonical penalty.[258]

As noted earlier in this chapter, the Eucharist is not to be given to those
who "obstinately presist in manifest grave sin." Canon 915 extends this obsti-
nancy status to the extremely rare cases of individuals who have been excommunicated or interdicted by a formal public declaration or imposition
(cf.Can.1341). This presents a formidable challenge to the chaplain and pastoral care personnel to probe discreetly for the cause of such obstinacy, and to
persuade such individuals to appreciate God's love and mercy with a view to
some sign of repentance. As mentioned previously, even doubtful and slight
signs of repentance (for example, accepting the priest's blessing) would justify
conditional absolution and conditional anointing. Only more certain signs of
repentance, however (for example, accepting and holding the crucifix, asking
for prayers, etc.) would justify the administration of Viaticum if there is no
danger of irreverence. The *Revised Roman Ritual* recommends praying for
them, and asking God to forgive their sins. While there is life, there is hope.
The power of prayer is greater than the power of persuasion.

The circumstances under which Catholics of the Latin Rite might receive
the sacraments of penance, anointing and Viaticum from priests of the Eastern or Oriental Rite (those in union with the Church), and under which non-
Catholics may sometimes receive these sacraments from a Catholic priest
were discussed at length in chapter two (2.2).

---

[258]*Ibid.*, n. 31.

> *Directive 41a:* All baptized Christians who can receive Communion are bound to receive Viaticum. Those in danger of death from any cause are obliged to receive Communion. The administration of this sacrament is not to be delayed, for the faithful are to be nourished by it while in full possession of their faculties.
>
> *Directive 41b:* For special cases, when sudden illness or some other cause has unexpectedly placed one of the faithful in danger of death, the continuous rite should be used by which the sick person may be given the sacraments of penance, anointing, and Eucharist as Viaticum in one service.

4.4 ADMINISTRATION OF THE SACRAMENT OF THE ANOINTING OF THE SICK

The anointing of the sick emphasizes a dual aspect of the mission of healing. The *Revised Roman Ritual* quotes the Council of Trent as follows:

A return to physical health may follow the reception of this sacrament if it will be beneficial to the sick person's salvation. If necessary, the sacrament also provides the sick person with the forgiveness of sins and the completion of christian penance.[259]

The sacrament is designed for those who have reached the use of reason and who begin to be in danger of death due to sickness or old age (Can.1004,1), and who request it at least implicitly while still in control of their faculties (Can.1006). This includes children "if they have sufficient use of reason to be strengthened by this sacrament."[260] In case of doubt as to the use of reason, and the degree of sickness or as to whether the person is living or dead, the sacrament nevertheless is to be administered (Can.1005). In case of necessity, a single anointing "on the forehead, or even on another part of the body" is sufficient while the full formula is recited. For a serious reason (for example, to avoid contagion, or the inability to get near to the victim at the site of an accident) an instrument may be used for the anointing (Can.1000). In one case (automobile hit by a freight train), the body of the

---

[259]*Ibid.*, n. 6.
[260]*Ibid.*, n. 12. Cf.

dying victim was on fire. It was impossible to extricate him from the front seat. The priest managed to anoint the victim by attaching a wad of cotton to a long stick. The sacrament can be repeated "whenever the sick person again falls into a serious sickness after convalescence or whenever a more serious crisis develops during the same sickness" (Can.1004,2). The sacrament is not to be administered to a sick person who obstinately persists in a "manifestly grave sin" (Can.1007).

The *Revised Roman Ritual* adds a few more directives: the sacrament may be administered before surgery "whenever a serious illness is the reason for the surgery;" elderly people may be anointed "if they have become notably weakened even though no serious illness is present; "the sacrament is to be administered" as soon as the right time comes"—delaying the reception of this sacrament is a "wrongful practice;" those who lack consciousness or the use of reason may be anointed if, as Christian believers, they "would . . . probably have asked for it were they in control of their faculties;" the sacrament is not to be administered to those who are dead, but may be given conditionally ("if you are living") if the priest is doubtful about the fact of death.[261]

Directive 41: Special care and concern should be shown that those who are seriously ill or are dangerously ill due to sickness or old age receive the Sacrament of Anointing. A prudent but probable judgment about the seriousness of the sickness is sufficient. If necessary a doctor may be consulted, although there should be no reason for scruples.

A sick person should be anointed before surgery whenever a dangerous illness is the reason for the surgery. Old people may be anointed if they are in weak condition although no dangerous illness is present. Sick children may be anointed if they have sufficient use of reason to be comforted by this sacrament.

The sacrament may be repeated if the sick person recovers after anointing, or, during the same illness, the danger becomes more serious.

Normally the sacrament is celebrated when the sick person

---

[261]*Ibid.*, nn. 10–15. Cf. also Canon 1005.

> is fully conscious. It may be conferred upon the sick who
> have lost consciousness or the use of reason, if, as Christian
> believers, they would have asked for it if they were in control
> of their faculties.

4.5   MINISTERING TO THE SPIRITUAL NEEDS OF NON-CATHOLIC PATIENTS

Due to the fact that discussion of the baptism of non-Catholics and of sacramental intercommunion with non-Catholics was included in chapter II on the Principle of Human Dignity (2.1 and 2.2), this section of chapter IV may be judged by the reader as remarkably brief. The problem with principles is that they overlap at times. This applies also to discussions of various aspects of the same principle. The aspect of respecting the religious beliefs of non-Catholics (the following section 4.6), for example, also refers to "ministering to the spiritual needs of non-Catholic patients" (4.5,above). It is a special topic, however, which calls for a separate discussion.

One remaining aspect of the application of the *Principle of Religious Freedom* which relates to the ministering to the spiritual needs of non-Catholic patients is the impropriety of efforts to "make converts" of adult non-Catholic patients during their stay in a Catholic hospital. Non-Catholic patients should be made to feel that their stay in a Catholic hospital will in no way expose them to the enticements of proselytism. They should be invited to express their religious affiliation or preference when registering so that their pastors or preferred ministers can be informed of their presence in the hospital. Non-Catholic pastors and ministers must be assured that the facilities of the hospital are at their disposal for any spiritual or sacramental ministrations. As mentioned in the chapter on the Principle of Human Dignity, such patients should be accommodated if they express an interest in having the chaplain or pastoral care personnel pray with them, read Bible passages, etc.

If a non-Catholic patient who is affiliated with some religious denomination voluntarily expresses an interest in hearing more about the Catholic faith with a view to becoming a Catholic, a distinction is in order. If a patient who is in danger of death and who had never received valid baptism manifests in any way ("quovis modo") an intention of receiving baptism and has "some knowledge of the principal truths of the faith . . . and promises to observe the requirements of the christian religion," he or she may be baptized (Can.865.2). In such situations it is assumed that any serious marital problems can be solved (for example, convalidating the marriage, promise to live as brother and sister if warranted, etc.). If the patient is not in danger of death, the proper approach would be to encourage that person to seek the "fullness of the faith," and put him or her in touch with the priest of his or her area of residence.

Father Karl Rahner's opinion with regard to ecumenical aspects of convert work is worthy of respectful consideration. Referring to Vatican II's *Decree on Ecumenism* (art.4) to the effect that both individual conversions and ecumenism "proceed from the wondrous providence of God," he states that the ecumenical efforts of Catholics "must take care not to aim at individual conversions to the Catholic Church, for this would bring that work into disrepute and make it impossible."[262] He admits that an individual who wishes to become a Catholic on genuinely religious grounds "must be afforded most attentive pastoral care," but he infers it would not be a case of interest on genuinely religious grounds if the non-Catholic prospect is motivated by a "purely negative attitude of protest" against his or her own religious denomination, or by a strong impression that everything is just perfect in Catholic parish life.[263] It does happen only too often that an ill-advised or improperly-motivated conversion ends in the abandonment of the Catholic faith or of all faith in God. The danger of "disrepute" in convert work enters an even more delicate area if the interested individual is a member of the Eastern Orthodox Church (2.2). This caution is not required, however, with regard to the Catholic approach to the vast field of fallen-away Catholics and of individuals with no religious affiliation at all.

> *Directive 42:* Personnel of a Catholic health facility should make every effort to satisfy the spiritual needs and desires of non-Catholics. Therefore, in hospitals and similar institutions conducted by Catholics, the authorities in charge should, with the consent of the patient, promptly advise ministers of other communions of the presence of their communicants and afford them every facility for visiting the sick and giving them spiritual and sacramental ministrations.

---

[262]Found in *Sacramentum Mundi*, 6 vols., II (New York, N.Y.: Herder and Herder, 1968), article on "conversion," p. 7.
[263]*Ibid.*, p. 7.

4.6 RESPECT FOR PERSONAL BELIEFS

Human freedom, while neither merely negative nor fully positive, does have a negative and a positive element. The former, which might be called "freedom from," or immunity from coercion, has been discussed above. The latter (the positive element) might be called "freedom for," or freedom to give external expression to inner beliefs and convictions. It could be called the core of human freedom, since it denotes a definite but limited self dominion. The first amendment to the American constitution reflects this dual relationship: "Congress shall make no law respecting an establishment of religion, or prohibiting the free exercise thereof." The positive element ("freedom for") is not absolute, except as it applies to the overriding dominium of Almighty God. As stated in Vatican II's Declaration on Religious Liberty (quotation, beginning of this chapter) this positive right and responsibility is limited by the moral obligation to seek the truth, especially religious truth, and to order their whole lives in accord with the demands of truth. Hence the exercise of this aspect of human freedom is qualified by the phrase "within due limits."

Religious freedom vindicates the right of the individual to externalize interior convictions in religious matters both in private and in public. Any deliberate failure on the part of others to recognize and respect such manifestations of internal belief amounts to restraint upon the individual. The same Declaration on Religious Liberty of Vatican II (nn.3 through 8) extends that freedom to externalize inner convictions both privately and publicly to groups and associations of individuals (since "the social nature of man itself requires . . . that he should profess his religion in community"), and insists that civil governments clearly transgress the limits of their power if they "presume to direct or inhibit acts that are religious" (n.3).

1) The Extent of Mankind's Dominion Over the Body

All patients, be they Christians, deists, atheists or non-believers (freethinkers, etc.) are subject to the primary principle of the natural moral law which tells them that they are to avoid evil (do not do evil) and do good. That *negative* obligation, "Do not do evil," is not under discussion at this time. The *positive* obligation to do good, which does not bind everywhere and at all times as negative obligations do, applies periodically to the extent that conditions and circumstances engage the conscience of the individual to take measures to satisfy that obligation. Included in that imperative ("Do good") is the obligation, incumbent upon each and every human individual, to preserve his or her life. Even though the individual is without religious convictions, or even opposed to religious values, his or her convictions with regard to the obligation to preserve life are, generally speaking, to be respected in the name of freedom of convictions—as a recognition of his or her responsibility as a participant in human dignity.

For Christian believers and other religious individuals, this sense of obligation to preserve life is reinforced by religious convictions. For Christians in particular, that obligation is viewed not as an absolute obligation but as a relative one. Such individuals share the conviction, as stated in Vatican II's document on *The Church* (Ch.II, opening quotation) that "an outstanding cause of human dignity lies in man's call to communion with God." Earthly life is a prelude, a proving ground for participation in eternal life. Human life is to be lived and preserved in testimony to love of God, love of neighbor, and proper love of self, with love of God as the basic and primary motivation. Thus Jesus said: "Whoever would save his life will lose it, and whoever loses his life for my sake will save it" (Luke,9:24. Cf. also Matthew,16:25; Mark,8:35; John,12:25). Each individual has a right to respect for his or her dedication and fidelity to personal convictions with regard to how this service of love contributes to the advancement of his or her moral and religious personality.

On several occasions, Pope Pius XII referred to the relative dominion of man over his body. In an address to a group of doctors on Jan. 30, 1945, he said: "For man is not really the absolute owner and master of his body, but only has the use of it; and God cannot permit him to use it in a manner contrary to the intrinsic and natural purposes which He has assigned as the function of its diverse parts."[264] The dominion of each individual over his or her body is relative as a right ("Your kingdom come, your will be done . . .," Matthew,6:10), as a duty ("Seek first His kingship over you, His way of holiness . . .," Matthew,6:33) and as a value ("Scripture has it: 'not on bread alone is man to live . . .,' " Matthew,4:4). Each individual's use of the body is limited by God's dominium over mankind, by the mandate of conformity to God's will and God's plan, and by the acknowledged superiority of spiritual concerns over the physical and material concerns of everyday life. It is within these parameters that man's proper dominion over self may justify a patient's personal option for refusing a medical or surgical procedure, for requesting the withdrawal of life-support equipment in certain circumstances, and for insisting on the right to "let nature take its course" in certain circumstances. The formal discussion of ordinary and extraordinary means is reserved for the following chapter on the Principle of Informed Consent. The

---

[264] *The Human Body* (cf. note 61), p. 67.

focus here is on the religious freedom factor, which can transform ordinary means of preserving life into subjectively-extraordinary and non-compulsory means.

2) Religious Freedom and the Refusal of Medical or Surgical Procedures

Every Catholic health facility is pledged to uphold its "faith obligations" which weigh heavily upon the corporate conscience. The obligation to prohibit and to have nothing to do with immoral procedures binds all who participate in the administration and operation of the health facility. The dedication to moral responsibility reads as follows:

Preamble, paragraph 5: The Catholic-sponsored health facility and its board of trustees, acting through its chief executive officer . . . carry an overriding responsibility in conscience to prohibit those procedures which are morally and spiritually harmful. The basic norms delineating this moral responsibility are listed in these *Ethical and Religious Directives for Catholic Health Facilities.* It should be understood that patients and those who accept board membership, staff appointment or privileges, or employment in a Catholic health facility will respect and agree to abide by its policies and these *Directives.* Any attempt to use a Catholic health facility for procedures contrary to these norms would indeed compromise the board and administration in its responsibility to seek and protect the total good of its patients, under the guidance of the Church.

The right to refuse to participate in any immoral treatments or procedures also applies to Catholic physicians, nurses and others who work in non-Catholic hospitals. If they make their opposition known kindly but firmly, they will win the respect of their professional co-workers. It could happen, in fact, that a physician or nurse in a Catholic hospital has doubts about the morality of a particular surgical procedure (for example, based on a personal conviction that the scheduled hysterectomy is not therapeutic but contraceptive), and requests that someone else be assigned to that particular surgical team. The hospital authorities should honor such a request without unfavorable comment of any kind.

The situation becomes far more sensitive if a non-Catholic patient refuses a medical or surgical procedure on the basis of religious convictions. The members of the Church of Christ Scientist ("Christian Science"), for example, hold that they can experience healing "to the degree that humans do understand God and follow His principles unswervingly," and that they may not be healed as a result of "their limitations in understanding and loving God."[265] A dedicated member of that denomination may insist on "leaving it all up to God," and refuse not only surgical procedures, but even routine life-saving treatments such as intravenous feeding, the use of oxygen, etc. In effect, therefore, such treatments subjectively become ethically extraordinary means of preserving life, and hence non-compulsory means.

If the physician cannot overcome possible misunderstandings and misapprehensions by patient explanation of the risks involved, the authorities of the hospital would have to respect the conscientious objections of the patient and refrain from proceeding with the treatment as required, even though the very life of the patient may be at stake. In some cases, the reluctance of the patient may be overcome by conferring with near relatives of the patient (spouse, parents, etc.) and asking them to use their powers of persuasion to convince the patient to submit to the treatment or procedure.

The members of the religious sect known as Jehovah's Witnesses are well known for their opposition to receiving blood transfusions. Despite some risks associated with blood transfusion, the procedure may be evaluated in many or most situations as an ordinary means of preserving life. Old Testament texts which forbid the "partaking of any blood" which are interpreted by scholars as a prohibition against the drinking or consuming of blood (for example, Genesis,9:4; Leviticus,3:17 and 7:26) are interpreted by the leadership of the Jehovah's Witnesses as including a prohibition against blood transfusions . . . a medical technique, incidently, which was unknown among people of biblical times. The penalty for members of that community for accepting a blood transfusion or for allowing a child of the family to be given a transfusion, is what is known as disfellowship. Such a person may attend Kingdom Hall meetings but may not speak or be spoken to by anyone. The penalty may be lifted after a year.[266]

If a competent member of the Jehovah's Witnesses refuses a life-saving blood transfusion on the basis of conscientious objection (or, if incompetent had so indicated when competent), the procedure would become a subjectively and ethically extraordinary and non-compulsory means of preserving

---

[265]Article by E.D. Canham in the *New Catholic Encyclopedia,* III (New York, N.Y.: McGraw Hill, 1967), p. 645.

[266]Whalen, William J., *Jehovah's Witnesses* (Chicago, Ill.: Claretian Publications, 1978), p. 18.

life for that patient. Surely such a person should be reminded of the risk involved, the social effects on spouse and children if death ensues, etc. If such efforts fail, however, it would be a violation of human rights if the transfusion nevertheless is given. It would also be wrong to seek a court order so as to force the patient to submit to the transfusion.

If the patient of the Jehovah's Witness sect is a pregnant mother who is in need of a life-saving blood transfusion, the right to life of the unborn child must be considered. The same would apply if the patient in need of the transfusion is an infant or young child of a Jehovah's Witness family *after* birth. In both cases, if the transfusion is rejected, the parents are failing in their objectively-serious obligation to provide ordinary care and protection for the child. Furthermore, in both cases, the religious-conviction issue which would make the transfusion a subjectively-extraordinary means for an adult, would not apply to the unborn or born child. If all efforts at patient persuasion do not overcome the opposition of the mother or parents to the blood transfusion, it would be appropriate (but not obligatory) for the hospital authorities to seek a court order to allow the transfusion. The attending physician might have additional reasons for seeking a court order. In addition to his concern for the right to life of the infant or child (who is untouched by the religious conviction issue), he may see the prohibition to transfusion on the part of the parents as a challenge to his dedication to the mission of healing. Furthermore, legal action might well be taken against him if the transfusion is not given and the infant dies. If the physician does decide to seek court action, the hospital administration should uphold his right to intervene. The trend in actual court decisions in such cases indicates that the freedom of conscience of the member of the Witnesses of Jehovah usually is upheld except in cases which conflict with the rights of the unborn and/or of the infant after birth.[267]

3) Religious Freedom and "Allowing Nature to Take Its Course"

Elderly patients in Catholic health facilities often manifest a resignation to "God's will be done" which is based on deep religious convictions. Knowing and accepting the fact that there is no cure for their condition, and that they are terminal, they may object to receiving treatments which can only provide a precarious and painful prolongation of life. They have reached the stage in life when all social and familial obligations have been fulfilled (all

---

[267]O'Donnell, Thomas J., S.J., *Medicine and Christian Morality* (cf. note 31), p. 58–61; cf. also McFadden, Charles, O.S.A., *The Dignity of Life* (cf. note 65), pp. 158–162. For additional cases, cf. *To Treat or Not to Treat* (St. Louis, Mo.: CHA, 1984), pp. 92–94.

children "on their own," etc.). Often they are patients who had asked to be transferred to a health facility not in order to receive costly life-prolonging *treatments* (renal dialysis, oxygen tents, respirator, etc.) but only because their nursing needs would make them somewhat of a burden to their loved ones at home. They are not rejecting *supportive nursing care,* but rather ineffective *treatments.*

The subject of ethically ordinary and extraordinary means will be discussed in the following chapter. It is fitting, however, to invoke the *Principle of Religious Freedom* in behalf of religiously-motivated terminal patients who wish to exercise their right to die with dignity, and without benefit of many of the life-prolonging and expensive means which might be judged as ordinary for the average, non-terminal patient. This proposal is well in line with the thought of Pope Pius XII as expressed on several occasions; for example, in an address dated November 24, 1957:

> But normally one is held to use only ordinary means—according to circumstances of persons, places, times, and culture—that is to say, means that do not involve any grave burden for oneself or another. A more strict obligation would be too burdensome for most men and would render the attainment of the higher, more important good too difficult. Life, health, all temporal activities are in fact subordinated to spiritual ends.[268]

Admittedly, such patients would have to oblige the attending physician by making their desires known clearly in some type of "living will," or preferably the statement recommended by the Catholic Health Association (1982) entitled "Christian Affirmation of Life." Without this assurance, the attending physician might feel remiss in his treatment of the patient, and could be subject to legal action from members of the patient's family. A well-functioning ethics committee could assist in tailoring hospital policy to include such "religious freedom" situations.

Directive 2: No person may be obliged to take part in a medical or surgical procedure which he judges in conscience to be immoral; nor may a health facility or any of its staff be obliged to provide a medical or surgical procedure which violates their conscience or these *Directives.*

---

[268]*The Pope Speaks,* spring, 1958, pp. 395, 396.

4) Religious Freedom and Cremation

Unfortunately the pro-abortion syndrome of our contemporary world has left little room for religious convictions with regard to the dignity of stillborns and dead fetuses. As early as 1795, state laws fully recognized the unborn child's personhood. This recognition came with the scientific discovery that the child was *alive* from the moment of conception, instead of at "quickening" as was once thought.[269] In the lamented Roe/Wade decision of Jan. 22, 1973, the U.S. Supreme Court stated: "Word 'person' as used in the Fourteenth Amendment does not include the unborn."[270] Ironically, Black Americans were excluded from legal personhood on the basis of the same Fourteenth Amendment in the Dred Scott decision 116 years earlier. In effect, the 1973 decision stated that the unborn child was the property of the mother and was not entitled to legal protection of the right to life.

The Catholic Church has always insisted on the dignity of every human individual from the moment of conception. If at all possible, stillborns and dead fetuses should be buried in a Catholic cemetery, especially if they have been baptized. The parents and their pastor can make the arrangements with a minimum of expense and ceremony. Cremation is allowed, however, if circumstances are such that a burial would place a heavy burden on the family, or if some danger of contagion is present.[271] If civil law allows it and the parents give their permission, a fetus may be retained for an autopsy or even be retained for research and teaching purposes. In such instances, cremation of the remains would be a more hygienic procedure. The ashes should be buried in a Catholic cemetery. Some cemeteries have special plots for such burials.

With regard to disposing of major body parts, that is, parts which retain human characteristics after amputation (arms, legs, feet, hands, etc.), cremation often is the only reasonable solution. Among the factors which justify such a solution are the unwillingness of patients or family members to assume that responsibility, civil health regulations, the expense involved, etc. Large hospitals usually have refrigerated storage facilities so that a preferred option for a mass burial in the hospital or parish cemetery from time to time can be scheduled (stillborns, fetuses, major body parts). If the option is for crema-

---

[269]Lippis, John, *The Challenge to be "Pro Life"*, revised ed. (Santa Barbara Pro Life Education, Inc., 1982), p. 5.

[270]*Supreme Court Reporter,* Vol. 93 (St. Paul, Minn.: West Publishing Co., 1974), Roe v. Wade, 93 S.Ct.705 (1973), p. 706, n. 12.

[271]Private response of the Sacred Congregation for the Doctrine of the Faith, Nov. 16, 1966, in *Canon Law Digest,* VI (cf. note 252), p. 669.

tion, however, it should also be done as a special mass cremation of such human remains ONLY. It would be an offense to human dignity to cremate such remains along with the usual cargo of hospital refuse (bandages, operating-room and pathology department tissues and organs, etc.). The ashes of such special cremations should also be buried in a reserved cemetery plot.

"The Church earnestly recommends that the pious custom of burial be retained; but it does not forbid cremation [of human cadavers], unless this is chosen for reasons which are contrary to Christian teaching" (Can.1176,3). Approved reasons for chosing cremation could be one of the following: high cost of transferring the remains to a distant place for burial; increased cost of standard burial as compared to cremation; national tradition or custom (as in India and other warm-climate countries); a haunting psychological or pathological fear of burial in the ground or in a tomb; remains disfigured due to ravages of a long illness, car accident, etc.

In the rare instance when a Catholic has made a decision to have his or her body cremated for reasons contrary to the Catholic faith ("ob rationes fidei christianae adversas"), and had not given some sign of repentance before death, Catholic burial rites are prohibited (Can.1184,1,n.2). According to a special instruction on cremation issued by the Holy See on May 8, 1963, such a prohibition would apply to an individual who had requested cremation because of a "denial of Christian dogmas, or because of a sectarian spirit, or through hatred of the Catholic religion and the Church," denying, that is, especially the Church's teaching on the resurrection of the dead and on the immortality of the soul.[272] There could be doubtful cases with regard to the reputation of the patient or the fact of "some sign of repentance." In such cases, the rule is "consult with the Ordinary and follow his judgment" (Can.1184,2).

The Church has also mitigated directives regarding burial rites in a crematory building. In a private response to the Cardinal Archbishop of Westminster (London) on July 9, 1966, the Holy See granted permission to allow funeral services in the chapel of the crematory.[273] The new *Rite of Funerals,* effective as of June 1, 1970, states that the rites ordinarily performed in the cemetery or at the grave may be celebrated in the crematory hall itself "if there is no other suitable place," provided that the danger of scandal and

---

[272]Instruction of the Holy Office, in *Canon Law Digest,* VI (as above), pp. 666 and 667, n. 2.

[273]*Canon Law Digest,* VIII (cf. note 38), p. 851. This rescript from the S. Cong. for the Doctrine of the Faith requires the "consent of the local Ordinary," and applies ". . . if appropriate and due precautions are taken, namely, if participation in sacred rites and if, insofar as possible, the danger of religious indifferentism are avoided."

religious indifferentism is avoided. Worthy of special note is the statement that such funeral rites (deceased cremated) should be celebrated "according to the plan in use for the region but in a way that does not hide the Church's preference for the custom of burying the dead in a grave or tomb, as the Lord Himself willed to be buried."[274]

Directive 43: If there is a reasonable cause present for not burying a fetus or member of the human body, these may be cremated in a manner consonant with the dignity of the deceased human body.

---

5) Policy Regarding Suicide Victims and "Manifest Sinners"

The individual's dominium over his or her body is limited. That limitation of human rights as indicated by the phrase "within due limits" (cf. Principle, beginning of this chapter) prohibits any efforts to "do away with oneself" (suicide). According to figures from the National Center for Health Statistics, there were 2,824 suicides in the U.S.A. in the 12-month period ending in August, 1984.[275] The un-recorded cases probably would amount to several times that number. In a hospital situation, debilitating factors such as deep depression, prolonged periods of intense suffering, etc., can explain why some patients may feel that they have a right to "end it all" by refusing nutrition and hydration, pulling out the feeding tube, etc. If death results from such incidents for reasons either pathological (depression, mental debility, etc.) or non-pathological (intense suffering, financial worries, etc.), the presumption should be that the patient is not morally responsible. In the words of an expert in pastoral medicine:

> Suicide committed in the state of endogenous depression is caused
> by a morbid (pathological) mental disturbance (psychosis), and

---

[274]*Rite of Funerals,* Revised Roman Ritual by decree of the Second Vatican Council (New York, N.Y.: Catholic Book Publishing Co., 1971), pp. 14, 15. It should be emphasized that the Church approves of the donation of the deceased body for noble purposes (for example for transplant of human organs, for medical study and research, etc.) Cf. Pope Pius XII's address to eye specialists on May 14, 1956, *The Human body* (cf. note 61), p. 381. Cf. also *Canon Law Digest,* IX (cf. note 44), pp. 701 and 715, for the application of such teaching to various guidelines for christian burial.

[275]*Monthly Vital Statistics Report,* U.S. Dept. of Health and Human Services, Hyattsville, Md., Dec. 26, 1984, p. 9.

hence is carried out without free determination of the will, without responsibility (imputability). Even so-called diminished imputability can reduce freedom of will to a point of eliminating almost all responsibility.[276]

The former code of canon law (Can.1240,3) denied Catholic burial rites to those who deliberately committed suicide, provided that they had not given some sign of repentance before death. It is significant that the present code of canon law (Can.1184) does not include suicide victims in a similar listing. Only strong evidence to the contrary (absolutely full knowledge, willfull determination, full deliberation) can militate against the presumption that the individual "did not know what he/she was doing." The element of scandal, however, must be given due consideration. The Holy See's *Declaration on Euthanasia* (May 5, 1980) provides appropriate guidelines:

> Although in these cases guilt may be diminished or completely lacking, such an error or judgment into which a conscience may fall, perhaps in good faith, does not change the nature of the death-dealing action, which is always impermissible

> The pleas of the very seriously ill as they beg at times to be put to death are hardly to be understood as conveying a real desire for euthanasia. They are almost always anguished pleas for help and love. What the sick need, in addition to medical care, is love: the warm human and supernatural affection in which all those around—parents and children, doctors and nurses—can and should enfold them.[277]

Directive 10: The directly intended termination of any patient's life, even at his own request, is always morally wrong.

With regard to "manifest sinners" who have not given some signs of repentance before death, Canon 1184,1, includes those "for whom ecclesiastical funeral rites cannot be granted without public scandal to the faithful," as well as "notorious apostates, heretics and schismatics." It would seem that an excommunicated person whose obstinacy was made public by a declared or

---

[276]Niedermeyer, Dr. Albert, *Compendium of Pastoral Medicine* (cf. note 89), p. 187.
[277]*The Pope Speaks,* 1980, p. 292.

imposed excommunication would be included among the manifest sinners. If giving them ecclesiastical burial would create a public scandal, therefore, and presuming that such a person had not given some signs of repentance before death, Catholic burial rites would be forbidden.[278] A more common situation is created by unmarried Catholics who are simply living together as man and wife, or living in an invalid marriage. Two responses of the Holy See in 1973 (May 29th and Sept. 20th) give evidence of a post-Vatican II spirit of leniency:

> . . . the celebration of religious obsequies will not be prohibited for the faithful who, although finding themselves before death in a situation of manifest sin, have preserved their attachment to the Church and have given some sign of penitence and on condition that public scandal on the part of other members of the faithful has been removed.

The recommendation for avoiding scandal is that pastors explain the meaning of "Christian obsequies" as an appeal to the mercy of God and a "testimony of the community's faith in the resurrection of the dead and eternal life."[279]

In the rare instances when Catholic burial rites must be denied, a priest may still visit the home of the deceased or the funeral parlor and say some prayers and present a few scriptural readings for the repose of the soul of the deceased and for the spiritual comfort of members of the family.[280]   In fact, unless the priest has definite reasons to believe that his presence in the home or funeral parlor would lead to an unpleasant encounter, he should perform this Christian kindness as a pastoral duty. In doubtful cases, a phone call in advance is recommended.

---

[278]*CLSA Commentary* (cf. note 45), p. 840.

[279]This quotation is from a private response of May 29, 1973, from the Sacred Congregation for the Doctrine of the Faith. The response referred to a forthcoming "new regulation" which actually was issued on Sept. 20, 1973. Cf. *Canon Law Digest,* VIII (cf. note 38), pp. 862–864.

[280]A similar recommendation is found in the Guidelines for Christian Burial of the Archdiocese of Newark, N.J. (Nov. 24, 1976) as found in *Canon Law Digest,* VIII (cf. note 38), p. 860.

CHAPTER V

The Principle of Informed Consent

> Hence man's dignity demands that he act according to a knowing and free choice. Such a choice is personally motivated and prompted from within. It does not result from blind internal impulse nor from mere external pressure. (*Pastoral Constitution on the Church Today*, n.17)

PRINCIPLE: IT IS THE RIGHT AND DUTY OF EVERY COMPETENT INDIVIDUAL TO ADVANCE "HIS HIGHER SPIRITUAL AS WELL AS HIS BODILY WELFARE" BY VOLUNTARILY CONSENTING OR BY REFUSING CONSENT (EITHER IMPLIED OR REASONABLY PRESUMED)—FREE OF ALL EXTERNAL PRESSURES—TO RECOMMENDED AND NECESSARY MEDICAL OR PSYCHOLOGICAL PROCEDURES AND/OR SPIRITUAL MINISTRATIONS, BASED ON A SUFFICIENT KNOWLEDGE OF THE BENEFITS, BURDENS AND RISKS INVOLVED. FOR INCOMPETENT INDIVIDUALS, THIS RIGHT AND DUTY IS TO BE INTERPRETED BY THE PARENTS, SPOUSE OR LEGITIMATE GUARDIANS IN ACCORDANCE (AS FAR AS POSSIBLE) WITH THAT INDIVIDUAL'S KNOWN OR REASONABLE WISHES.

The principle of informed consent is grounded on the dignity and inviolability of the human person. It is designed to protect the autonomy and integrity of the individual. Due to human factors and limitations (less than total freedom, barriers to adequate understanding, etc.), there are those who look upon the concept of informed consent as something of an impossible dream.[281] The admitted difficulties of arriving at perfection with regard to this principle should serve to increase the determination to pursue the ideal with dedication and ingenuity. Based on the moral principle that "no injury is done to one who possesses knowledge and exercises free will," it is more appropriate to regard informed consent as a process rather than as an event. The implementation of this principle requires both continuous informing and consenting and continuous efforts to achieve the desired aim.

5.1   THE CHALLENGE OF SELF-DETERMINATION

A competent patient is an adult, or an emancipated minor patient, who is conscious, able to understand the nature and severity of his or her illness and the relative risks and alternatives, and able to make informed and deliberate choices about the treatment of the illness. In civil law, an emancipated minor is a young man or young woman under the age of 18 who has been released from parental control. If they do not have court-appointed guardians, such emancipated minors "speak for themselves."

Unless the civil law rules otherwise, it must be admitted that in some cases those who are minors in Church law (less than 18 years of age, cf. Can.97) are competent to consent or to refuse consent to a significant surgical or medical procedure. This often is true of young boys and girls who are "on their own" and earning their own living. Father Gerald Kelly, S.J. mentions that the natural law would uphold the right of an intelligent 15-year-old boy to give consent to an operation even against the unreasonable refusal of his parents.[282] As to children who have not reached the teen-age category, the presumption is that they have not arrived at the degree of perception and experience required for giving or refusing consent to a medical procedure. In most cases of young folks in the lower teen-age category, the consent of the parents or guardians should be obtained and should suffice, although a child's *assent* may be appropriate and advisable.

---

[281]In an article entitled "The Fiction of Informed Consent," Eugene Laforet, MD states: "Informed consent is a legalistic fiction that destroys good patient care and paralyzes the conscientious physician. It hedges the experimental situation with barriers that cannot be surmounted. It is not applicable, even by definition, to a large segment of the involved population. The term has no place in the lexicon of medicine." Cf. *Journal of the American Medical Association,* April 12, 1976, pp. 1584, 1585. However difficult of application, the moral *right* to informed consent must be defended to whatever extent possible.

[282]*Medico-Moral Problems* (cf. note 22), p. 40.

The word "incompetent" (one who is NOT "able to understand . . ,"
cf.definition) applies as a general rule to minors and to all who are delirious,
unconscious, comatose, or in such an advanced state of confusion or agitation
that they are unable to properly understand, appreciate and evaluate recommended life choices. Procedure in such cases will be discussed in the final
section of this chapter.

The *duty* to give or withhold consent depends for its exercise on a proper
realization of the corresponding *right*. Since the competent individual exercises that right in large measure through the physician, the physician-patient
relationship must be clarified. It begins with a type of informal but binding
contract when the physician accepts the individual (usually without limitation
as to the duration of the contract), as one of his or her patients. This contract
ends or is breached when the patient voluntarily terminates the contract or
agreement or chooses another physician, or when the physician announces
from inner conviction that the choice of another physician would be in the
best interests of the patient. Once a treatment or medical procedure has been
initiated, however, the physician may not abandon the patient. He may resign
or withdraw from the case, however, after having arranged for an appropriate
interim or follow-up treatment, pending the choice of another physician on
the part of the patient.[283]

Informed consent is grounded on the proposition that the patient has a
right to make choices about the type of care to be received. No matter how
competent the patient may be, however, consent to choices will be far from
ideal unless adequate information is provided (to be discussed in section 5.6
of this chapter); and adequate information depends upon open lines of *communication* between patient and physician. The obstacles to open communication are many. Unfortunately, many adult patients have no personal
physician. With the spread of Health Maintenance Organizations (HMO's)
and other health care provider agencies, the patient reports to the physician
on duty rather than to a physician of choice. Other obstacles to ongoing
communication are associated with the very nature of the illness, the degree
of pain, the effects of drugs, etc., so that competency itself becomes a fluctu-
ating factor, and depends heavily upon a close patient-physician relationship.

The basic key to an effective patient-physician relationship is communication. In these days of multiple testing and high technology, the "bedside
manner" in establishing rapport with the patient is a neglected art. Test
results, no matter how extensive, cannot substitute for "getting to know you

---

[283]Horan, Dennis J., JD, "Euthanasia, the Right to Life and termination of Medical Treatment: Legal Issues," in *Moral Responsibility in Prolonging Life Decisions,* Donald G. McCarthy and
Albert S. Moraczewski, O.P., eds. (St. Louis, Mo.: Pope John Center, 1981), p. 155.

and your condition." All admit that the patient is primary. Yet, without open lines of communication, the right of the patient to "speak up" (before diagnosis, after prognosis, etc.) is a tenuous and illusory right. An example of how such lines of communication are neglected was given in a 1981 survey in a university teaching hospital in Boston, Mass., with regard to the critical subject of cardiopulmonary resuscitation. Although the physicians involved in the survey claimed to have formed an opinion about the patient's attitude on CPR in 68% of the cases, the patients actually had discussed the subject of CPR with their private physician or house office (or both) in only 19% of the cases.[284] With such clogged lines of communication, words such as "patient autonomy" and self-determination are almost without meaning.

Self-Determination and "The Spiritual as well as Bodily Welfare"

Attending to the spiritual needs of all patients in a Catholic health facility has been discussed at length in chapters II and IV. The connection between spiritual welfare and communication must be emphasized. The period preliminary to treatments and prognosis must be utilized insofar as possible not only to comfort them with reminders of God's grace, goodness and mercy, but also, in due time, to sound out their ideas on suffering, resignation to God's will, having recourse to cardiopulmonary resuscitation and life-prolonging treatments and techniques, etc. If the chaplain and pastoral care personnel use the initial days or weeks of complete competency to get to know the patient and his or her wishes and preferences also in medical matters, they may be of consoling help to family members in interpreting the mind and will of the patient if and when the patient turns unconscious, comatose or delirious. Their spiritual welfare is of prime importance, and their views on spiritual matters (especially on resignation to God's will and providence) will color their views on life, suffering, extent of the obligation to submit to life-prolonging treatments, etc. Helping them to bring such unpleasant subjects out into the open, with all due caution, charity and diplomacy, can contribute to their spiritual growth and to their ability to face the future with faith and confidence in God.

So little can be done for seriously-ill patients when debility has brought them close to delirium, unconsciousness and incompetency—or even to a state of prolonged depression. Waiting until they are unwilling or unable to talk, is to deprive them of occasions to face the realities of life and life-

---

[284]Bedell, Susanna E., MD, and Delbanco, Thomas L., MD, "Choices About Cardiopulmonary Resuscitation in the Hospital," in *The New England Journal of Medicine*, April 26, 1984, pp. 1089–1092.

threatening situations at a crucial period in their lives. These are all basic preliminaries to "shaping up" both their spiritual and physical welfare as a prelude to persuading them to make peace with God, to seek reconciliation by having a marriage revalidated, by restoring familial or domestic peace, etc. The sad fact is that for many of them, this may be their last chance for reconciliation and peace within. "Small talk" in getting to know seriously-ill patients should lead to "big talk" communication.

A spiritually-motivated physician is a powerful ally to the chaplain and pastoral care personnel in their efforts to prepare patients for reconciliation with God and for embracing God's will. In an address to the 1978 meeting of the National Federation of Catholic Physicians' Guilds, the Most Rev. Lawrence J. Riley, D.D., Auxiliary Bishop of the Archdiocese of Boston, reminded the assembly that Our Divine Lord's touching Parable of the Good Samaritan "has been preserved for mankind by the pen of St. Luke, the Physician," and added:

> I have said that the physician must imitate Christ's profound appreciation of the dignity of the human personality. He must imitate Christ's gentleness and tenderness and understanding. But also he must imitate Christ's inflexible and uncompromising opposition to evil . . . For a physician to imitate Christ's opposition to evil demands a profound and deep-rooted conviction and a conscientious implementation of the fundamental truths of medical ethics.[285]

With close cooperation between an attending physician of such professional stature and the hospital chaplain in particular, the best interests of the patient, both physical and spiritual, usually will be secured well before the patient lapses into incompetency. The element of informed consent will not be neglected.

The word "self-determination" as a guarantee of autonomy is closely related to a patient's sense of personal well-being. It is defined as a person's capacity to form, revise, and pursue his or her own plans for life in keeping with personal values and goals and in fidelity to personal convictions of dignity and self-worth. It is dangerous to chart one's course in life in accord with

---

[285]"The Catholic Physician and Morality in Contemporary Society" in *Linacre Quarterly*, February, 1979, p. 12. Catholic physicians will be strengthened in their resolve to project Catholic moral standards in their professional lives by joining the National Federation of Catholic Physicians' Guilds. Contact can be made by writing to *Linacre Quarterly*, 850 Elm Grove Road, Elm Grove, Wis., 53122.

the popular dictum: "All is well as long as I feel good about myself as I am."[286] That "feeling good about oneself" must be based on a realistic appraisal of personal strengths and weaknesses. Without such an effort to "know thyself," an unfavorable diagnosis or prognosis can be a damaging experience. This emphasizes the challenge to everyone who is engaged in the mission of healing to enhance the individual patient's *internal* potential in making the right choices with regard to the appropriate type of medical care and treatment.

5.2 INFORMED CONSENT AND ORDINARY—EXTRAORDINARY MEANS

It is more difficult to realize the extent to which "good must be done" than it is to realize the extent to which "evil must be avoided." The distinction between *ordinary* and *extraordinary* means grew out of a consciousness among moralists that there must be reasonable and proportionate limits to one's duty to do good.[287] Promoting health and preserving life is a primary human good. Especially in cases of prolonged illness and of terminal illness, a patient has a right to ask: "To what extent am I obligated to preserve this bodily life?" The Church responds in the *Declaration on Euthanasia* as issued by the Sacred Congregation for the Doctrine of the Faith on May 5, 1980:

> It is always licit to be content with the ordinary remedies which medical science can supply. Therefore, no one may be obliged to submit to a type of cure which, though already in use, is not without some risks or is excessively burdensome. This rejection of a remedy is not to be compared to suicide; it is more justly to be regarded as a simple acceptance of the human condition or a desire to avoid the application of medical techniques that are disproportionate to the value of the anticipated results or, finally, a desire not to put a heavy burden on the family or the community.[288]

---

[286]Kilpatrick, William Kirk, in his book entitled *Psychological Seduction* (New York, N.Y.: Thomas Nelson Publishers, 1983), writes: "If psychology's great optimism about raw human nature is correct, then Christianity is not necessary; Christ's redemptive action on the cross becomes superfluous." p. 39.

[287]Kelly, Gerald, S.J., *Medico-Moral Problems* (cf. note 22), p. 131.

[288]*The Pope Speaks,* 1980, p. 295.

It comes down to a weighing or balancing of *benefits* that can be reasonably anticipated against the extent of *burdens* which are inherently associated with the remedies as recommended or proposed. Naturally the *associated burdens* usually are more clearcut than the *anticipated benefits*. In a pastoral letter in 1976, the U.S. Catholic Bishops spoke of a similar "reasonable hope of recovery" as opposed to "excessive burdens."[289] With regard to both benefits and burdens, non-medical factors must be included in themselves and in their relationship to both patient and to family members and the community. From an ethical point of view, there is no list of procedures which are always and everywhere *ethically* ordinary or extraordinary. The distinction depends upon a prudential weighing of the associated benefits vs the anticipated burdens in each particular case as experienced by the patient.

An unusual case involving family members in the weighing of benefits vs burdens appeared in the American press in late 1984. Padwel Sitarz, 16, son of a "Solidarity" leader who was freed from prison on condition that he leave his native Poland, was seriously ill with a condition which later was diagnosed as prostate cancer. Knowing that his parents had no money for medical treatment, and convinced that they depended heavily upon his knowledge of English in their difficult period of adjustment to life in a new country (parents unable to speak English), he did not tell them about his illness. On Dec. 12, 1984, he was rushed to the hospital; the cancer had spread to his lungs and stomach; he died on Dec. 15th, 1984.[290] Treatment for prostatic cancer would rate *medically* as an ordinary means of preserving life. For Padwell ("Paul" to his friends) Sitarz, age 16, subjectively considered with all due implications for his loved ones, it was an *ethically* extraordinary and non-compulsory means of preserving his life.

Several factors must be clarified with regard to weighing *reasonably anticipated benefits* against *associated burdens* in applying the distinction between ordinary and extraordinary means:

1) *MEDICAL vs THEOLOGICAL TERMINOLOGY:* The general rule is that what *physicians* consider as ordinary means (*customary* or *usual* in a given case) are not necessarily what *theologians* consider as ordinary means of preserving life. Whereas physicians rate such means from the viewpoint of medical practice, theologians rate them from the moral viewpoint of the extent of the burdens placed on the patient and others. The example mentioned above, unusual though it may be, is an illustration of that difference of viewpoint. Another example could be the situation of an elderly

---

[289] *Pastoral Letters of the U.S. Catholic Bishops,* Hugh J. Nolan, ed., vol. IV (Washington, D.C.: United States Catholic Conference, 1984), p. 183, n. 58.

[290] *St. Louis Post-Dispatch,* Dec. 22, 1984, p. 9A.

woman with advanced kidney dysfunction, whose children are all married and "on their own." She may choose to regard the prospect of renal dialysis several times each week in a hospital 50 miles distance from her place of residence as an excessive burden—hence as an extraordinary and non-compulsory means of preserving her life. The decision regarding the choice of such a means of preserving life lies with the patient and not with the physician.

2) *The IMPORTANCE of the "OVERALL" VIEW:* The choice of the recommended means of preserving life must be looked upon as an *"all things considered"* decision—including due consideration of non-medical factors such as cost, imposition on a strained marriage or family relationship, dedication to religious values and ideals, etc. Again, an enlightening quotation from the Holy See's *Declaration on Euthanasia:*

> In any case, a correct judgment can be made regarding means, if the type of treatment, its degree of difficulty and danger, its expense, and the possibility of applying it are weighed against the results that can be expected, all this in the light of the sick person's condition and resources of body and spirit.[291]

This would find application especially in cases involving the group of patients who are classed as the "hopelessly ill,"—especially, but not exclusively. Especially with regard to "excessive burden" situations, it is probable that a religious-motivated elderly single man with chronic diabetes, who had no caring relatives left in this world, would regard the surgical removal of his only good leg (one already removed) as an excessive burden, and hence an ethically extraordinary and non-compulsory means.

3) *"QUALITY OF LIFE" CONSIDERATIONS* do not limit the right or duty to preserve human life. The preservation of life, *as an end,* is as precious for a handicapped person (mentally or developmentally retarded individual) as for individuals who are not handicapped. *As a means* of preserving life, however, a competent person with Down Syndrome, for example, would be justified in regarding the prospect of renal dialysis (until "if and when" a kidney transplant is available) as adding an *additional* handicap which might constitute an excessive burden; hence, as an ethically extraordinary means of preserving life and non-compulsory. There definitely is a limit as to how much burden a person is expected to take upon himself. He would be refusing renal dialysis not primarily because of the limitation of "qual-

---

[291] *The Pope Speaks,* 1980, p. 294.

ity of life" brought on by his original handicap (Down Syndrome), but because of the additional and excessive burden of renal dialysis *as a means* of preserving his life.[292]

The right to make a decision as above belongs to the patient only. A proxy for a handicapped person who is incompetent could interpret the will of that patient as being in favor of refusing the recommended procedure as an ethically extraordinary (excessive burden added to his handicap) only if the handicapped patient, if and when competent, had indicated clearly that he would reject such a means of preserving his life. The proxy is obligated to make the decision (based on knowledge of and communication with the patient) which the patient himself would have made in the state of competency. If the patient never had been competent, or, when competent, had not expressed his or her wishes or preferences in the matter, the proxy would have to be guided by an honest appraisal of the best interests of the patient.

4) *UNFULFILLED MORAL OR RELIGIOUS OBLIGATIONS* of considerable significance would obligate the patient to consent to an ethically extraordinary means of preserving life until such obligations have been discharged. The fact that the patient has yet to make his peace with God, or has not settled some major controversial matter of family inheritance are two examples of such moral or religious obligations. The patient would, in general, be obligated to continue the use of life-supporting equipment (respirator, renal dialysis, etc.) as a means of obtaining peace with God or (in the second example) as a means of assuring peace and justice in the family.

5) *USEFUL vs USELESS MEANS:* If the probability of a particular treatment benefiting a patient is reduced to little or nothing, the patient would not be obligated to consent to the treatment even though otherwise it might be considered as an ethically ordinary means of preserving life. This could apply also to non-terminal cases when the treatment proposed is of very dubious beneficial effect. In order to identify such cases, one has only to take seriously an estimate of the American Medical Association which indicates that *additional treatments* and *extra diagnostic testing* as prescribed by physicians "add from $15 billion to $40 billion to the national health-care cost."[293] If a terminal patient is near death, otherwise medically ordinary life-sustaining treatments such as oxygen, renal dialysis, etc., would not

---

[292]Connery, John R., S.J., "Prolonging Life: The Duty and Limits," in *Moral Responsibility in Prolonging Life Decisions* (cf. note 283), pp. 132–134.

[293]*Time,* Jan. 28, 1985, p. 75.

be obligatory if they were useless in sustaining life. The principle involved is that no one is held to what is useless ("nemo ad inutile tenetur"). The application of this principle calls for "tender, loving care" in treating patients who are terminally ill.

The variety of factors and considerations which go into a realistic definition of ethically "extraordinary means" are assembled well in Father Edwin Healy's definition of the phrase: "We may define as an extraordinary means whatever here and now is very *costly* or very *unusual* or very *painful* or very *difficult* or very *dangerous,* or if the good effects that are to be expected from its use are not proportionate to the difficulty and inconvenience that are entailed."[294] The time-honored distinction between ethically ordinary and extraordinary means has suffered from undue expectations. Contemporary advances in medical technology have served to emphasize the impossibility of establishing "cut and dried" and "hard and fast" categories based on that distinction. The distinction never was intended as a panacea in taking the anguish out of decision-making with regard to medical treatment.

Although the *President's Commission* does see some "moral significance" in the distinction "if . . . understood in terms of usefulness and burdensomeness of a particular therapy," their conclusion is that it would be better to avoid the use of the ordinary-extraordinary distinction, and to "speak instead in terms of the proportionate benefit and burdens of treatment as viewed by particular patients."[295] The Declaration on Euthanasia also refers to the distinction as "less evident today because of its vagueness or because of rapid advances in the treatment of illness."[296] Yet, in the definition of ethically extraordinary means by Father Healy above, the distinction is based precisely on the proportion or disproportion between benefits and burdens. Changing the terms to proportionate/disproportionate, or to obligatory/non-obligatory, or to compulsory/non-compulsory is not going to arrest the factor which makes the ordinary/extraordinary difficult to apply in contemporary life—and that is the "rapid advances in the treatment of illness" as noted above. It is only realistic to assume that Catholic moralists will continue to speak of ethically ordinary and extraordinary means. One dividend of such a continued practice is that recourse to that distinction will avoid identification with those who are disposed to decide right and wrong on the basis of "proportionalism."

---

[294]*Medical Ethics* (cf. note 46), p. 67.

[295]*Deciding to Forego Life-Sustaining Treatment* (cf. note 215), pp. 88, 89 and note 132. They also quote Paul Ramsey as calling the distinction "no longer useful." *Ibid.*

[296]*The Pope Speaks,* 1980, p. 294.

5.3 INFORMED CONSENT AND LEVELS OF HOSPITAL CARE

In varying degrees, levels of hospital care correspond to levels of the competency of the patient. When the patient is fully competent and enjoys open lines of communication with his or her physician, choices can be made for medication and treatment which approach the ideal. Most patients are in fairly good health when they check in at a hospital. Some mysterious pain or puzzling lapse of memory, balance or consciousness may have led to the familiar physician's refrain: "You had better check in the hospital for a few tests." Within weeks, many of these patients will be back in the hospital because of the test results. If the physical condition which brought them back to the hospital is of a serious or potentially-serious nature, the average physician would want to use that occasion to "sound out" the patient on critical questions which simply could not be answered with full satisfaction after full competency has been diminished by worries, tiring treatments, sedatives, etc.—questions such as their preferences with regard to cardiopulmonary resuscitation, expensive life-prolonging treatments, etc.[297] Undoubtedly this would have to be done in a caring, diplomatic manner without creating excessive anxiety in the patient. The argument that it is "just in case" and "for your own good" should put the average patient at ease.

This would be done normally during the first level of hospital care which is the *level of general care*. Although the comparison limps badly, this stage of the physician-patient relationship might be compared to the prescribed "reading of rights" to a suspected criminal soon after having been apprehended by police officers. In both cases, it could be a matter of life or death. The patient must be made to understand that he or she has the last word in consenting to treatments, in discontinuing treatments, in requesting professional consultations, in deciding to entrust his or her medical care to another physician, etc. However shocking it may appear to initiate such discussions early in the patient's illness, it is far more considerate and caring than waiting until diminished competence has rendered the patient less capable of understanding crucial rights and making critical decisions.

1) The Level of Emergency Resuscitation Care

Resuscitation refers to the ability to rescue a person from the brink of death by restoring life-giving heartbeat and breathing. The Prophet Elisha's revival of the young son of a Shunamite woman is the first recorded account

---

[297]Wanzer, Sidney H., MD, et al., "The Physicians's Responsibility Toward Hopelessly Ill Patients," in *The New England Journal of Medicine*, April 12, 1984, p. 957.

of such a marvel: ". . . placing his mouth upon the child's mouth, his eyes upon the eyes, and his hands upon the hands . . . the boy . . . now sneezed seven times and opened his eyes" (II Kings, 4:34,35). Resuscitation was developed initially for otherwise healthy persons whose heartbeat and breathing failed following surgery or near-drowning. Today it is used on virtually everyone who is a victim of cardiac arrest in a hospital. The *President's Commission* evaluates this procedure as follows:

> The initial success rate for in-hospital resuscitation is about one in three for all victims and about two in three for patients hospitalized with irregularities of heart rhythm. Among patients who are successfully resuscitated, about one in three recovers enough to be discharged from the hospital eventually. Especially when used on the general hospital population, long-term success is fairly rare. In the past decade, health care providers have begun to express concern that resuscitation is being used too frequently and sometimes on patients it harms rather than benefits.[298]

Cardiopulmonary resuscitation (CPR) is considered to be a medically ordinary means of preserving life. There are situations, however, when it should not be administered: a) when it cannot be done within a few minutes (3 to 5 minutes) after cardiac arrest (useless, hence non-compulsory); b) in cases of irreversible terminal illness when death is imminent and the patient is beyond any hopeful prognosis (useless, hence non-compulsory); c) when the patient, while still competent, definitely decided against it and did not later reverse that decision. It is unreasonable to predict any hope of the successful application of CPR unless the critical time element can be anticipated by an early physician-patient discussion of the likelihood or possibility of the need of it. This discussion, adapted time-wise to the age of the patient, nature of the illness, etc., should include an honest evaluation of the risks and benefits involved. Even if the discussion is not considered opportune (young patient, strong heart, etc.), the patient may bring up the subject.

Although the cost of CPR should not, in itself, rule out the application of CPR as a matter of policy, individual patients have a right to know that resuscitation efforts "commonly cost over $1000 and usually entail substantial derivative costs in caring for the surviving patients who suffer side effects." Those "derivative costs" could include additional weeks in intensive care due to side effects (for example, a fractured rib).[299]

---

[298]*Deciding to Forego Life-Sustaining Treatment* (cf. note 215), pp. 234, 235.
[299]*Ibid.*, p. 244 and note 44.

A DNR order ("Do Not Resuscitate"), also known as "No Code," means that the "resuscitation team" shall not be called to reverse cardiac arrest. If the team is to be called into action, a "Code Blue" announcement (or some other suitable expression) is made over the hospital's public address system. Hospital policies should require adequate physician-patient communication about a resuscitation decision (cf.5.1 as evidence of this need). Another standard requirement is that any DNR order must be written in a patient's chart, duly signed by the physician, and include sufficient documentation of the supporting reasons for the DNR. Physicians must also keep in mind the ongoing need of frequent revisions of the DNR order (every 24 to 48 hours recommended).

The *President's Commission* recommendations might be summarized as follows: If the patient expresses a preference for resuscitation and the physician likewise (even when unclear as to whether it would benefit the patient), the decision should be in favor of resuscitation; if the patient is hesitant or has no preference, and the physician favors resuscitation (even when unclear as above), the presumption still should stand in favor of resuscitation. Meanwhile, before the possibility of cardiac arrest must be faced, efforts should be made to enlist family members and others (pastor, priest-friend) to help break down barriers to understanding and to encourage the patient to come to a definite decision, either pro or con. If the patient decides against resuscitation, his decision must be respected. Ongoing efforts to re-examine the situation should be continued—it is a case of life or death if cardiac arrest occurs. In some instances, the climate of disagreement between physician and patient may become so unpleasant that it would be for the best interests of the patient if the physician withdrew from the case and helped the patient find a new physician.[300]

If the patient is incompetent, the recommended procedure is the same except that the proxy (spouse, parent, guardian) must speak for the patient. If the patient had made a definite decision while competent, that decision must prevail. Disagreement may break out between the physician and the proxy, however, over whether or not CPR would benefit the patient. Either the physician or the proxy could be opposed to CPR. Here is where an "Ethics Committee" or similar group could be of significant help in a consultative capacity. The other alternative to settling the problem within hospital walls could be court action. In the meantime (court action pending), if the patient suffers cardiac arrest, CPR should be administered. Both hospitals and indi-

---

[300]*Ibid.*, pp. 244–247.

vidual physicians have a right to be wary of court-rendered solutions. Hospitals are uncertain about their liability under the law; physicians often are torn between "DNR" or "Code Blue" for fear of being sued for making a wrong decision. The *President's Commission* concludes that "decision-making about life-sustaining care is rarely improved by resort to courts."[301]

Finally, with regard to incompetent patients, CPR should not be administered if the physician decides that it would not benefit the patient and the proxy is opposed to CPR in behalf of the patient. The general rule for CPR (for both competent and incompetent patients) might be stated as "In case of doubt, bring the team out." Considering the life-or-death nature of the procedure and the hovering prospects of legal liability, such a rule is both prudential and practical. A special plea must be added for both charity and justice in omitting CPR (whatever the fictioned legal consequences) for near-death and beyond-hope patients who are lingering in an irreversible terminal illness. All too often, measures taken by the resuscitation-team add to the misery, the injuries and the suffering of defenseless souls and constitute a flagrant violation (however well-intended) of "Above all, cause no harm" ("Primum, non nocere"). It is unjust and unkind to prolong needlessly the dying process of hopelessly ill patients. What can be done if the patient is incompetent, and no friends or loved ones are available who could interpret what the wishes of the patient would have been when competent? If the hovering alternative of court intervention is to be avoided, the recommendation of the *President's Commission* should be considered:

> When a patient's likely decision is unknown, however, a surrogate decision-maker should use the best interests standard to choose a course that will promote the patient's well-being as it would probably be conceived by a reasonable person in the patient's circumstances.[302]

2) The Level of Intensive Care and Life-Support

The contemporary practice of medicine manifests a definite trend to make the most of the phenomenal progress in medical science and technology so as to sustain and support human life to the absolute limit. There are over 7000 acute-care hospitals in the U.S.A. The spiral of continuous upgrading in medical services in scope, variety and intensity seems to have escaped ade-

---

[301] *Ibid.*, p. 247. For guidelines for incompetent patients with regard to CPR, cf. pp. 246–248.
[302] *Ibid.*, p. 136.

quate control. This is one of the prime factors responsible for the frightening rise in medical costs. Other contributing factors such as the growth of the "senior citizen" category, the rising costs of goods and services (especially labor costs) and of insurance liability premiums have proven to be elusive targets of effective control. In the words of one qualified observer, science and technology must respond to reasonable control:

> . . . like it or not, sooner or later we will be left with only one choice. Either we will accept the continued rise of hospital costs that result from full exploitation of technological advances, or we will start to ration hospital care.[303]

The patient who is in need of acute or intensive care is caught in this spiral. Informed consent becomes less and less valid when sustaining and supporting life is conceived as depending upon vigorous and aggressive treatment in the "expensive care" unit. Since time is of the essence, formidable options often are presented to the confused patient as "brooking no delay;"— more diagnostic tests, organ transplant, by-pass cardiac surgery, etc. A further discussion of this subject will require a few definitions. The following definitions are found repeatedly in the publication of the *President's Commission* entitled *Deciding to Forego Life-Sustaining Treatment:*[304]

"Terminal Condition" means an incurable condition caused by injury, disease, or illness, which, regardless of the application of life-sustaining procedures, would, within reasonable medical judgment, produce death, and where the application of life-sustaining procedures serve only to postpone the moment of death of the patient.

"Life-sustaining Procedure" means any medical procedure or intervention which utilizes mechanical or other artificial means to sustain, restore, or supplant a vital function, which, when applied to a qualified patient, would serve only to artificially prolong the moment of death and where, in the judgment of the attending physician, death is imminent whether or not such procedures are utilized.

"Qualified patient" means a patient diagnosed and certified in writing to be afflicted with a terminal condition by two physicians, one of whom shall be the attending physician, who have personally examined the patient.

"Imminent Danger of Death" means that death probably will occur, in the ordinary course of events, within two weeks.

---

[303]Schwartz, William, MD, "The Most Painful Prescription," *Newsweek*, Nov. 12, 1984, p. 24.
[304]Cf. note 215; Appendix D, review of "Natural Death Statutes," pp. 324 ff.

The phrase *"irreversible condition"* can refer both to patients who are in a terminal condition (as defined above), or to patients who are not terminally ill (persons who are acutely psychotic, mentally retarded or senile) but who are in a permanent comatose state or in a permanent vegetative state (as far as it is possible to predict the condition as permanent), and (a) there is no reasonable medical possibility that the patient will avoid death and return to a normal cognitive and sapient state, and (b) life can be sustained only through the use of medically extraordinary life-sustaining procedures. The term *"hopelessly ill"* must be used with due caution. It cannot be applied to severely retarded or psychotic individuals or to others of a diminished "quality of life" condition as a basis for denying them life-sustaining treatment. Such patients could be in a "hopeless" condition, but they are not terminally ill.

a) Informed Consent and Life-Sustaining Treatment

The present discussion concerns those who can still cherish a reasonable hope of returning to an improved-health status. As long as that hope is alive, life-sustaining treatment, including the use of a respirator, oxygen tent, chemotherapy, etc. are medically ordinary means of preserving life. In particular cases, however, such life-sustaining treatments could be considered as ethically *extraordinary* and hence non-compulsory means of preserving life. *Aggressive* treatments, unless clearly established as medically indicated for a particular individual, can become ethically extraordinary, non-compulsory means of preserving life in a particular case. The *Declaration on Euthanasia* (to be quoted presently) apparently was referring to aggressive treatments in the following passage: ". . . the most recent medical techniques, even if these are not yet fully tested and are not free of risk."

It is said that the malpractice scare has made some physicians wary of legal complications to the extent that they are tempted to practice "defensive medicine." That means adding tests and treatments which the patient could very well refuse simply because they are not needed. The patient usually has confidence in his or her attending physician, and will not object. One survey of the American Medical Association indicated that 27% of the physicians who responded to the survey admitted that they had "prescribed additional treatment," and 40% said that they had "ordered extra diagnostic tests" because of their concern about possible legal complications. The multi-billion increase in health-care cost, like the increased price of health insurance, is passed on to the patient.[305] Both the additional cost and the additional inconvenience (and suffering, in many cases) should have prompted the average

---

[305] *Time,* Jan. 28, 1985, p. 75.

well-informed patient to refuse consent to such unwarranted treatments. No patient, either in general medical care or in intensive care, is obligated to consent to such treatments. If consent is given on the basis of "Doctor knows best," it is neither well-informed nor valid consent in the strict sense of the phrase. Whenever such additional treatments are proposed, either the patient or (if incompetent) the patient's proxy must be made to feel free to ask pertinent and pointed questions such as: "Is this medically indicated?," and "If not, why do you propose it?"

If the patient is well-informed by the physician, consent to some additional treatments may be given either in the hope of a beneficial outcome or for higher motives. The *Declaration on Euthanasia* states: "If other remedies are lacking, it is permissible, with the consent of the sick person, to use the most recent medical techniques, even if these are not yet fully tested and are not free of risk. The sick person who agrees to them can even give an example thereby, of generous service to the human race."[306] Aggressive treatment must be distinguished from *unnecessary* treatment, which will be discussed under the Principle of the Double Effect.

When the burdens of a life-sustaining treatment (expense, suffering, danger, etc.) outweigh the hoped-for benefits, there is no obligation to continue the treatment. The role of the physician in determining when the burdens outweigh the benefits must guide the patient (or proxy, if the patient is incompetent) in arriving at a decision to discontinue the treatment. The quotation from the *Declaration on Euthanasia* (below) would seem to recommend a helpful distinction both in initiating ethically extraordinary treatment and in withdrawing such treatment—a distinction between a prudential *judgment* with regard to the ethically extraordinary nature of the treatment, and a definite *decision* to initiate or to discontinue the treatment. Examples of the latter (discontinue treatment) might be questions as to writing a Do-Not-Resuscitate order, or taking a patient off the respirator, or transferring the patient to a nursing home, etc. The *judgment* (that the treatment is ethically extraordinary) would be made by the patient or proxy (patient incompetent) with heavy reliance on the explanations and expertise of the physician; the *decision*, made by the patient or proxy, would direct that the treatment be discontinued. If the patient is incompetent, the decision must be based on the patient's previously expressed and reasonable wish or (if that is impossible), on a deliberated conclusion as to the best interests of the patient.[307]

---

[306] *The Pope Speaks,* 1980, p. 295.

[307] This helpful distinction is proposed by Father Donald G. McCarthy in a chapter entitled "The Responsibilities of Administrators," in *Moral Responsibility in Prolonging Life Decisions* (cf. note 283), pp. 248–251.

The advantage of this distinction is that it delineates clearly the heavy responsibility both of the physician and of the patient or proxy, and provides some protection against confusing those two responsibilities. Naturally the distinction applies as well to initiating or withdrawing treatment in life-*prolonging* treatments (where there is no hope of recovery). The quotation from the *Declaration of Euthanasia* would seem to apply to many proposed extraordinary procedures or interventions:

> It is also licit to discontinue the use of these means [most recent medical techniques, even if these are not yet fully tested and are not free of risk] as soon as results disappoint the hopes placed in them but, in making this decision, account should be taken of the legitimate desire of the sick person and his or her family as well as of the opinion of truly expert physicians. The latter are better placed than anyone else for judging whether the expense of machinery and personnel is disproportionate to the foreseeable results and whether the medical techniques used will cause the sick person suffering or inconvenience greater than the benefits that may be derived from them.[308]

b) Care of Developmentally-Disadvantaged Newborns

The most defenseless of all handicapped individuals are the developmentally-disadvantaged newborn infants. Usually they have parental love in their favor. Some would say, however, that if parents really loved seriously-handicapped infants, they would allow them to die. The attention of the nation was focused recently on three developmentally-disadvantaged newborns: Baby Doe of Bloomington, Ind., in 1982 (allowed to die), Baby Jane Doe of New York State in 1983 (eventually received medical treatment), and Baby Stephanie Fae of Barstow, California in 1984 (lived three weeks with the implanted heart of a baboon). Those who suggest that such infants should be allowed to die are saying, in effect, that "quality of life" considerations can constitute a restriction of the dignity of life and of the right to life. Eventually, in the wake of publicity over the Baby Doe case (1982), the federal government moved into action in defense of handicapped newborns.

The federal regulations on this subject, however, had a short and stormy history. On May 18, 1982, in response to a directive from President Reagan,

---

[308] *The Pope Speaks,* 1980, p. 295.

the Director of the Department of Civil Rights of the U.S. Department of Health and Human Services (HHS), reminded health care providers receiving federal assistance that newborn infants with handicaps such as Down syndrome were protected under section 504 of the Rehabilitation Act of 1973. Subsequent HHS regulations, known as the "Interim Final Rule" (March 7, 1983), courted opposition from hospital personnel by insisting on conspicuous posted notices in hospitals (to the effect that the regulations were covered by section 504 of the Rehabilitation Act of 1973), a telephone "hotline" to report violations of the regulations, and expedited access to hospital records and facilities when judged necessary to protect the life or health of a handicapped individual. Various medical associations had recourse to legal action to challenge the validity of the HHS regulations. The new "Proposed Rules" as issued by the HHS on July 5, 1983, and the "Final Rules" as promulgated on December 30, 1984, did not halt the efforts of various medical associations to have the courts declare the regulations to be invalid.[309]

The case eventually reached the U.S. Supreme Court on certiorari (that is, a writ requesting the proceedings of a case of a lower court for review). The decision of the U.S. Supreme Court, under date of June 9, 1986, affirmed the judgment of the District Court for the Southern District of New York, and of the United States Court of Appeals for the Second Circuit, to the effect that the investigative actions as alleged by the Secretary of the HHS (posted notices, "hotline," onsite inspection of hospital records, etc.) were not authorized by section 504 of the Rehabilitation Act of 1973, "and that the regulations which purport to authorize a continuation of them are invalid."[310]

It must be admitted that if the U.S. Supreme Court had upheld the validity of the HHS regulations, disabled infants who need medically-indicated treatments would be given extensive protection. Much of what could not be accomplished by HHS regulations was accomplished by legislation. President Reagan signed the "Child Abuse Amendments of 1984," on October 9, 1984. The most significant paragraph of this legislation reads as follows (indentations added so as to emphasize appropriate distinctions):

> The term "withholding of medically indicated treatment" means
> the failure to respond to the infant's life-threatening conditions by
> providing treatment (including appropriate nutrition, hydration,
> and medication) which, in the treating physician's or physicians'

---

[309]Cf. Bowen v American Hospital Assn., in *United States Supreme Court Reports, Lawyer's Edition*, July 17, 1986, under "opinion of the court," pp. 592 ff. This discussion is, in part, a review of the "Discrimination against human life" section of chapter III.

[310]*Ibid.*, p. 610.

reasonable medical judgment, will be most likely to be effective in ameliorating or correcting all such conditions, except that the term does not include the failure to provide treatment (other than appropriate nutrition, hydration, or medication) to an infant when, in the treating physician's or physicians' reasonable medical judgment,

(A) the infant is chronically and irreversibly comatose;

(B) the provision of such treatment would (i) merely prolong dying, (ii) not be effective in ameliorating or correcting all of the infant's life-threatening conditions, or (iii) otherwise be futile in terms of the survival of the infant; or

(C) the provision of such treatment would be virtually futile in terms of the survival of the infant and the treatment itself under such circumstances would be inhumane.[311]

Three other features of this legislation are worthy of special mention: it establishes a new requirement for state participation in federal child abuse grant programs (including mechanisms for responding to instances of medical neglect of disabled infants, programs for appropriate coordination and consultation, authority to pursue legal remedies); it authorizes federal grants to states and to public or private nonprofit groups for information clearing houses, social services, etc.; it requires the secretary for Health and Human Services to issue regulations implementing all aspects of the law, including model guidelines to encourage the establishment of (hospital) committees for educational, advisory, and counseling purposes on the subject of handicapped infants.[312]

Interpretation of "Child Abuse Amendments of 1984"

The legislation clearly extends "child abuse" to the withholding of "medically indicated treatment" from disabled infants with life-threatening conditions. The phrase "life-threatening condition" is not defined, but as indicated in provision (B), the legislation would not apply to infants who are dying (i), nor to all cases of infants who are victims of more than one life-threatening condition (ii) (see below), nor to situations where treatment would serve no

---

[311]*Child Abuse Amendments of 1984,* Pub. L, No. 98-457, Oct. 9, 1984. Cf. Conference Report, Title I, Part B, Sec. 121, Section 3.

[312]*Ibid.,* Title I, Part B, Sec. 122 (3), Sec. 123 (2)(A), Sec. 124 (b)(1).

useful purpose (iii). The "more than one life-threatening condition" is explained as follows: "Under the definition, if a disabled infant suffers from more than one life-threatening condition, and, in the treating physician's or physicians' reasonable medical judgment, there is no effective treatment for one of those conditions, then that infant is not covered by the terms of the amendment (except with respect to appropriate nutrition, hydration, and medication) concerning the withholding of medically indicated treatment." It is logical to assume that "life-threatening condition" means simply "in some danger of death." That it is NOT restricted to "imminent death" is indicated in the "Joint Explanatory Statement" that the amendment "may include older infants (than one year) who have been continuously hospitalized since birth, who were born extremely prematurely or who have long-term disabilities."[313]

The legislation makes it very clear that "appropriate nutrition, hydration, and medication" may not be withheld even with regard to dying infants. Naturally this imperative is subject to the rule of "primum, non nocere" ("above all, cause no harm") which would apply if efforts at any of the "comfort measures" (nutrition, hydration, medication) could not be tendered without adding to the suffering of the infant. The phrase "reasonable medical judgment" is explained as "a medical judgment that would be made by a reasonably prudent physician, knowledgeable about the case and the treatment possibilities with respect to the medical conditions involved." The phrase "virtually futile" in section (C) apparently means "useless" or "worthless for all practical purposes" (as opposed to "absolutely futile"). The full sense of that final section (C), however, is stated as "virtually futile in terms of the survival of the infant and the treatment itself under such circumstances would be inhumane."[314] The inference seems to be: "it would be lacking in compassion if the treatment would lead to a mere tenuous survival" (see comment below).

Application of This Legislation to Actual Cases

Interpreted in the light of Catholic moral principles, the guidelines furnished by the *Child Abuse Amendments of 1984* can serve to vindicate the right to life and to life-saving treatments for developmentally-disadvantaged newborns. This category, includes not only approximately 130,000 infants born

---

[313]"Joint Explanatory Statement by Principal Sponsors of Compromise Amendment Regarding Services and Treatment for Disabled Infants," *Appendix, Congressional Record,* July 26, 1984, S9309-9310, p. 41.

[314]*Ibid.*

each year who have readily detectable congenital abnormalities, but also some 230,000 low-birth-rate infants (usually premature). Many of these infants have both a correctable life-threatening disorder or condition and a permanent, irremediable handicap that is not life-threatening such as mental retardation. A prime example is the Down Syndrome infant. A minority of Down Syndrome infants may have a life-threatening complication such as a gastro-intestinal blockage or a congenital heart defect. It is of prime importance to stress that section (B) (ii) of this legislation ("more than one life-threatening condition") must not be applied to infants with a mental retardation handicap. Mental retardation is not a life-threatening condition, and the infant is fully entitled to any treatment which might be effective in ameliorating or correcting an accompanying life-threatening condition. Diminished "quality of life" in no way diminishes the rights of the handicapped.

Developmentally-disadvantaged newborns might be divided into three groups. First, there are the many cases where treatment is not morally indicated except for "comfort care" (nutrition, hydration, medication). These are the infants who are born dying. The charming Baby Stephanie Fae of Barstow, Cal., was born dying on Oct. 12, 1984 (three weeks premature) with an incurable condition known as hypoplastic heart syndrome. She was transferred to the hospital at Loma Linda, Cal., the same day. According to an interview with the mother of this infant, the physician told her at Loma Linda the following day that Baby Fae was dying and that "there was nothing they could do for her."[315] There was every indication that the parents of the infant, Teresa and Howard, were not rushed or pressured into agreeing to the transplanting of a baboon heart as a means of saving the life of the infant. In fact, Dr. Leonard Bailey spent hours with Teresa and her mother—long into the night—to explain possible options (the two-stage Norwood procedure, a human heart transplant, an artificial heart). He even showed them slides of the Norwood procedure and told them that they could take the infant to Philadelphia for that procedure. The decision was left up to the parents. Howard, the father, emphasized this when he said: "They gave us all kinds of chances to back out of the whole thing—we could have stopped it right up to the time she was in surgery—but I can tell you I never once considered that."[316]

The distinguished Dr. Leonard T. Bailey and his colleagues made medical history on October 26, 1984, by implanting the heart of a healthy baboon in the chest cavity of Baby Fae. In view of the dying condition of the infant, this was the procedure of choice for Dr. Bailey and for the parents. Baby Fae succumbed to the odds and died 21 days later.

---

[315]*People Magazine,* Dec. 3, 1984, "Baby Fae: A Child Loved and Lost," p. 54.
[316]*Ibid.,* pp. 54 and 57.

A second group of developmentally-disadvantaged newborns have life-threatening conditions which clearly must be treated. Such was the case of Baby Doe of Bloomington, Ind. (1982) who was born with a handicap (NOT a life-threatening condition) and also a life-threatening esophageal blockage which prevented the intake of food and water. A frequently-performed surgical procedure would have removed the threat of death by starvation. The parents refused to consent to have the surgery done. Their decision was upheld by a circuit court judge, and eventually by the Indiana Supreme Court. Ostensibly because of her handicap (Down Syndrome), the infant was deprived of food and water and even of intravenous nourishment and hydration. She died within 6 days. It must be added, however, that civil courts rose to the defense of infants in similar situations: the Baby Houle case in Maine in 1974 (virtually identical to the Baby Doe case); the Chad Green case in Massachusetts in 1978 (victim of leukemia); the Cicero case in New York City in 1979 (victim of spina bifida).[317] In all three cases (as in the Baby Doe case), the infants were not born dying and the treatment was life-saving. If the treatments as medically indicated had been judged futile or useless "in terms of the survival of the infant," consent to such treatments would not have been obligatory either civilly or morally.

The third class of developmentally-disadvantaged newborns could challenge the wisdom of a Solomon. Due to the variety of life-threatening conditions (often multiple) and the uncertainty of the effectiveness of possible treatments, the recommendation of seeking the help of ethics committees or infant care review committees is amply justified. A case in point is that of Baby Jane Doe of New York. This infant was born on Oct. 11, 1983, with multiple birth defects including meningomyelocele or spina bifida (sometimes called "open spine") and a hydrocephalic condition (fluid on the brain). After adequate medical and spiritual consultation, the parents opted for conservative care of the infant (nutrition, hygiene, antibiotic treatment, etc.). They did not consider surgical repair of the spina bifida condition to be in the best interests of their infant at that time. A pro-life attorney, unrelated to the family, brought an action in state court seeking the appointment of a guardian for the infant so that the hospital could be directed to allow the surgery. The decision of the court in favor of the surgery was reversed by an appellate court the following day. The decision of the parents was upheld as founded on responsible medical authority and as representing the best interests of Baby Jane Doe. That decision later was affirmed by the highest court of the State of New York.

---

[317]Horan, Dennis, JD, and Grant, Edward R., JD, "Prolonging Life and Withdrawing Treatment: Legal Issues," in *Linacre Quarterly*, May, 1983, pp. 159–160.

To infer that the parents of Baby Jane Doe refused to consent to surgery for their child initially because of the infant's handicap ("quality of life considerations") would have been unfair. The reason for their initial refusal was because at that time, surgery presented serious risks and promised few benefits for the infant.[318] They did permit surgery in March, 1984, when a shunt was installed for her hydrocephalic condition. Her spinal lesion healed without need of surgery. On April 4, 1984, the happy parents took the infant home.[319] The infant also has appeared on national T.V. with her parents. This case provides an occasion to interpret section (B) (ii) of the Child Abuse Amendments of 1984. The morally-acceptable interpretation would have to be that the amendments would still apply (favoring treatment of the infant) if one or more life-threatening conditions could be *treated at a later date*. There must be many cases when ameliorating or corrective treatments would be opportune only after an infant had reached a certain age, or after another life-threatening condition had been corrected.

With all due praise for the Child Abuse Amendments of 1984, it must be admitted that they have substantial limitations. Those limitations are listed in an enlightening article in the September, 1985 issue of *Issues in Law and Medicine*. First, the five states which do not receive child abuse grants (Alaska, Arizona, Indiana, Oregon, Pennsylvania) need not comply with the Act and regulations; second, only child abuse agencies are authorized to bring an action to protect disabled infants in these circumstances (excluding the federal government and even the parents); third, the Child Abuse Amendments address only actions to protect a child then alive and in need of medical treatment (not if the child is dead or so debilitated by medical neglect that medical treatment is no longer beneficial); Finally, the Amendments deal with denial of treatment only on a case by case basis and are ineffective against an institutionally-adopted policy of discrimination.[320]

The Role of Ethics Committees and Infant Care Review Committees

The rules which justify the refusal of ethically extraordinary means for developmentally-disadvantaged children basically are the same as those which apply to adults. Due to the wide variety of possible congenital defects in

---

[318]Cf. a thoughtful analysis of this case entitled "Baby Jane Doe: The Ethical Issue," by John J. Conley, S.J., in *America*, Feb. 11, 1984, p. 86.

[319]*Linacre Quarterly*, Feb., 1985, p. 54; article by Dennis J. Horan and Burke J. Balch.

[320]Bopp, James, Jr., JD, and Balch, Thomas J., JD, "The Child Abuse Amendments of 1984 and Their Implementing Regulations: A Summary," in *Issues In Law and Medicine*, September, 1985, p. 130.

newborns (more than 3000) and the aggressive type of treatment which might be tried with parental approval, handicapped newborns naturally would receive a wider range of treatments which would rate as useless or futile as well as a wider range of increased burden cases (vs. anticipated benefits) both for the infant and for the family as represented by the proposed treatment (NOT for the original handicap). A newborn with spina bifida, for example, may also have a brain tumor which could respond to a treatment which would put the infant in a vegetative state for life. It would seem that this would be an example of what the Child Abuse Amendments of 1984 refer to as "futile in terms of the survival of the infant;" in other words, the question of "what kind of burden of survival?" following treatment must be kept in mind as a *humane* consideration.

This is mentioned as an illustration of the need of ethics committees and, with regard to developmentally-disadvantaged newborns, *Infant Care Review Committees* (ICRC's) as proposed by the federal government. The subject of such committees had to be introduced in chapter III on the Principle of the Right to Life (pp.113 ff.) and will come up for further discussion in chapter VII on the Principle of the Common Good. Presuming that the ICRC committee (in behalf of such newborns) can well be incorporated into the scope and purpose of the hospital ethics committee, it must be stressed that the recommendation of goals and policies based on the review of actual cases does not amount to decision-making. Particularly with regard to developmentally-disadvantaged newborns, decision-making rests with the parents of the infant. As proxies for such infants, they are exercising a right that belongs to the infant. They are not justified in denying treatment for such infants based on their own unwillingness to care for the handicapped infant, but based rather on what is in the best interests of the infant. It bears repeating, however, that there are limits to the burdens which the infant and even the parents and family members must bear in cases where the burdens far outweigh the benefits of a proposed treatment.[321]

3) The Level of Supportive Nursing Care (Comfort Measures)

Patients who require this level of care *only* usually are those who clearly are in a terminal condition or in an irreversible condition. With regard to their physical condition, attention is focused on eliminating pain and in assuring comfort to the highest degree possible. From the spiritual and psychological viewpoint, however, this final phase in the healing mission presents the

---

[321]Fleischman, Alan R., MD, and Murray, Thomas H., Ph.D, "Ethics Committees for Infants Doe ?," in *Hastings Center Report*, Dec., 1983, p. 9.

Catholic hospital with the grand opportunity to prove in tender, caring ways that catering to the "higher spiritual welfare" of every terminal patient is the "specialty of the house"—the distinguishing feature of a Catholic health facility.

Little "Martha" routines of on-the-dot pulse-taking, blood-pressure readings, lab returns, etc., can be tempered or even omitted in favor of "Mary" manifestations of hushed anticipation of the moment of truth and the hour of liberation. Freedom from *treatment* tubes and from testing and monitoring might even advance to the stage where the patient could be taken home to die amid familiar things and among loved ones as the "hospice movement" might propose. Whether at home or in the hospital, however, the treasures of the Catholic faith (Mass when possible, sacraments, crucifix, rosary, bible quotes, praying together, holding hands, etc.) must be used by the chaplain and pastoral-care personnel as well as by hospital workers and volunteers so as to project the expectation of the transfer to eternity and salvation of one of God's pilgrim people.

These are "Come, Lord Jesus" days (Revelation,22:20) for God's fervent people. Medical science should not be allowed to mar the dignity and sacredness of the occasion with unnecessary medical *treatments*. The fact is that 80% of Americans die in hospitals or in nursing homes. The truth is that Catholic teaching does not favor the pathetic and expensive prolongation of life by the marvels of medical *treatments* once the summons to eternity is clear and final. Again, to quote the Declaration of Euthanasia: "In our day it is very important at the moment of death to safeguard the dignity of the person and the Christian meaning of life, in the face of a technological approach to death that can easily be abused."[322]

Medical Treatment vs Supportive Nursing Care

The agonizing problem of withholding or withdrawing nutrition and hydration from a patient in a terminal condition or in an irreversible condition is less complicated if a distinction is made between *medical treatment* and *supportive nursing care*. The former would include artificial *substitutes* for irreversibly broken-down body functions such as kidney dialysis, respirator, installation of a mechanical heart, intravenous feeding when used as a substitute for a completely broken-down alimentary system, etc. Such *treatments* can be renounced "when death is imminent and cannot be prevented" because they can "only yield a precarious and painful prolongation of life" (cf.note 323). *Supportive nursing care* would include pain relief, hygiene, medication, as

---

[322] *The Pope Speaks,* 1980, p. 294.

well as hydration and nutrition. These cannot be renounced except to the extent that administering them is useless, or brings excessive pain or burden to the patient (that is, they have become ethically extraordinary means). This is an application of the "primum non nocere" guideline ("above all, cause no harm") which has special application to a patient who is in a terminal condition or in an irreversible condition (cf.definitions, pp.168,169).

It is noteworthy that the *Declaration of Euthanasia* (1980) in the Latin text uses the word "curationibus" (well translated into English as "healing" or "cure") when speaking of the *treatments* which a patient may renounce in good conscience in appropriate circumstances, but uses the word "ordinariis curis" ("carefulness, solicitude, attention") when speaking of the "ordinary *cares* due to the sick in such cases" which may not be interrupted.[323] The Latin derivation of the words "medicinus" and "medicus" from the Latin verb "medicare" ("to heal, cure") indicates that a *treatment or remedy* is designed to allay or cure the physical condition of the patient; whereas nursing *care* (concern, solicitude, attention) is not a remedy or treatment designed to heal or cure any particular disease, but rather something which every human person needs basically to support the struggle for human life. In support of his contention that nutrition "is not, in any strict sense, medical treatment, even if provided in a hospital," one contemporary author writes:

> It gives what all need to live; it is treatment of no particular disease; and its cessation means certain death, a death at which we can only be said to aim, whatever our motive.[324]

Writing well before the publication of the Holy See's *Declaration on Eutha-*

---

[323]The Latin text of this portion of the Declaration on Euthanasia reads as follows: "Semper licet satis habere communia *remedia,* quae ars medica suppeditare potest. Quapropter nemini obligatio imponenda est *genus curationis* adhibendi quod, etsi in usu jam est, adhuc tamen non caret periculo vel nimis est onerosum . . . . . Imminente morte, quae *remediis adhibitis* nullo modo impediri potest, licet ex conscientia consilium inire *curationibus renuntiandi,* quae nonnisi precariam et doloris plenam vitae dilationem afferre valent, haud intermissis tamen *ordinariis curis,* quae in similibus casibus *aegroto debentur"* (emphasis ours). Cf. *Enchiridion Vaticanum, vol. VII, Documenti Ufficiali Della Santa Sede 1980-1981* (Bologna: Edixioni Dehoniane, 1982), p. 348, nn. 370, 371. The same distinction between "treatment" and "care" clearly is made in the *Report of the Pontifical Academy of Sciences* on "The Artificial Prolongation of Life and the Exact Determination of the Moment of Death" as released by the Vatican on Oct. 30, 1985. Cf. The *St. Louis Review,* Nov. 8, 1985, p. 11; also found in *Origins,* Dec. 5, 1985, Vol. 15, p. 415.

[324]Meilaender, Gilbert, Professor of Religion at Oberlin College, "On Removing Food and Water: Against the Stream," in the *Hastings Center Report,* December, 1984, p. 13. Cf. also Meyers, David W., JD, LL.M., "Legal Aspects of Withdrawing Nourishment from an Incurably Ill Patient," who compares the *Barber* case (California) and the *Conroy* case (New Jersey), in *Archives of Internal Medicine,* Jan., 1985, pp. 127, 128.

nasia in 1980, Father Gerald Kelly, S.J. wrote two articles for *Theological Studies* on the subject of the duty to preserve life. Although the main focus in both articles concerned the right to renounce or refuse to submit to medical *treatments* or artificial *substitutes* for broken-down body functions, he also voiced his opinion with regard to providing nutrition and hydration—an opinion in harmony with the 1980 Declaration on Euthanasia. Using the word "treatment" in a broad sense, he wrote:

> Proper treatment certainly includes the use of all natural means of preserving life (food, drink, etc.), good nursing care, appropriate measures to relieve physical and mental pain, and the opportunity of preparing for death.[325]

He was saying, in effect, that receiving basic nutrition and hydration is an ethically *ordinary* means of preserving life which, as a general rule, cannot be denied to the sick. In the words of a contemporary theologian, the denial of such basic support would be "a *direct* killing of a person through the deliberate omission of an act which is obligatory, namely, to feed the person."[326] As emphasized in chapter IV on the Principle of Religious Freedom, no human individual has such a complete dominium over his body that he could say "let me starve to death" (IV,4.6); and no fellow human being is allowed to intervene in such a situation where the patient himself is devoid of such a right.

Whereas tube feeding can be regarded as supportive nursing care, however, intravenous feeding should be classified as medical *treatment* if it is used not as a supplement to tube feeding, but rather as a *substitute* for a broken-down alimentary system. In other words, if administrating nutrition through

---

[325]His articles appeared in the June, 1950, and December, 1951 issues of *Theological Studies,* pp. 203–220 and 550–556 respectively. The quotation appears in the latter article, p. 556, and is repeated in his book, *Medico-Moral Problems* (cf. note 22), p. 141.

[326]McFadden, Charles J., O.S.A., *The Dignity of Life* (cf. note 65), p. 150. Similar sentiments as to principle are found in the following: Ashley/O'Rourke, *Health Care Ethics* (cf. note 80), p. 388, n. 4 (These authors seem to have modified their opinion in their recent book entitled *Ethics of Health Care,* p. 203, as published by the Catholic Health Association, St. Louis, Mo., 1986); *To Treat or Not to Treat* (cf. note 267), p. 53; Callahan, Daniel, Director of the Hastings Center, "On Feeding the Dying," in the *Hastings Center Report,* October, 1983, p. 22; Lynn, Joanne, MD, and Childress, James F., Ph.D., "Must Patients Always be Given Food and Water?," *ibid.,* pp. 17–21. Two recent documentary sources which favor the administration of nutrition and hydration to patients who are in imminent danger of death, are the statement of the U.S. Bishops' Committee for Pro-Life Activities (cf. *Origins,* "The Rights of the Terminally Ill," Sept. 4, 1986, pp. 222–224) and the brief of the New Jersey State Catholic Conference (*Origins,* "Providing Food and Fluids to Severely Brain Damaged Patients," Jan. 22, 1987, pp. 582–584).

a gastrostomy or by nasogastric tube is impossible or has become totally ineffective, the recourse to intravenous feeding could be rejected by a competent patient who is in a terminal condition, or by one who has been designated to interpret the will of such a patient who is incompetent (or of a patient who is in a permanent irreversible condition). When the normal process of ingesting and digesting food is facilitated by means of tube feeding, the alimentary system as a system is impaired, but still in working order. Assisting or *facilitating* that process is within the range of supportive nursing care. Providing an artificial *substitute* for a broken-down alimentary system (known as "hyperalimentation") should be classified as a medical *treatment*.

Several excellent Catholic theologians insist that nutrition and hydration become a medical *treatment* if they are provided not by way of mouth, but by medical procedures. It is difficult for this writer to understand just how "what must be done" (feeding the patient) can be so readily canceled out by "how it is done." Both alternative procedures (nasogastric and by gastrostomy) have their disadvantages, but both are rated as relatively simple, tolerable and inexpensive procedures (comparable to oral feedings after installation). Although the latter (gastrostomy) involves minor surgery performed under local anesthesia, it is described as "quite comfortable for the patient once the incision for insertion is healed;" and both procedures are rated as "excellent" for efficacy in providing fluids and nutrition with a low cost factor. The "acceptability" factor for both patient and others is higher for a gastrostomy (which has a "good" rating) than for the nasogastric.[327]

Unacceptable Solutions From the Medical Community

An article entitled "The Physician's Responsibility Toward Hopelessly Ill Patients" appeared in the April 12, 1984, issue of *The New England Journal of Medicine* (sometimes referred to as the *Wanzer Report*). A footnote (p.955) explains that the report was formulated at a meeting of Sidney H. Wanzer, MD, and nine other physicians of prestigious medical institutions throughout the nation on October 28–30, 1982, under the auspices of the Society of the Right to Die.[328]

---

[327]Cf. article by David Major, MD, in *By No Extraordinary Means* (Bloomington, Ind.: Indiana University Press, 1986), Joanne Lynn, MD, ed., pp. 21–27).

[328]Cf. pp. 955–959. The declaration of the 7-member council on ethical and judicial affairs of the American Medical Association at their March, 1986, meeting in New Orleans, was of similar liberal proportions. They declared that it was "not unethical" to withdraw all life-prolonging measures, including "artificially or technologically supplied" food and water, from patients determined to be irreversibly comatose, "even if death is not imminent." Cf. *Time*, March 31, 1986, p. 60.

This report of Dr. Wanzer and his distinguished colleagues recommends the following procedures for three categories of *incompetent* patients (always, however, with due consideration for the patient's prior wishes and the "understanding and agreement of the family" as it may apply): (a) *Patients in a persistent vegetative state:* "it is morally justifiable to withhold antibiotics and artificial nutrition and hydration, as well as other forms of life-sustaining treatment, allowing the patient to die;" (b) *Severely and irreversibly demented patients:* "it is ethically permissible for the physician to withhold treatment that would serve mainly to prolong the dying process . . . If such a patient rejects food and water by mouth, it is ethically permissible to withhold nutrition and hydration artificially administered by vein or gastric tube. Spoon feeding should be continued if needed for comfort;" (c) *Elderly patients with permanent mild impairment of competence* (often "pleasantly senile"): "freedom from discomfort should be an overriding objective in the care of such a patient. If emergency resuscitation and intensive care are required, the physician should provide these measures sparingly . . ."[329]

The concern of these medical authorities to provide guidance in a very sensitive area of medical practice must be commended. Many of their recommendations, however, clash with basic Catholic moral standards. This is not surprising, since there is no evidence of the active participation of any experts in ethics or theology in the process of formulating the report. There are also reasons to suspect that "quality of life" figured prominently in their considerations. Patients who are severely and irreversibly demented, elderly patients of the "pleasantly senile" category and, in some cases, patients who are in a persistent vegetative state are not necessarily in a terminal illness. Their status as handicapped individuals in no way diminishes their right to appropriate care and treatment. Finally, these recommendations are a sample of what can be expected if attorney George P. Fletcher is right in saying that "doctors are in a position to fashion their own law to deal with cases of prolongation of life."[330] The fact that the project was undertaken under the auspices of the Society of the Right to Die validates the suspicion that at least some of the participants were motivated by a pro-euthanasia philosophy of life.

An Interpretation of "Primum Non Nocere"

As noted earlier in this chapter (cf.note 323), when death is imminent, the ordinary care which is due to the sick person (that is, supportive nursing

---

[329]*Ibid.* (Wanzer Report), p. 959.

[330]"Legal Aspects of the Decision Not to Prolong Life," in *Moral Problems and Medicine,* Samuel Gorovitz, ed. (Englewood Cliffs, N.J.: Prentice-Hall, Inc., 1976), p. 266.

care) may not be interrupted. Although the *Declaration on Euthanasia* (1980) does not expressly mention nutrition and hydration as among those "ordinary cares," the directive has been understood and interpreted quite universally as including nutrition and hydration. The recent report of the Pontifical Academy of Sciences on "The Artificial Prolongation of Life and the Exact Determination of Death," however, explicitly mentions "feeding" in their proposed medical guidelines: "If the patient is in permanent coma, irreversible as far as it is possible to predict, treatment is not required, but care, including feeding, must be provided."[331] Although this report has not as yet received the official approval of the Holy See, it does complement the *Declaration on Euthanasia* of 1980 to a remarkable degree.

When speaking of patients who are in imminent danger of death, two categories come to mind: those who are in a *terminal condition* with no reasonable medical possibility of survival, and those who are in an *irreversible condition* (permanently comatose or in a permanent vegetative state) with no reasonable medical possibility of survival (cf.definitions, pp.168,169). The latter category (irreversible condition) *might* also include persistent cases of the rare condition known as a "locked-in" state (consciousness without movement).[332] The teaching of the Church, as evidenced in the documents mentioned in the above paragraph, is that patients in either of these two categories, even when in imminent danger of death, must not be denied the supportive care of nutrition and hydration. It is in keeping with Catholic moral principles to add, "unless there is evidence that the administration of nutrition and hydration is practically useless, or that the administration of same is excessively painful or burdensome for the patient." The latter phrase is an application of the medical axiom "primum, non nocere."

It must be emphasized that difficult and disturbing cases such as that of Karen Quinlan, who lived nine years on tube feeding after the respirator had been removed, are comparatively rare. Such cases truly present an agonizing challenge to fidelity to traditional convictions with regard to human dignity in life and in dying. There is some consolation in saying "they are exceptional

---

[331]*St. Louis Review,* Nov. 8, 1985, p. 11. This report was published as "prepared for Pope John Paul II." Also found in *Origins,* Dec. 5, 1985, p. 415.

[332]Listed under "irreversible coma" in *Defining Death,* a report of the *President's Commission* (Washington D.C.: U.S. Gov. Printing Office, July, 1981), p. 87. The "locked in" syndrome, first described in medical literature less than 20 years ago, is not necessarily a hopeless condition. An article entitled "Who Speaks for the Patient With the Locked-in Syndrome?" in the Dec., 1985 issue of the *Hastings Center Report,* by Grant E. Steffen, MD and Cory Franklin, MD, pp. 13–15, describes a "locked-in" patient who was able to understand and to communicate (ineffectively, however) through eye movements. There are documented cases of such patients who later recovered. The authors present opposing views as to whether or not such a patient should be given vigorous life-sustaining treatment.

cases." It is safe to say, for example, that over 90 percent of all patients on respirators or ventilators receive life support in that manner for two weeks or less. Usually, within that brief period, the patient either recovers or dies. As to comatose or vegetative-state patients who are not on respirators but who are kept alive by tube feeding, their number is estimated at anywhere between 5000 and 10,000 throughout the nation.[333] It may seem harsh and even heartless to say that all patients, even those in imminent danger of death, who are being kept alive by mouth feeding or by tube feeding, may not renounce such supportive nursing care—or be denied the same if incompetent. There is a qualifying phrase, however, which makes such a moral standard intelligible, tolerable, and even consoling. That phrase is: "Provided that such supportive care does not become excessively painful or burdensome for the patient." In other words: "Above all, do no harm" ("Primum, non nocere").

Presumably this axiom, "primum, non nocere," can be traced back to the famous Hippocratic oath. Whether or not this oath was written by the celebrated physician whom Aristotle called "the Great Hippocrates" (born about 460 B.C.), it projects a standard of professional moral conduct which could be called Christian. A portion of that oath reads as follows:

> Into whatsoever houses I enter, I will enter to help the sick, and I
> will abstain from all intentional wrong-doing and harm, especially
> from abusing the bodies of man or woman, bond or free.[334]

Applying this axiom to supportive nursing care, the difficulty lies in knowing just when the administration of nutrition and hydration becomes excessively painful or burdensome to the patient. Another respected axiom must be mentioned: the administration of food and hydration also can be rejected or discontinued if it is practically useless (futile, without effect). This axiom is "nemo ad inutile tenetur" ("No one is bound to what is useless"). Obviously such very crucial judgments (useless, excessively painful or burdensome) are made by the physician in conjunction with the patient or proxy.

In the phrase "excessively painful or burdensome," the "painful" aspect would refer to the patient only. The "burdensome" aspect also refers primar-

---

[333]The case of Paul E. Brophy, a retired firefighter of Easton, Ma., claimed national attention from December, 1983 (when he failed to regain consciousness after surgery for a ruptured brain aneurysm) until his death on October 23, 1986—8 days after nutrition was discontinued pursuant to a 4–3 decision of the Massachusetts Supreme Judicial Court (Sept. 11, 1986). This decision reversed the decision of a lower court (Oct. 21, 1985) which had denied the request of Mrs. Brophy to discontinue artificial feeding. Cf. review of this case, *The Boston Globe*, Oct. 24, 1986, pp. 1 and 39.

[334]*Ethics in Medicine*, Stanley Joel Reiser et al., eds. (Cambridge, Ma.: The MIT Press, 1977), Introduction, p. 5.

ily to the patient. There is a limit, however, to how much burden others, such as concerned family members, can be expected to bear in extremely trying circumstances. This could apply especially in the home-care of severely and irreversibly demented patients in some circumstances. For the patient, the burden cannot be the burden of continued existence. It could be some excessively burdensome aspect of the supportive nutrition and hydration process itself. With regard to those who are responsible for the care of the patient, the burden could not be the burden of keeping the patient alive, but rather the burden of constant concern and vigilance in maintaining the supportive nutritive care (patient repeatedly pulling out the feeding tube, effectively resisting efforts to re-instate the process, etc.). Even severely psychotic patients can be brought under control, however, with a properly prescribed regimen of drugs and sedatives. The case is mentioned as an example of how a very rare situation of excessive burden might possibly develop.

The Church's teaching on nutrition and hydration is based on respect for human dignity. There can be an additional dividend, however, for persons who are in a terminal condition or irreversible condition but are not in imminent danger of death. With contemporary advances in medical technology, an illness considered terminal today, or a condition considered irreversible today, could become non-terminal and reversible with the passage of time. A competent patient who is terminal but not advanced in age might well wish the supportive nutrition and hydration process to be continued in the hopes of some discovery in the field of medicine. Such could be the attitude of a victim of the AIDS epidemic in his or her 30's or 40's who is determined to survive until a cure is discovered. Such could be the attitude of a young victim of advanced renal failure who has learned about the efforts of several medical centers throughout the nation to control renal disease through "individually tailored, low-protein diets and food supplements."[335]

As a logical basis for such expectations, such hopeful patients could be encouraged by the dramatic management of Hodgkin's Disease in the past decade, or the phenomenal advances in drug therapy in returning many seriously-afflicted victims of mental illness to a healthful future. Family members and health-care workers should be encouraged to feel that putting up with the burden and tedium of administering supportive care is a ministry of love which could amount to "buying time" for the physical or mental recovery of many patients.

---

[335]"Low Protein Diet for Kidney Patients," in *The Boston Globe*, Sept. 9, 1985, p. 42. In rare cases, this can also apply to comatose patients such as Sgt. David Mack of Minneapolis, Minnesota who regained consciousness after 22 months of coma, and testified that he had been aware of happenings around him for six months. Cf. *Minneapolis Tribune*, April 25, 1982, p.1.

In the following discussion of supportive nursing care with regard to various categories of patients, the presumption is (in all categories) that the patient is in *imminent danger of death,* and that a tube-feeding apparatus (naso-gastric or gastrostomic) had been installed before the patient arrived at that imminent-death status. The moral position taken is that it would be wrong to discontinue that tube-feeding process except on the basis of "primum, non nocere." There are many situations, however, where patients have not been subjected to a nutrition-hydration device right up to the time of diagnosis as being in imminent danger of death (still able to take sustenance by mouth, etc.). This is true of most situations where patients are being treated in their homes or in a modest hospice-type health facility which lacks adequate facilities for feeding by nasogastric tube or by the gastrostomy procedure. The legendary Mother Theresa of Calcutta, in her inspiring concern for the dying, must often forego the possibility of making such procedures available to the patients in her humble hospices. This introduces the question as to whether or not there is a moral obligation to provide patients who are in imminent danger of death with a nutrition apparatus (not previously pro-vided) even in health facilities which are equipped to provide such proce-dures.[336]

Presuming that the *conscious* patient who is in *imminent* danger of death is incapable of receiving nutrition by way of mouth, and presuming further-more that he had not been provided previously with a tube-feeding appa-ratus, that patient's very status as "in imminent danger of death," as a general rule, should militate *against* any efforts to install a tube-feeding system—and this on the basis of "above all, do no harm" (Primum, non nocere). The very process of installing and maintaining the system could be disproportionately painful and burdensome for a patient who is destined to die within the near future (two weeks or less). There could be exceptions—for example, a conscious patient in imminent danger of death who is well-sedated, and who is willing to sustain the added burden and pain which the procedure would involve.

If the patient in the scenario above (not previously intubated for nutri-tion) is permanently *unconscious,* such as those in a comatose or vegetative state, however, the excessive pain or pain factor would not be a significant consideration. Even in such cases of patients in imminent danger of death, however, the potential unfavorable consequences of the very process of install-ing tube-feeding at such a stage of human debility (for example, pneumonia

---

[336]For an extended discussion of the subject of "withholding" vs "withdrawing" treatments, cf. report of the *President's Commission* entitled *Deciding to Forego* (cf. note 215), pp. 73–77.

in the nasogastric procedure, infection in the gastrostomy procedure, etc.) would constitute arguments against the effectiveness of the procedure. "Primum non nocere." In these circumstances, the *usefulness* of the installation procedure would also have to be questioned. "Nemo ad inutile tenetur." The situation is quite different if the tube-feeding mechanism has been operative and effective previous to the "imminent danger of death" diagnosis. In tube-feeding previous to the "imminent danger of death" diagnosis, physicians undoubtedly encounter situations where the tube-feeding process is harmful or no longer effective. Authors Joanne Lynn and James Childress mention, for example, that terminal pulmonary edema, nausea, and mental confusion are more likely "when patients have been treated to maintain fluid and nutrition until close to the time of death."[337] If there is definite evidence to warrant such a medical judgment, there would be no moral objection to discontinuing the feeding process or to removing the apparatus. Precisely because the feeding and hydration process refers to *supportive nursing care* and not to *medical treatment,* however, this writer cannot share the view of those who would approve of withdrawing tube feeding on the basis of a decision to "let him or her die."[338]

If the withdrawal of the nutrition and/or hydration process is justified for patients who are in imminent danger of death, it is unfair to present the spectre of "dying of thirst or starvation" in gruesome tones. Oncologists have made giant strides in the past decade in perfecting pain-killing drugs and sleep-inducing medications.[339] In addition to pain relief, comfort measures such as proper hygiene, bed comfort, the "glucose drip" if the patient still has

---

[337]"Must Patients Always be Given Food and Water?," by Joanne Lynn, MD and James F. Childress, Ph.D., in the *Hastings Center Report,* Oct., 1983, p. 19. As examples of "futile treatment" in the effort to install or continue the intubation process, they mention: a patient with a severe clotting deficiency and a nearly total body burn; a patient with severe congestive heart failure who develops cancer of the stomach with a fistula that delivers food from the stomach to the colon without passing through the intestine and being absorbed; an infant with infarction of all but a small segment of bowel. *Ibid.,* p. 18.

[338]Cf. *Medical Ethics,* by Fathers Kevin D. O'Rourke, O.P., JCD, and Denis Brodeur, Ph.D. (St. Louis, Mo.: The Catholic Health Association, 1986), pp. 212–215. These authors state: "It seems then that tube feeding could be withdrawn from a patient when a decision has been made to let him or her die, because this is a life-support system rather than a comfort device." They would explain this as not "starving to death," but rather "dying of a malfunction of the digestive system and it is time to let nature take its course." *Ibid.,* pp. 213, 214.

[339]Veatch, Robert M., in *Death, Dying and the Biological Revolution* (New Haven, Conn.: Yale University Press, 1976) quotes several medical authorities to the effect that pain and suffering can be controlled in virtually every case by the administration of pain-killing drugs and sleep-inducing medications, p. 94. Directive 29 of the *Catholic Hospital Directives* allows the administration of such sedatives and analgesics to the dying "for the alleviation of pain when such a measure is judged necessary." Cf. Chapter III, p. 118.

a swallowing reflex, and above all, T.L.C. (tender loving care) must be continued. Sponging out the mouth and moistening the lips should also be continued.[340] The following quotation from the *Declaration on Euthanasia* is also a source of comfort to family members and loved ones of the patient:

> Many concordant testimonies persuade us that nature herself has taken steps to ease separations at the moment of death, which could be extremely bitter if they involved a person in good health.[341]

Various Categories of Patients in Imminent Danger of Death

The following categories are modeled after the ones listed in the *Wanzer Report* (cf.p.183) with appropriate comparative observations. It should be understood that, except for the application of the "primum, non nocere" guideline, the withdrawal of nutrition-hydration mechanisms from patients who are in imminent danger of death would also be immoral at any time before that diagnosis (imminent danger of death) has been made.

Competent patients in a terminal condition who are generally alert and conscious: Comfort care should include continued mechanical nutrition and hydration even if the patient is inclined to reject such ministrations. Neither intensive care, nor aggressive treatment, nor emergency resuscitation are indicated unless the patient insists upon one or the other of such ministrations and compliance with the request is medically feasible and warranted. Hence it is possible to agree with the following recommendation of the *Wanzer Report:*

> When the facilities provided by an acute-care hospital are not essential to the comfort and dignity of the dying patient, he or she should be moved to a more appropriate setting, if possible. Care at home or in a less regimented environment, such as a hospice, should be encouraged and facilitated.[342]

Attention to this recommendation would decrease dramatically the horrendous cost of maintaining such patients in a hospital setting. The continued

---

[340]Cf. Lynn and Childress (cf. note 337), p. 21, note 14.
[341]*The Pope Speaks,* 1980, p. 292.
[342]*The New England Journal of Medicine,* April 12, 1984, p. 958.

administration of nutrition and hydration by gastrostomy or nasogastric tube (if still effective) as well as the precisely-calculated administration of narcotics can be handled by a visiting nurse or by a properly-instructed member of the family. In most cases, the patient would be comforted by the prospect of living out his or her final days among loved ones and amid familiar faces and places.

Incompetent patients in a persistent vegetative condition: According to the *Wanzer Report,* it would be morally justifiable to withhold artificial nutrition and hydration, "allowing the patient to die," if the neocortex of the brain is largely and irreversibly destroyed ("although some brain-stem functions persist"), and if this neurologic condition has been established with a high degree of medical certainty and has been carefully documented. From the context of the report, it appears that this would apply also to *withdrawing* nutrition and hydration; that is, discontinuing the administration of food and water through the tube mechanism. Such a proposed standard is morally wrong. The patient is not brain dead, and is deserving of all of the comfort care which is due to a living human individual. This is clear from the Holy See's *Declaration on Euthanasia.* The unofficial 1985 report of the *Pontifical Academy of Sciences* is somewhat more specific:

> If the patient is in permanent coma, irreversible as far as it is possible to predict, treatment is not required, but care, including feeding, must be provided.[343]

There would be no question of an added *treatment* if there were indications that the tube-feeding mechanism was becoming ineffective, and the physician decided to *supplement* the failing system by adding a peripheral entry of nutrition intravenously (through a small needle). If the nutrition-hydration system became totally ineffective, however, there would be no obligation (as mentioned previously) to install a *substitute* nutrition-hydration intravenous system (hyperalimentation) whereby a special catheter is placed into one of the veins of the chest. This would be contraindicated not only because it exceeds the limits of supportive nursing care (actually is a *medical treatment*), but also on the basis of "primum, non nocere." Such an invasive intravenous procedure is not only risky, considering the state of debility of the patient, but also renders the patient vulnerable to infection and to technical errors.[344] It must be emphasized that in the event that the tube-feeding mechanism has to be discontinued, every effort must be made to respond to the hydration needs of patients who are in imminent danger of death (sip of water or the "glucose

---

[343] *The St. Louis Review,* November 8, 1985, p. 11
[344] Lynn and Childress (cf. note 337), p. 18.

drip" if possible, sponging out the mouth, etc.—cf. pp.188,189). Death by dehydration is more to be feared than death by starvation.

Severely and irreversibly psychotic or mentally-retarded patients: The statement of the *Wanzer Report* that "it is ethically permissible to withhold nutrition and hydration artificially administered by vein or gastric tube" if such patients reject food by mouth betrays "quality of life" considerations. There is no justification for discontinuing nutrition and hydration by gastrostomy or by nasogastric tube for such patients. If such patients simply refuse to accept food and drink by way of mouth, nutrition and hydration by means of the previously-installed gastrostomy or nasogastric tube would provide the only means of sustaining life.

It cannot be denied that the burden for the health-care worker or for the family members in attending to the nutrition and hydration needs of such a patient can be close to intolerable at times. Such patients may succeed in pulling out the feeding tube despite the restraints which are required to keep them from harming themselves. In most cases, the problem can be mitigated by requesting the attending physician to prescribe appropriate sedation. If such drug therapy is not successful, and the patient requires constant vigilance and monitoring, there is no choice but to have the patient transferred to a facility which is equipped especially for such patients.

Elderly patients with permanent mild impairment of competence: In saying that "Freedom from discomfort should be an overriding objective in the care of such a patient," the *Wanzer Report* implies that they should continue to receive nutrition and hydration. As noted above, however, that obligation to provide nutrition and hydration by mechanical means would cease (according to the *Wanzer Report*) if the patient becomes severely and irreversibly demented and rejects food and water by mouth. Again, "quality of life" considerations makes such a proposal contrary to Catholic moral standards.

For all patients who are in an irreversible condition due to terminal illness, permanently comatose, or in a permanent vegetative state, it is safe to say that *treatment* with antibiotics for an intercurrent illness is not recommended or obligatory once they are diagnosed as in imminent danger of death. If needed for comfort care, however, such ministrations should be continued. An example of such an "intercurrent" illness would be if such a patient developed pneumonia as a consequence of the prolonged regimen of nasogastric feeding. The answer and the reason for the answer is stated in the *Declaration on Euthanasia:* "When death is imminent and cannot be prevented by the remedies used, it is licit in conscience to decide to renounce treatments that can only yield a precarious and painful prolongation of life" (cf.note

323). The report of the *Pontifical Academy of Sciences* (1985) supplements the quotation above by stressing the obligation of administering all due *medical care* to a victim of such an intercurrent illness—*treatment* not required since there is no prospect of cure or recovery.[345]

Another important observation is appropriate with regard to the rather common contention that, as a general rule, dying patients are impervious to pain and the pangs of thirst and hunger especially if they are comatose. Undoubtedly this could be true in many cases, depending upon the nature of the illness and the extent to which sections of the brain may have been deprived of the very potential for functioning. To the extent that such a conclusion is based on a general presumption rather than clinical evidence, however, the withdrawal of nutrition and hydration would be a violation of human dignity. Furthermore, for patients who are not deeply unconscious, the mere fact that efforts are being continued to maintain nutrition and hydration (even, at times, against the will of the patient) is a precious comfort factor which should not be underestimated.

Priests, nurses and others who administer to the needs of dying patients can relate unusual incidents when the unconscious patient was considered to be incapable of hearing or of feeling pain,—patients who later returned to consciousness and told of pain they had experienced and conversations they had heard. With regard to semi-conscious patients, this writer will never forget an experience at the death bed of a grand lady who had been in the final stages of a terminal illness for several interminable weeks. Right after having received the Eucharist, she was given a sleeping pill and a few sips of cream to ease the swallowing process. Her last words were: "God, that was good." She expired just minutes later.

On the subject of the elderly who are not in poor health, a word must be said about the wisdom of *preventive* measures to protect them from premature senility and impaired competence. Senile deterioration can be due, in many cases, to psychological causes rather than somatic ones,—factors such as compulsory retirement, ineligibility for employment, rumors of curtailed benefits for the elderly and retired, etc.[346] It is especially important that the elderly be

---

[345]The same report of the *Pontifical Academy of Sciences* continues: "If some prospect of recovery is medically established, treatment is also required and pursued. If treatment may bring no benefit to the patient, it can be withdrawn, care being pursued." *St. Louis Review,* Nov. 8, 1985, p. 11.

[346]Rizzo, Dr. Carlo, article on "Geriatrics," in *Dictionary of Moral Theology,* Francesco Cardinal Roberti and Msgr. Pietro Palazzini, editors (Westminster, Maryland: The Newman Press, 1962), p. 536.

made to feel useful and needed in a family setting. Families in America are to be commended for "caring for their own" among the elderly. The problem is bound to increase, however, with the "graying of America." According to U.S. Census Bureau figures, the number of men and women 85 or older will double by the turn of the century (from 2.5 million or 1.1% of the population in 1982, to 5.1 million or 2.5% of the population in the year 2000). The problem is increased by the high incidence of incapacitating chronic conditions such as Alzheimer's Disease and various types of mental impairment.[347] The home front will be expected to respond to this challenge with even greater generosity.

5.4 CONSENT—EITHER IMPLIED OR REASONABLY PRESUMED

In the words of Pope Pius XII: "The doctor has only that power over the patient which the latter gives him, be it explicitly, or implicitly and tacitly."[348] Tacit or presumed consent is qualified in the *Hospital Directives* (n.1) as a "reasonably presumed" consent. If a victim of attempted suicide is brought to the hospital and refuses medical attention, it is reasonable to presume that, once restored to a stable condition, the individual would be grateful for the restorative procedures. If a psychiatric patient resists therapeutic procedures which are medically indicated, and the next of kin cannot be contacted in time, it is reasonable to presume consent in emergency situations. In fact, if the treatment is urgent and there are no other more acceptable but recommended alternative treatments to bring about the desired results, consent can be presumed in some cases even against the unreasonable objections of the next of kin.[349]

Medical procedures for individuals who are brought to the hospital in an unconscious state are also reasonable presumed-consent cases provided that such procedures are necessary and cannot be postponed until the person has regained consciousness. It also happens that a surgeon may see the critical need of more extensive surgery in the course of an operation. Usually there would be no time to contact the spouse, parents or proxy of the incompetent

---

[347] *Wall Street Journal*, July 30, 1984, pp. 1 and 10. The prediction for the year 2050 is that 16 million men and women will be 85 or over—some 5.2% of the population.

[348] Address to the First International Congress of Histopathology, Sept. 13, 1952, in *The Human Body* (cf. note 61), p. 198, n. 358.

[349] O'Donnell, Thomas J., S.J., *Medicine and Christian Morality* (cf. note 31), p. 44. He adds, however: "In such cases the physician should be careful that legal requirements are fulfilled."

patient. Consent can be presumed. The surgeon would have to proceed, however, on the basis of an interpretation of what the patient himself or herself would want him to do in the circumstances. Patients who are not psychiatric, but who are in such an advanced state of emotional anxiety and confusion as to be clearly unreasonable in opposing recommended procedures, can be considered to be temporarily incompetent. Unless the medical procedure is absolutely critical and cannot be postponed, however, the physician should contact the spouse, parents or proxy before proceeding with the treatment. Finally, there are situations when the objections of a competent patient seem unreasonable and unacceptable to the physician. He could enlist the help of next of kin (spouse, parents, etc.) or of close friends of the patient. If all efforts at persuasion fail to convince the patient, however, he would have no right to proceed with the treatment or procedure even in the event that the patient lost consciousness. He could withdraw from the case after having used his influence to have another physician assigned to the case.

The phrase "implied consent" refers to the propriety of submitting to customary diagnostic and therapeutic procedures as implied in the physician-patient relationship. The patient may not be familiar with some of the procedures, but can be presumed to know that his or her desire for medical attention must involve submitting to the "means to the end." The physician should be caring and patient in explaining procedures which are unfamiliar to the patient. If the patient expresses reasonable objections to certain procedures—for example, objections to too many x-rays—and the physician fails to convince him or her of the value or importance of the procedure, the decision of the patient must prevail. If the patient is a child, or an adult who is not fully competent, the spouse, parents or proxy should be brought into the decision-making process.

"Natural Death Acts,"—Living Wills

The State of California led the way in passing a "Natural Death Act." It was signed into law on Sept. 30, 1976. Similar legislation has been enacted in many other states and in the District of Columbia (37 as of March 6, 1986, when South Carolina enacted a "Death with Dignity" act). In the California law, an adult can sign a directive (co-signed by two witnesses) for a five-year period, stating (in part) as follows:

> If at any time I should have an incurable injury, disease, or illness
> certified to be a terminal condition by two physicians, and where
> the application of life-sustaining procedures would serve only to

artificially prolong the moment of my death and where my physician determines that my death is imminent whether or not life-sustaining procedures are utilized, I direct that such procedures be withheld or withdrawn, and that I be permitted to die naturally.[350]

As a mere re-reading of the paragraph above would indicate, such a declaration could justify many arbitrary decisions about treatment, and tilt the scales against the senile, the helpless, the very ill and the very aged. The physician would have a rather free hand after having confronted the patient with the chilling news: "we have decided that you are terminal and your living will now goes into effect!" The very concept of such a "natural death declaration" ignores the fact that many people think differently about the struggle for continued life when they are laid low by serious illness, than when they were in robust health. Often the determination to cling to life is significantly responsible for rescuing a very seriously ill patient from the ravages of suffering and disease. The "living will" can destroy the legitimate will to live which is endemic to all mankind.

Other objections to the "living will" concept is that physicians do not want such a "carte blanche" in their relationship with their patient,—that caring for the sick according to the letter of such a declaration is contrary to their solemn Hippocratic oath which stresses health, life and healing,—that such a declaration often ties the hands of a dedicated and innovative physician who is anxious to promote the best interests of the patient. It should be noted that the "living will" campaign is encouraged by the Society for the Right to Die, which is closely related to the Euthanasia Society and the Euthanasia Educational Council. As to the legal aspects of such a directive, attorney Dennis Horan has the following comment: "If anything . . . it adds officious burdens to the death bed, encumbers medical decisions with unnecessary additional consultations and creates, rather than clarifies, legal problems."[351] Futhermore, the state has no jurisdiction to grant the "right to die."

The reference here is to what is known as passive euthanasia, which might be defined as a voluntary *omission* of an ethically obligatory action which is designed to preserve the life of a person, but with the intention or desire of thus hastening the death of that person. The proponents of euthanasia insist that a terminal patient in an irreversible condition has a right to request such benign medical neglect as a "merciful release" from suffering, in

---

[350]"The 'Right to Die': Legislative and Judicial Developments," in *Linacre Quarterly*, Feb., 1979, p. 67.

[351]*Ibid.*, p. 57. Mr. Horan was referring specifically to the California "Natural Death Act."

the interests of "death with dignity." In the Catholic tradition, however, any removal of life-sustaining and life-prolonging measures (nutrition and hydration included) would be justifiable only if such measures are either useless or causing excessive pain or burden for the patient,—but not with the intention of hastening the death of the patient. If the euthanasia mentality prevails, it would be only a question of time before *active* euthanasia would be advocated; that is, allowing the physician to inject a bubble of air into the circulatory system or to administer a death-dealing drug at the request of the patient in order to provide an "easy death." This would be a flagrant violation of "Thou shall not kill."

A recommended alternative to a "living will," is the *Christian Affirmation of Life, A Statement on Terminal Illness* (1982 version) as proposed by the Catholic Health Association (4455 Woodson Rd., St. Louis, Mo., 63134), which incorporates Christian concepts of the value of suffering and the prospect of the reward of eternal life. It is addressed "To my family, friends, clergyman, physician and lawyer," and reads as follows

> Because of my Christian belief in the dignity of the human person and my eternal destiny in God, I ask that if I become terminally ill I be fully informed of the fact so that I can prepare myself emotionally and spiritually to die.
>
> I have a right to make my own decisions concerning treatment that might unduly prolong the dying process. If I become unable to make these decisions and have no reasonable expectation of recovery, then I request that no ethically extraordinary means be used to prolong my life but that my pain be alleviated if it becomes unbearable. ("Ethically extraordinary means" signifies treatment that does not offer a reasonable hope of benefit to me or that cannot be accomplished without excessive expense, pain, or other grave burden.) No means should be used with the intention of shortening my life, however.

5.5 FREEDOM FROM EXTERNAL PRESSURE

In consenting or in refusing consent, freedom is an essential element. If consent or refusal of consent is clouded by undue inducement or by any element of force, fraud, deceit, duress or other form of constraint or coercion, the patient cannot be in control of the decision process. The lack of freedom robs the patient of his or her ability to consider all of the pros and cons so as to make it a valid decision.

It is the physician above all who provides the information, the explanations, the risks, the alternatives, so that the patient can evaluate the benefits and the burdens in arriving at that free act of choice. The difficulty of crossing the fine line between proper professional influence and even an unintentional posture of undue pressure or subtle duress is somewhat inherent in a confidential patient-physician relationship. If the physician is unduly comprehensive in listing all of the possible risks associated with a treatment, for example, he could be contributing to an improper decision by playing on the patient's fears. Some patients are fortunate in having such an open, friendly and confidential relationship with the physician that they can feel free to discuss not only their fears and misapprehensions, but also non-medical matters such as cost, home conditions, etc. The danger of abusing that confidence must be kept in mind. Frankly expressing his opinion in matters both medical and non-medical is commendable; using his position of authority and confidence to sway or manipulate the sentiments of the patient or of family members could constitute undue pressure.

A conscientious physician will keep in mind certain factors endemic to his professional background which should make him cautious in his advisory role: the professional tendency to want to do more, not less, for the patient; the lack of any guarantee of infallibility in diagnosis and prognosis; the influence of fear of legal liability in prescribing appropriate treatments and procedures; the tendency to equate the limitation of a patient's recovery with professional failure; undue consideration of the monetary costs to society in the use of scarce treatment resources for the hopelessly ill, etc.[352] Unfortunate personality traits can also mar the physician-patient relationship. If the physician is inclined to show resentment if his recommendation for treatment is questioned by the patient, for example, the patient may be reluctant to ask questions or to seek the advice of others.

The vast majority of physicians are dedicated to high professional ideals. Contemporary surveys indicate, however, that the caution "patient be wary" ("caveat aegrotus") can apply to all professions. In his book *Aborting America,* Dr. Bernard Nathanson has scathing remarks for many of his fellow gynecologists in misrepresenting facts and figures, and even in inventing reasons for recommending abortions.[353] The advisory role of the physician is enhanced if he has taken the time to develop a confidential bond of open, frank and

---

[352]Cf. Wanzer Report, *The New England Journal of Medicine,* April 12, 1984, pp. 956, 957.
[353]*Aborting America* (cf. note 115), pp. 39–41.

friendly communication with the patient. He cannot afford to forget that when it comes to the final decision with regard to medical treatment, the patient must remain firmly secured in the driver's seat.

Influence of Spouses, Parents, Family Members

The role of proxies and guardians will be discussed in the final section of this chapter. Since they represent the interests of incompetent patients, their potential weakness is not in exercising an undue influence over the patient, but rather in forgetting that they are obligated to decide as the patient himself or herself would decide if competent.

Spouses and family members can exert undue pressure on patients particularly with regard to initiating or withdrawing extraordinary means. How can an elderly husband make his own choice to discontinue an expensive, long-standing regimen of renal dialysis (with no hope of recovery or of obtaining a kidney transplant) if his devoted wife keeps crying and saying "How can I get along without you?" How can an elderly wife prevail in her desire to submit to a very complicated cardiac bypass operation if the husband says: "You know, of course, that if the operation fails, I cannot take care of you," or "How could I afford a decent nursing home for you?" In too many cases, complaints of married children ("We have our own families to support!") have influenced a loving, widowed mother to refuse consent to a serious but potentially life-saving operation.

If their children are minors, the parents as guardians are obligated to decide as the child himself or herself would decide. Otherwise, they are deciding against the best interests of their children. As Father John Connery, S.J. wrote, parents do not have the right to "determine a child's lifespan."[354]

5.6   ADEQUATE INFORMATION

Informed consent to spiritual ministrations was discussed adequately in previous chapters. The focus here is on the third prerequisite for valid, informed consent (in addition to competency and freedom from coercion) which is adequate information, intelligibly communicated to the patient. As mentioned above, a full recital of all of the possible risks involved in a medical procedure could restrict freedom of consent. Ordinarily it should suffice to

---

[354]"Prolonging Life: The Duty and its Limits," in *Moral Responsibility in Prolonging Life Decisions* (cf. note 283), p. 135.

mention only the possible risks which are substantial and probable. A person can enter a valid marriage contract without being informed of all of the significant risks to marital happiness. In the physician-patient relationship, the conscientious physician is faced with a variety of challenging questions: How much should I tell?; when is the patient capable of both absorbing and understanding the information? Can the information be given without destroying all hope?; what if I am morally certain that the illness is fatal? There are no pat answers to such questions in particular cases. It should be possible, however, to establish certain parameters of response.

How much to tell? It is unfair to the patient to provide merely a litany of medical facts, risks and options without a realistic assessment of the alternative courses of giving or of withholding consent. The emotional and psychological state of the patient must be kept in mind. Usually, the anxiety over the suspected and the unknown is more difficult to handle than the anguish of knowing the truth. Many patients are expressing that conviction when they say "Give it to me straight, Doc." A comprehensive explanation of the various alternatives of treatment is not required. As mentioned above, substantial and probable risks should be mentioned and explained. The patient's right (and duty) to make choices about the type of care or treatment must be emphasized. The manner of communication must conform to the patient's educational level, and create an atmosphere favorable to asking questions.

When is the patient able to "take it?" A bit of light conversation before communicating a definite diagnosis or prognosis often can establish whether or not the patient is "open" to the message—that is, able to both absorb and understand the information. A definite diagnosis or prognosis should not be given, of course, until all facts and test results have been assembled and evaluated (with professional consultation if necessary). It is far better to communicate such information earlier in the illness (if at all possible) rather than later on when the patient has been debilitated by the illness. The question "What should I do, Doctor?" must be handled with caution, and with a kind reminder that "the final decision must be your very own." It is also of prime importance that the patient must be made to feel free to seek a second opinion.

Can the information be given without destroying all hope? The reminder that "while there is life, there is hope," can defuse irrational fears. Even if the illness definitely is terminal in nature, the word "terminal" often can be explained as still offering a considerable lease on life (slow-growing prostate cancer, for example). Hope can be nursed also on the possibility of a timely medical breakthrough (advances in the treatment of Hotchkin's Disease, for example). A positive attitude enhances any treatment process—diagnosis and prognosis often have turned out to be wrong. A second opinion is often a proper course of action. In even the most hopeless situations, a patient with high spiritual values and ideals can be motivated to leave the matter in the hands of God.

What if the illness definitely is fatal in the sense of "so many weeks or months to live?" The Catholic position is that the physician is obligated to inform the patient at the appropriate time either personally or through another. The obligation is mitigated somewhat time-wise if there is definite evidence that the patient is well prepared for death both as to spiritual and temporal obligations. This obligation to inform the patient of the approach of death is based on the right of every patient to know the truth so as to prepare for the solemn moment of death. In many cases, the physician approaches this obligation with trepidation, and is relieved to find out that the patient has already "figured it out" for himself or herself.

The information that death is near should be given, if at all possible, before the physician judges that death is imminent. At the same time, he should communicate the information to family members so that the chaplain or pastor of the patient can be called in to administer the sacrament of the anointing of the sick and Viaticum. Father Edwin Healy, S.J. mentions that the obligation of the physician to inform the patient of the approach of death (which binds in charity) would not exist in the following circumstances: if it is entirely unnecessary (for example, the patient is well aware of his condition); if the warning would prove useless (because the patient would ignore it completely); if the warning would prove harmful because it would deeply disturb a patient who is already well prepared to die, or would drive the patient to despair or risk his committing suicide.[355] In the last two instances (harmful to patient; lead patient to despair), the physician should tell the hospital chaplain and the near-relatives of the patient of his decision NOT to inform the patient so that they might devise a proper approach to informing the patient. Father Felix Cappello, S.J. insists that the physician would still be bound by the obligation to inform the patient of the approach of death if others do not want to do so, or if they are not able to do so, or if the patient simply would believe no one but the physician. He would also recommend such cases (no one willing or able to inform the patient who has not as yet received the last rites) to the kindness of the pastor or confessor (or chaplain) who could do it in a manner which would not disturb the patient, but rather inspire "comfort and the greatest confidence."[356] Surely no dedicated chaplain or priest would turn down a physician who approached him with such a request.

---

[355]*Medical Ethics* (cf. note 46), pp. 378, 379.

[356]*De Sacramentis*, III, 4th. ed. (Rome, Italy: Marietti, 1944), n. 279.

> *Directive 8:* Everyone has the right and the duty to prepare for the solemn moment of death. Unless it is clear, therefore, that a dying patient is already well-prepared for death as regards both spiritual and temporal affairs, it is the physician's duty to inform him of his critical condition or to have some other responsible person impart this information.

5.7 INCOMPETENT PATIENTS

The role of parents in using their "authority to act for" or become proxies for minor children who are patients, and of a spouse in doing likewise for an incompetent husband or wife has been referred to frequently throughout this chapter. In other cases, a competent person may designate someone to speak and act in his or her behalf in the event of incompetency; and necessity sometimes requires that a proxy be appointed by a civil court. Whatever the term may be (sometimes also called a "surrogate"), these individuals must remember that they exercise a right which belongs to the patient. They are obligated to make decisions based on what the patient may have expressed as his or her personal wishes or, in absence of such directives, based on their honest interpretation of how the patient would decide if he or she were still competent. This presumes some degree of closeness and familiarity with the patient as a basis for such an interpretation. This presents no special problem when the proxy designated by the competent patient is a close relative or friend. To the extent that such an interpretation is less likely (parents deciding for small children, for example), they must decide on the basis of what they have reasons to consider to be the best interests of the patient.

In the same illness, the patient may be competent at certain times (and speak for himself or herself), and doubtfully competent or incompetent at other times. Caution is required. The mere fact that a patient who is terminal and incurable may refuse life-sustaining treatment is not, in itself, a reason for questioning that patient's competency. If there are additional reasons for questioning the competency of such an individual, however, it may be necessary to decide the issue of competency by consulting with the physician, family members, close friends and, if necessary, a psychiatrist. Anything close to unanimity among such resource persons should settle the issue (competent or incompetent). Competency can be reduced by the illness, prolonged or intensive pain, administration of drugs, etc. In such situations, the presence of a patient-directive while competent such as a "Christian Affirmation of Life" or similar document can be a source of relief to the physician (cf.5.4).

Father John Connery, S.J. mentions the possibility that the physician may suspect that the patient's signature on the consent form does not really represent an understanding and acceptance of the treatment. He suggests that if recourse to a proxy would not solve the issue, the physician himself might have to act as proxy as a means of guaranteeing the best interests of the patient.[357] Another alternative for the physician (when no proxy has been designated) would be to attempt to learn of the attitudes and wishes of the incompetent patient by consulting with family members and close friends of the patient. If the known wishes of the patient cannot be ascertained in this manner, the physician may have to proceed on the basis of what he knows to be the reasonable wishes of the patient as communicated to him in the physician-patient relationship. If the physician is practically a stranger to the patient, however, consultation with a professional colleague would be advisable. This may give him the assurance that his own judgment of the best interests of the patient is not being obscured by his own prejudgment of the best treatment.

Since the usual power of attorney, whereby a person can designate someone else to act in his or her behalf, becomes inoperative when that person (the principal) becomes incapacitated or incompetent, it is important to find out whether or not the state wherein the health facility is located has legislated *durable* powers of attorney. Durable powers of attorney are effective even after the person has lost competence. Over 40 states in the U.S.A. have passed such legislation.

In order to assure the effectiveness of this type of "advance directive" (appointment of a proxy with durable powers of attorney), and especially if the person chosen as proxy is not a natural choice such as a spouse, parent, or close relative, several important factors must be given consideration: to specify just when the directive takes effect (for example, only after a definite diagnosis has been made, or, only when the patient is designated as "terminal," etc.); to avoid the appointment of individuals, especially non-family members, who may have a conflict-of-interest problem (in line for a substantial inheritance, has borrowed a substantial amount from the patient, patient owes him a substantial amount, etc.); to insist on a discussion with the physician or other health-care professional regarding the patient's condition as well as a discussion with the patient (if competent) to learn of his or her wishes, goals, and values; to specify that the directive is to be renewed periodically

---

[357]"Patients' Informed Consent Requires Understanding of Treatment Risks" in *Hospital Progress*, May, 1984, p. 40.

(every few years, or every few months, depending upon the principal's state of health).[358] Naturally, when the principal (patient or patient-to-be) is competent, he or she makes the decisions.

The question as to whether or not the proxy should have access to the medical records may pose some problems. On the one hand, it is somewhat of an invasion of privacy. If the proxy is a close relative or close friend, however, the principal is more likely to agree to the requirement. If it is likely that the proxy may not be available when needed, the directive might specify another to act in the principal's interest during such periods—or even empower the proxy to designate such a substitute. The directive should also specify just how and when the directive might be revoked—presuming that it can be done so that the principal, if incompetent, is not abandoned without a proxy. If it should happen that the patient, when incompetent, countermands or changes earlier competent directives, the matter may have to be submitted to some type of independent review. In extreme cases, this may well involve judicial proceedings.

> *Directive 1: The procedures listed in these Directives* as permissible require the consent, at least implied or reasonably presumed, of the patient or his guardians. This condition is to be understood in all cases.

---

[358]*Deciding to Forego Life-Sustaining Treatment* (cf. note 215), pp. 149–153.

CHAPTER VI

The Principles of Integrity and Totality

This article n.61 of *The Church Today* consists of an appeal for the whole human person, which demands a balanced development of the various human faculties in accordance with a just hierarchy of values, permitting both the enrichment of knowledge and the integration of this increased information in a unifying process which brings a personal growth and true cultivation (*Commentary on the Documents of Vatican II*, V, p.275).

PRINCIPLES: "INTEGRITY" REFERS TO EACH INDIVIDUAL'S DUTY TO "PRESERVE A VIEW OF THE WHOLE HUMAN PERSON . . . IN WHICH THE VALUES OF INTELLECT, WILL, CONSCIENCE, AND FRATERNITY ARE PRE-EMINENT" (*The Church Today*, n.61). "*TOTALITY*" REFERS TO THE DUTY TO PRESERVE INTACT THE PHYSICAL COMPONENT OF THAT INTEGRATED WHOLE, WHEREBY, IN THE WORDS OF ST. THOMAS AQUINAS, EVERY MEMBER OF THE HUMAN BODY "EXISTS FOR THE SAKE OF THE WHOLE AS THE IMPERFECT FOR THE SAKE OF THE PERFECT. HENCE A MEMBER OF THE HUMAN BODY IS TO BE DISPOSED OF ACCORDING AS IT MAY PROFIT THE WHOLE. . . . IF . . . A MEMBER IS HEALTHY AND CONTINUING

IN ITS NATURAL STATE, IT CANNOT BE CUT OFF TO THE DET-
RIMENT OF THE WHOLE" (II-II, q.65, art.1, corp.)

The Principle of Integrity and the Principle of Totality, as two interpene-
trating and interdependent aspects of total personhood, should be viewed as
complementary. The latter contributes to the realization of the former as a
means to an ultimate common end, which, in the Christian value system, is
summarized by the Lord Jesus as "Thy kingdom come, thy will be done."
Although the immediate end or purpose of preserving health traditionally has
been confined to physical well-being (totality), it is oriented, by God's will
and plan, to the ultimate end of human integrity. For this reason, the Principle of Totality is oriented, indirectly, to respect for the "values of intellect,
will, conscience, and fraternity" which are considered preeminent (text
above) in the pursuit of human integrity.

Human birth and human life is the basis for all other human rights and
obligations. Even on the purely human level, there is wisdom in the saying:
"oportet primo vivere, deinde philosophari" (rough translation: "attention to
physical well-being comes first—then, the pursuit of your goal in life"). St.
Francis of Assisi was realistic when he referred to his body as "brother ass,"
and thereby inferred the basic importance of the subservience of a healthy,
disciplined body (totality) to the higher goals of life (integrity). St. Paul emphasized a similar challenge when he said: "What I do is discipline my own
body and master it, for fear that after having preached to others I myself
should be rejected" (I Cor.,9:27). This is not to infer that "discipline" and
"mastery of the body" falls directly within the province of totality, but rather
that the pursuit of such ideals presupposes at least a modicum of physical
well-being.

The point is that the pursuit of the high, coordinating goals of human life
is rendered far more difficult (integrity) if there is a lack of coordination in
the physical functioning of the individual. The sad fact that many individuals
are at a disadvantage through no fault of their own (handicapped, in poor
health, denied the basics of life, etc.) only emphasizes the importance of
preserving the possibilities of physical well-being which are at hand. To the
degree possible to each individual, the saying "mens sana in corpore sano"
("a healthy mind in a healthy body") presents a challenge which cannot be
rejected if the duty to "preserve a view of the whole human person" is to be
fulfilled in the pursuit of the higher goals of life.

One thoughtful analysis of the interpenetration of the Principles of Integrity and Totality insists that the subordination of the lower functions to higher
functions must exclude the total sacrifice of any of the lower functions either
within the limits of personhood or by any means external to personhood. As

an example, the ability to produce babies in test tubes or "in vitro" "does not of itself justify the elimination of the reproductive power of human persons as no longer necessary."[359] The will and plan of the Creator as stamped on the purpose, finality and interdependence of each human function, is an indication that the pursuit and perfection of human integrity in keeping with human dignity must be done "humano modo" (in a "human way"). This is the working capital for salvation, the matrix of human perfection, which must be "transformed" by the renewal of the human mind and offered "as a living sacrifice holy and acceptable to God, your spiritual worship" (Romans,12:1–2).

6.1   THE PRINCIPLE OF INTEGRITY AND THE WHOLE HUMAN PERSON

Pope Pius XII's views on the Principle of Totality will be discussed later. In his address to the *First International Congress of Histopathology* on Sept. 13, 1952, he referred to *integrity* as follows: "For man, and for the Christian, there exists a law of integrity and personal purity, of personal esteem for himself, which forbids him to plunge himself thus wholly into the world of sexual representations and tendencies. The 'medical and psychotherapeutical interests of the patient' find here a moral limit."[360] The reference to unrestricted medical research and techniques in the "world of sexual representations and tendencies" is but one example of moral frontiers which medical science may not transgress even in the interests of the patient. Ethical considerations must be taken into account:

> Here, well-defined frontiers present themselves which even medical science cannot transgress without violating higher moral values. The relationship of confidence between doctor and patient, the right of the patient to life, physical and spiritual, and its psychic or moral integrity—here, amongst others, are values which rule scientific interests.[361]

The Holy Father's emphasis on the "interests of the patient" could well serve as a source of the quotation from Vatican II's *The Church Today* (above): to preserve a "whole human person" view of intellectual ("intellect"), moral

---

[359]Ashley-O'Rourke, *Health Care Ethics* (cf. note 80), p. 42.
[360]*The Human Body* (cf. note 61), p. 200.
[361]*Ibid.*, p. 197.

("will, conscience"), social ("fraternity") and spiritual values. The "spiritual" is stressed in the text of article 61 of *The Church Today* as referred to above (Principle), which continues as follows: "These values are all rooted in God the Creator and have been wonderfully restored and elevated in Christ."[362]

It is right and proper to conceive high expectations of the medical profession, and to inquire as to just how far mankind might go in expecting medical science and technology to facilitate the pursuit of human integrity. Again in the words of Pope Pius XII, members of the medical profession face a stimulating challenge in this regard:

> What does the doctor do who is worthy of his vocation? He takes command of these forces [he mentions the curing power of radioactivity, the ability to turn poisons into healing agents, the use of deadly germs to prepare serums], these natural qualities, to employ them for purposes of healing, to give health and strength, and what is still more worthwhile, to preserve men from sickness and contagion and epidemics.[363]

Today, with laser technology, computerized equipment, fiberoptics, the wonders of microsurgery, etc., the professional arsenal of the medical world has been expanded beyond expectations. Leaving aside for now the medical profession's ability to correct, repair, cure and heal, it might be well to focus attention on that "still more worthwhile" ability,—that is, "to preserve men from sickness and contagion and epidemics." The focus is on preventive medicine.

Integrity and Preventive Medicine

The *President's Commission for the Study of Ethical Problems in Medicine and Biomedical and Behavioral Research* (referred to throughout this book as *President's Commission*) was created by an act of Congress during the presidency of Jimmy Carter in 1978 to "study the ethical and legal implications of problems in medical practice and research." It was not empowered to regulate or to enforce, but exercised a wholesome power of persuasion so as to raise the consciousness of the nation to the urgent need of using the fantastic growth in medical technology more humanely and effectively in response to expanding

---

[362]Abbott, Walter, S.J., *The Documents of Vatican II* (cf. note 50), p. 267.

[363]Address to the Fourth International Congress of Catholic Doctors, Sept. 29, 1949, *The Human Body* (cf. note 61), p. 117.

medical needs.[364] If, in the effort to meet every possible medical challenge, the aggressive use of advanced medical technology (which is the only controllable factor in the interests of "cost containment," cf. chapter II, p.63), could be tempered, and channelled instead to reach the maximum number of prospective victims of the more widespread afflictions of mankind (heart disease, cancer, malaria, cholera, malnutrition, etc.), emphasis on aggressive preventive medicine would be seen as a national priority. As a consequence, physicians would be on the forefront of health education as a natural prelude to a better world.

It is said that some of the populous developing nations such as China do a creditable job of meeting the medical needs of their citizens by training and dispatching a veritable army of nurses and medical technicians (for lack of physicians) to visit hundreds of towns and hamlets to attend to the common ills and diseases of the citizens and to instruct them in the basic principles of avoiding illnesses, diseases, contagion and epidemics.[365] Since even a nation as wealthy and resourceful as America cannot guarantee all the medical care that may be needed to everyone who is in need, a more vigorous national program of promoting health through health education and the promotion of preventive-medicine programs should be given top priority. "Health education" may be defined as follows:

> The ultimate goal of health education is the improvement of the nation's health, and the reduction of preventable illness, disability, and death . . . Health education is that dimension of health care that is concerned with influencing behavioral factors and is therefore complementary to those components of health care that are concerned more with the organic factors of health and disease. As such, health education is a vital and indispensable component of health care delivery in which virtually all health care professions must be involved.[366]

Basic to effective health education is the one-to-one relationship between the physician and the patient. Unfortunately, this line of communication is

---

[364]Abram, Morris B., JD, LL.D, and Wolf, Susan M., JD, "Public Involvement in Medical Ethics," in *The New England Journal of Medicine*, March 8, 1984, pp. 627 and 629. The original 11 commissioners were appointed by President Carter, but by the time the commission terminated its work in 1983, 8 of the 11 members were appointees of President Reagan. *Ibid.*, pp. 629, 630.

[365]Fox, Stephen, MD, "China: Dairy of a Barefoot Bioethicist," in *The Hastings Center Report*, Dec., 1984, pp. 18–20.

[366]Somers, Anne R., ed., *Promoting Health* (Germantown, Md.: Aspen Systems Corp., 1976), p. 105. The author of the above definition is Dr. S.K. Simons.

open only after symptoms of illness have appeared and the individual "goes to the doctor." Physicians should lead the way in using their professional influence to initiate and encourage school health programs, occupational health and safety programs in commerce and industry, community health projects, national health programs such as the excellent work of the American Heart Association, media participation in making citizens health-conscious, etc. Progress in preventive dentistry has been nothing less than spectacular.[367]

Much remains to be done to prepare students of medicine for effective leadership in health education. With regard to undergraduate requirements for entry into one of the 126 medical schools in America (1982–1983 figures), only 11% of the schools required courses in the humanities, only 9% required courses in behavioral science, and only 8% required courses in social science. In the curriculum directory of medical schools (1981–1982 figures), courses are offered in subjects on the general area of behavioral and social science such as courses in community medicine, death and dying, ethical problems in medicine, health care delivery, and patient education, but only on an *elective* basis. Members of the medical profession admit this deficiency in medical schools: "Medical schools generally do not teach the skills necessary for the practice of health promotion. Concepts of risk assessment, behavior change, exercise physiology, and nutrition are visibly absent from medical school curricula."[368]

The basic task is not only information but motivation—to motivate the citizens of American communities to assume responsibility for their own health and to want to change to more healthful life styles. "Health education" as a special objective could be traced back either to 1919 when the term was first used at a conference of the Child Health Association, or to 1921 when the first graduate fellowship was awarded for study in health education.[369] Progress over the past 65 years has been moderate at best. The efforts at health education must be vigorous, for the obstacles are many: unfavorable social conditions, economic restraints, environmental problems, resistance to change, apathy, etc.

As an illustration of the rich dividends of preventive medicine, the Jan., 1984 report of an extensive study of the National Heart, Lung and Blood

---

[367]One Chicago dentist with 40 years experience in the practice of dentistry is quoted as follows: "We are one of the few professions in history that has done everything in its power to put itself out of business." Cf. *Time*, Sept. 9, 1985, p. 73.

[368]Dismuke, S. Edwards, MD, and Miller, Stephen T., MD, "Why Not Share the Secrets of Good Health?," in *Journal of the American Medical Association*, June 17, 1983, p. 3182. For information on actual course requirements, cf. *Making Health Care Decisions*, a publication of the *President's Commission* (Washington D.C.: U.S. Gov. Printing Office, 1982), p. 131, note 6, and p. 141.

[369]Somers, Anne R., *Promoting Health* (cf. note 366), p. 106.

Institute is deserving of special mention. This $155 million study of the connection between heart disease (the nation's No. 1 killer) and high cholesterol levels tracked the incidence of heart disease in 3,806 men (ages 35–59) over a period of seven to ten years. None of these men had overt signs of heart disease when recruited for the study. All had abnormally high cholesterol levels. All of the men were put on a low-cholesterol diet (limiting the intake of fatty meat, eggs and dairy products), and realized a reduction of their cholesterol level by 4%. More significant results emerged from another part of the study, however, in which half of the men were treated with cholestyramine (a powerful drug which lowers cholesterol) and the other half received a placebo (an inactive substance—not a medication). Those on the low-cholesterol diet who had received the drug experienced a drop of from 18% to 25% in their cholesterol levels. They also had 20% fewer episodes of angina (heart condition) and 21% fewer coronary by-pass operations than those who had received the placebo.[370] This is but one illustration of the extent to which preventive medicine can contribute effectively to the pursuit of human integrity.

Integrity and the Behavioral Sciences

One study of behavioral habits reveals that 44% of admissions to hospitals were related to preventable causes, primarily to alcohol and cigarette abuse. The same source states that 70% of heavy smokers state that they would stop smoking if urged to do so by their physicians.[371] If physicians did issue strong advice and even warnings when warranted to patients who are heavy users of alcohol and tobacco, they apparently would be preaching what most of them practice personally. One survey of American physicians indicates that 64% who formerly smoked quit the habit. Articles in medical journals in several areas of the nation indicate that the majority of physicians have reduced saturated fat in their diets, exercise regularly, wear seat belts, and, if they indulge in alcohol, take no more than one or two drinks per day.[372] Only

---

[370]Reported in *Time*, January 23, 1984, p. 30. Popular publications seem to have joined the campaign to warn the public of the need of "preventive medicine" by reporting on studies of various medical agencies, as indicated by the following articles in *Time* magazine: "Hold the Eggs and Butter," March 26, 1984, pp. 56–63; "The Fatty Diet Under Attack," December 24, 1984, p. 58; "Gauging the Fat of the Land," February 25, 1985, p. 72; "Dieting: The Losing Game," January 20, 1986, pp. 54–63. It must be noted, however, that the effectiveness of such reporting is curtailed by the fact that the medical community is divided on many aspects of appropriate diet control. Cf. "Diet Advice, with a Grain of Salt and a Large helping of Pepper," by Eliot Marshall, in *Science*, February 7, 1986, pp. 537–539.

[371]Dismuke-Miller, "Why Not Share the Secrets of Good Health?," (cf. note 368), p. 3181.

[372]*Ibid.*, p. 3181.

the physicians who "speak up" can exercise their professional potential to slow the advance of major silent killers which take the lives of hundreds of thousands each year. Cancer alone, usually detected too late, claims 450,000 lives annually.

Evidence of a definitive relation between alcohol consumption and smoking and cancer (the number 2 "killer" in America, after heart disease) is not as clear as the relation between high cholesterol levels and heart disease (above). A report of a study of alcohol consumption and cancer, as published in the March 8, 1984 issue of *The New England Journal of Medicine,* involved an analysis of information on diet, alcohol consumption, smoking history, socio-economic factors and demographic variables of 8006 Japanese men. These men, born between 1900 and 1916, submitted to a physical examination from 1965 to 1968, and also to a follow-up contact period of approximately 14 years. The final analysis, adjusted for the effects of age and cigarette smoking, revealed a positive association between the consumption of alcohol and rectal cancer. This was accounted for primarily by an increased risk in men whose usual monthly consumption of beer was 500 oz. or more (an average of 3.5 cans of beer per day) as compared to those who did not drink beer. It also revealed a significant positive relation between alcohol consumption and lung cancer, accounted for primarily by an increased risk for those who consumed larger amounts of wine or whiskey, as compared with those who did not drink those beverages. This realistic report ended with the following cautionary statement: "Nevertheless, more work is needed to determine whether alcohol actually increases the risk of cancer of the rectum and lung."[373]

Even outside of premature poor-health and death statistics, the misery dimension stemming from excessive drinking (violence, wife beating, child abuse, broken marriages, car accidents, etc.) is beyond calculation. From a financial viewpoint, the amount involved in hospitalization, rehabilitation, supportive social programs, absenteeism in employment, etc., is considered to be in the tens of billions of dollars per year. Especially pathetic is the suffering caused to children born of women who are chronic, heavy drinkers. These children are victims of what is known as the fetal alcohol syndrome (FAS). The abnormalities attributed to FAS include malformations of the head and face, and mental retardation. Experts admit that little is known about the fetal effects of moderate consumption of alcohol on the part of pregnant mothers. Dr. Kutay Taysi, MD of the St. Louis Children's Hospital in St. Louis, Mo. inspires caution in this regard in his statement that "Most

---

[373]Pollack, Earl S., Sc.D.et al (4 physicians), "Prospective Study of Alcohol Consumption and Cancer," *The New England Journal of Medicine,* March 8, 1984, p. 621.

babies with full-blown clinical features of the fetal alcohol syndrome have been born to women whose alcohol intake is 8 to 10 hard drinks per day."[374]

A two-part presentation on "Smoking: Health Effects and Control" in the August 22nd and August 29th, 1985 editions of *The New England Journal of Medicine* reveals some success in the U.S. Government's campaign to emphasize the dangers of cigarette smoking. A definite trend to a change in social norms is evidenced by the militancy of the nonsmokers in demanding smoke-free air, by the civility of smokers in some social groups in requesting group-permission before lighting up, by reports that many ex-smokers mention social pressure as the reason why they gave up smoking.[375] Among heavy smokers (25 or more cigarettes per day), however, a 1984 report of the U.S. Department of Agriculture announced an increase in heavy smoking of 35% among men smokers, and 24% among women smokers.[376] Statistics continue to validate the arguments for giving up the habit of cigarette smoking in particular—although cigar and pipe smokers who inhale also rate high in some categories (for example, oral cancer, and also lung cancer if they inhale deeply).

A partial list of the disastrous effects of cigarette smoking includes the following: 30 to 40% of the 565,000 deaths from coronary heart disease each year can be attributed to cigarette smoking; smoking is the leading cause of cancer mortality in the U.S.A. and between 80 and 85% of deaths from lung cancer are directly attributable to smoking; one case-control study estimated that 84% of all cases of cancer of the larynx among men could be attributed to smoking; the estimated percentage of bladder cancers attributable to smoking is between 40 to 60% for men and 25 to 35% for women. Women smokers who use oral contraceptives are at a double risk. In one case-control study of women smokers not using oral contraceptives, the risk of stroke (especially subarachnoid hemorrhage and thromboembolic events) was 5.7 times greater than for a nonsmoker, whereas for a woman who smoked and used oral contraceptives the relative risk increased to 21.9 times greater. Smoking during pregnancy leads to direct retardation of fetal growth. Infants born to such women weigh an average of 200 grams less than those born to nonsmokers. Futhermore, the proportion of preterm deliveries attributed to smoking ranges from 11 to 14% of all live births, and the risk of prematurity is directly

---

[374]Chapter entitled "Genetic Disorders," in *Genetic Medicine and Engineering*, Albert Moraczewski, O.P., Ph.D., ed. (cf. note 188), p. 9.

[375]By Jonathan E. Fielding, MD of the University of California, Los Angeles; Issue of Aug. 29, 1985, pp. 555–561. P. 560.

[376]Same author, *Ibid.*, issue of Aug. 22, 1985, pp. 491–498. P. 496.

associated with the smoking dose.[377] Such statistics "cry out" for changes in norms of human social behavior.

Integrity and a Prime Social Problem—Diet Control

Some aspects of diet control have been mentioned above (cholesterol levels, alcoholic excess, etc.). There is more than a grain of truth in the saying that health wise "you are what you eat and drink." There is a vast array of major illnesses and diseases of the human body which can be traced to improper diet as a contributing cause. The subject of diet control and obesity gets much attention in the popular press. The scientific community, however, recommends that reports on surveys and studies on this subject be read with caution and discernment. The associations between per capita consumptions of total fat, saturated fat, and cholesterol and national incidence rates of colon cancer, for example, are remarkably high. In Japan, recent increases in fat consumption have been associated with a striking increase in rates of colon cancer. Case-control studies of fat intake and cancer in individual subjects as conducted in Israel and in the United States, however, failed to find any material association between fat intake and colon cancer.[378] Although these studies, as well as others as conducted among individual subjects in Canada, the Hawaiian Islands and Greece, provide inconsistent support for the hypothesis that fat intake is related to colon cancer, the fact remains that experiments in animals and data relating to the effects of bile acids suggest that such a relation may exist. The situation calls for additional epidemiologic studies on the relationship between diet and cancer.

> Since meat is the most important source of dietary fat in the United States, it will be important to determine whether it has any relation with colon cancer that is independent of its fat content; at present there is little such evidence.[379]

The danger is real enough to make individuals concerned as to whether or not they are to be classified as obese. The tables on obesity which are based

---

[377]*Ibid.* (issue of Aug. 22, 1985), pp. 491–493 and 496. As to *passive* smoking (defined as the exposure of nonsmokers to tobacco-combustion products in the indoor environment), one study reported that children of mothers who smoked had a 70% greater chance of being hospitalized for respiratory conditions than the children of nonsmoking mothers. *Ibid.*, p. 495.

[378]"Diet and Cancer—An Overview," by Walter C. Willett, MD, and Brian MacMahon, MD in *The New England Journal of Medicine*, March 15, 1984, pp. 697–701. Reference on p. 698.

[379]*Ibid.*, p. 699.

on height over weight are less than reliable. They are based on averages, and do not take into account body-fat distribution, concurrent risk factors, social, economic and ethnic status and age. Physicians are advised to assess such factors, and to use *body-mass index* in evaluating overweight patients. The body mass index is obtained by dividing the weight in kilograms by the square of the height in meters. Treatment for obesity is indicated if the body-mass index is more than 27.8 in men and 27.3 in women, or if the individual has non-insulin-dependent diabetes mellitus, hypertension or hypercholesterolemia (excess of cholesterol in the blood).[380]

One indication for anticipating the "battle of the bulge" relates to the obesity of the biologic parents of an individual. In a recent study conducted in Denmark (using the body-mass index), detailed information obtained about 3580 male and female *adoptees* (mean age, 42 years) provided "unequivocal findings" of a clear relation between the body-mass indexes of the adoptees and those of their biologic parents and of a "lack of any relation" between the body-mass indexes of the adoptees and those of their adoptive parents.[381] This project was made possible because the Danish Adoption Register provides data about both adoptive and biologic parents. This is not to deny that environmental conditions can contribute to the obesity-tendency of adopted children whose biologic parents were obese (for example, the adoptive parents are thin, but "big eaters"), but to forewarn such children as to the importance of diet control, physical exercise, and a wholesome regimen of what might be called "defensive eating" (not only "how much," but avoiding high-fat snack foods).

Americans who inherit obesity from their biologic parents face a double challenge inasmuch as they are surrounded by a culture which is oriented to high-fat foods, frequent snacks and drinks, and a more or less pervasive tendency to a sedentary life-style. Even though the science community is not as yet in a position to issue many specific guidelines on the damages of the neglect of diet control, it has demonstrated the importance of successful management of obesity in improving the quality of life and in reducing the risk of illness and premature death. Of particular interest to obese individuals who are inclined to heart trouble, it is important to note that a small weight loss is

---

[380]"Consensus Panel Addresses Obesity Question," in *The Journal of the American Medical Association*, Oct. 11, 1985, p. 1878.

[381]"Bad News and Good News About Obesity" by Theodore B. Van Itallie, MD in *The New England Journal of Medicine*, Jan. 23, 1986. pp. 239 and 240. The actual study by A.J. Stunkard et al. entitled "An Adoption Study of Human Obesity," is found in the same issue, pp. 193–198.

beneficial in "unloading the heart from the double burden of obesity and hypertension."[382]

The Oct. 11, 1985 issue of *The Journal of the American Medical Association* published a brief report of a Consensus Development Conference which was assembled by the National Institutes of Health to review decades of research findings on the subject of obesity and health. A panel reviewed the literature and listened to 1 1/2 days of expert testimony. The following response to the question of whether or not obesity affects health merits serious consideration:

> Studies have determined that persons who ranked above the 85th percentile in terms of body mass index . . . have a significantly higher prevalence of hypertension, hypercholesterolemia and non-insulin-dependent diabetes mellitus. Mortality from cancers of the colon, rectum, and prostate is higher in obese men and from cancers of the breast, uterus, ovaries, gallbladder, and biliary passages in obese women than it is in normal-weight persons the same age.[383]

It would be beyond the purpose of this chapter to include a discussion of other aspects of helping the individual to protect "the integrity of the body together with all its bodily functions" (for example, environmental deterrents to good health). Enough has been said to construct a persuasive argument that the general public has a right to look to medical and health-care professionals to lead the way in making stepping stones out of stumbling blocks which impede the individual's pursuit of personal integrity.

Directive 4: Man has the right and duty to protect the integrity of his body together with all of its bodily functions.

6.2   TOTALITY AND INJURIOUS MEMBERS OF THE BODY

"Totality" refers to the duty to preserve intact the physical component of that integrated whole, whereby, in the words of St.

---

[382]"Cardiopathy of Obesity—a Not-So-Victorian Disease," by Franz H. Messerli, MD, in *The New England Journal of Medicine,* Feb. 6, 1986, pp. 378 and 379. Reference on p. 379.

[383]*The Journal of the American Medical Association,* Oct. 11, 1985 (cf. note 380), p. 1878.

Thomas Aquinas, every member of the human body "exists for the sake of the whole as the imperfect for the sake of the perfect. Hence a member of the human body is to be disposed of according as it may profit the whole" (cf.chapter heading).

An important distinction must be made between the physical organism, "the man," and the moral organism known as "humanity." As St. Thomas points out (above), it is permitted, when necessary, to sacrifice directly a particular member of the human body (hand, foot, eye, ear, kidney, etc.) for the good of the whole body, "the man," but it is not permitted to sacrifice directly a human individual for the good of "humanity." Pope Pius XII clarified this distinction in his address to a group of eye specialists on May 14, 1956:

> The physical organism of "the man" is one complete whole in its being. The members are parts united and bound together in their very physical essence. They are so absorbed by the whole that they possess no independence. They exist only for the sake of the total organism and have no other end than that of the total organism.
>
> It is an entirely different matter in the case of the moral organism that is humanity. This constitutes a whole only in regard to act and finality; individuals, insofar as they are members of this organism, are only functional parts. The "whole" can make demands on them only in what pertains to the order of action. In their physical being individuals are not in any way dependent on one another or on humanity.[384]

The neglect of this basic distinction has led authoritarian governments to claim the right to sacrifice individuals directly in behalf of the nation or community (medical experiments in concentration camps, for example). As citizens of a nation, individuals can be obligated to do all that is required for the true common good such as keeping laws, paying taxes, responding to the call to military service, etc., but they cannot be sacrificed directly in behalf of the state or nation. Again, quoting the words of Pope Pius XII: ". . . man, as a person, in the final reckoning, does not exist for the use of society: on the contrary, the community exists for man."[385]

---

[384]*The Human Body* (cf. note 61), pp. 375 and 376.
[385]Address to the First International Congress of Histopathology, Sept. 13, 1952. *Ibid.*, p. 204.

Pope Pius XII On the Principle of Totality

As a preliminary observation, the Principle of Totality should be understood as referring not to the *anatomical* wholeness of the body (as if cutting the hair or fingernails or donating a pint of blood would mar that wholeness), but rather to the *functional* wholeness of the human body. Thus the proper functioning of the body in the performance of acts which are important to a person's well-being would be diminished only if a medical procedure involved the excision or suppression of some organ of the body (a lung, kidney, prostate gland, etc.) or the amputation of some member of the body (an arm, leg, hand, etc.).[386] Nature has provided some organs in pairs (kidneys, lungs, eyes, etc.) so that the removal of one of the pair would not destroy that particular function unless something had happened to weaken or destroy the remaining organ of that pair; other organs (heart, liver, prostate, etc.) cannot be removed without causing death or unfortunate consequences for the individual. The Principle of Totality is limited to preserving the physical perfection of the human body. It could not justify the donation of an organ of the body to another person (for example, a kidney). Another principle would have to be applied to justify such a noble gesture.

Pope Pius XII mentions three conditions which would be required in allowing a surgical procedure to deprive an individual of the physical wholeness of his or her body: 1) That a continuing preservation or functioning of a particular organ presents a serious damage or constitutes a threat for the whole organism; 2) That the damage cannot be avoided or at least notably diminished except by the proposed mutilation, with good assurance as to its effectiveness; 3) That there is a reasonable basis for counting on a compensation of the negative effect (the mutilation and its consequences) by the positive effect (elimination of the danger for the whole organism, easing of pain, etc.).[387]

The first condition does not mean that the organ to be removed is diseased or useless, but that its presence or normal functioning is harmful or injurious in a manner which makes it a serious threat to the entire body. The organ itself may be healthy and normal both in form and in function as the responses of Pius XII (to follow) well demonstrate. It would also seem unwar-

---

[386]This helpful observation of Father Charles McFadden, O.S.A. is found in his book, *The Dignity of Life* (cf. note 65), p. 186.

[387]*The Human Body* (cf. note 61), pp. 277, 278. In the original French, the second condition could be interpreted as meaning "the only reasonable alternative" or "last resort" procedure: "que ce dommage ne puisse être évité que par la mutilation en question." Cf. *Acta Apostolicae Sedis,* XLV (1953), n. 14, p. 674.

ranted to interpret the second condition as meaning that the operation or mutilation is allowed *only* if there is no other available way of preserving life. Such an interpretation could mean that a man with a painful gall bladder condition or with a very serious stomach ulcer would have to forego the surgery in favor of a long and costly series of non-surgical treatments. If an alternative way of removing the danger to the whole body was available, it would seem reasonable to be free to select the proposal which is most likely to eliminate that danger—the one with the best "assurance as to its effectiveness" ("que l'efficacité de celle-ci soit bien assurée"). In other words, as stated in the third condition, the proposal which will best compensate (danger eliminated, pain eased, etc.) for the means used.[388] In many cases, surgery may be the only choice which would eliminate the danger to the whole body on a life-long basis. Finally, the word "mutilation" should be understood not in the Latin sense of "to maim, to damage," but in the medical-moral sense of the removal of an organ or the suppression of its function.[389]

Practical Application of the Principle of Totality

Pope Pius XII applied the Principle of Totality to two cases; one in reply to a case presented by his audience (Congress of Urologists), and the second of his own volition. On the affirmative side, he approved of castration ("removal of the seed-producing glands") in two possible situations: either when the removal of a healthy organ and the suppression of its normal function may remove from the disease (cancer, for example) its potential for spreading, or may change the damaging effect of the disease on the whole body;—or, when a healthy organ, by its normal function, exercises such a harmful effect on a diseased organ as to aggravate the disease and its repercussions on the whole body. In both cases, a surgical operation to remove the organ would be permissible "if there is no other alternative available."

On the negative side, he did *not* allow a procedure whereby the fallopian tubes would be "removed or put out of action" if a woman has unhealthy organs (kidneys, heart, lungs) and her condition would be aggravated in the event of another pregnancy. In explaining this response he stressed that the danger threatening the mother does not derive at all—directly or indirectly—

---

[388]O'Donnell, Thomas J., *Medicine and Christian Morality* (cf. note 31), p. 71. Cf. also Connell, Francis J., C.SS.R., STD, "Surgery for the Healthy," in *American Ecclesiastical Review*, 1947, pp. 143, 144.

[389]O'Donnell, Thomas J., S.J., *Ibid.*, p. 65, 66.

from the presence of normal functioning of the oviducts, nor from the influence they exercise over the diseased organs (kidneys, heart, lungs):

> The danger comes only when free sexual intercourse causes a conception which can menace the organs mentioned, because these are too weak or diseased. But the conditions which permit a part to be disposed of in favor of the whole, in virtue of the principle of totality, do not exist.[390]

His decision with regard to the section or ligation of the fallopian tubes caused some consternation among theologians inasmuch as he mentioned only the Principle of Totality as a basis for his response. Based on the natural teleology of the reproductive organs of the body, the Church teaches that such organs are not only subordinated to the total good of the whole organism, but that they also serve a prime *social* function inasmuch as they are oriented to the good of the human species. Any attempt to remove directly that capacity to have children can be justified in a particular case only if it is both therapeutic (thus satisfying the Principle of Totality) and also *indirect* (thus satisfying the Principle of the Double Effect) inasmuch as it involves the destruction of a function which possesses a finality independent of the good of the individual.[391]

Pius XII clarified the issue some 5 years later (Sept. 12, 1958) in his address to the hematologists. On this occasion, he referred to the previous address of Oct. 8, 1953, and said: "The same principles apply to the present case." The "present case" involved his *disapproval* of the "removal of glands or of sexual organs for the purpose of impeding the transmission of defective hereditary characteristics," as well as his *approval* of taking anovulant pills upon the advice of a doctor so as to remedy "the condition of the uterus or of the organism." He mentioned expressly that the principles he was referring to were "the general principles governing acts with a double effect."[392] This is interpreted as meaning that he had taken into consideration both the Principle of Totality and the Principle of the Double Effect.[393]

---

[390]Address to the 26th Congress of Urology, Oct. 8, 1953, in *The Human Body* (cf. note 61), pp. 278, 279.

[391]Ford-Kelly, *Contemporary Moral Theology*, II (cf. note 65), p. 327. Cf. also "Fertility Control by Hormonal Medication," by Denis O'Callaghan, in *The Irish Theological Quarterly*, XXVII (1960), pp. 1–15, especially pp. 8 and 9; Kelly, Gerald, S.J., *Medico-Moral Problems* (cf. note 22), pp. 6–11.

[392]*The Pope Speaks*, VI (1959–1960), p. 395.

[393]Ford-Kelly, *Contemporary Moral Theology*, II (cf. note 65), pp. 321–327.

Application to Uterus Weakened by Repeated Cesareans

There are women whose wombs have been so weakened by repeated cesarean sections that a physician could have valid reasons for fearing, in a particular case of cesarean delivery, that the womb will very likely rupture in a subsequent pregnancy. After completing the delivery process, would that physician be allowed to remove that irreparably damaged womb as a seriously pathological organ? That physician had repaired the weakened walls of the womb after each previous cesarean section on that patient, and is convinced that further repair, sufficient for the woman to sustain a future pregnancy to term without a serious danger of rupture, would be highly improbable.

In 1978, 510,000 women had abdominal or cesarean-section deliveries in U.S. hospitals (15.2% of hospital deliveries) as compared to 195,000 women in 1970 (5.5% of hospital deliveries).[394] The dictum "once a cesarean always a cesarean" is being questioned in contemporary medical circles. An article in the Feb. 8, 1985 issue of the *Journal of the American Medical Association* states that that no deaths from a ruptured cesarean scar have been reported for more than 20 years. The article also states that the consensus of a panel convened by the National Institutes of Health in 1981 was "to question seriously the validity of automatic repeat cesarean section."[395] The author of this article lays considerable stress on the propriety of the "current practice" of what he describes as "the low cervical cesarean section with transverse [as opposed to 'vertical'] uterine incision," because of its great strength and diminished danger of rupture. His summary reads as follows:

> However, a significant decline [in cesarean sections] may be expected in two areas: many of the midforceps operations that are now medicolegally unsound will be permissible and appropriate if the definitions become more precise, and the more frequent use of trial labor after a prior cesarean section should eliminate at least 30% of the currently performed automatic repeat cesarean sections.[396]

The "cesarean section" case as sketched above is quite different than the "Fallopian tube" case which received a negative response from Pope Pius XII; that is, the case of a woman with a disease (heart, lung, kidneys) which

---

[394]Danforth, David N., MD, "Cesarean Section," in the *Journal of the American Medical Association,* Feb. 8, 1985, pp. 811–817. Reference, p. 811.

[395]*Ibid.,* p. 813.

[396]*Ibid.,* pp. 813, 814.

might be aggravated in the event of another pregnancy. Resection or ligation of the fallopian tubes would have deprived the woman directly of her capacity to have children. In both cases ("cesarean section" and "fallopian tube") the woman would face the danger only if she became pregnant again. The difference is that in the "cesarean section" case, the woman does have a serious pathological condition of the reproductive system itself. The situation is not as "clear cut" as that of a woman with a cancerous uterus which endangers her life *independently* of pregnancy. The fact remains, however, that the serious pathological condition of the uterus does endanger the whole organism.

As to the application of the *Principle of Totality* (whereby the procedure is therapeutic), Pope Pius XII outlined the parameters as follows:

> . . . in virtue of the principle of totality, of his right to employ the services of the organism as a whole, [the person] can give individual parts to destruction or mutilation when and to the extent that it is necessary for the good of his being as a whole, to assure its existence or to avoid, and naturally to repair, grave and lasting damage which could otherwise be neither avoided nor repaired.[397]

As to the application of the *Principle of the Double Effect* (whereby the evil effect, sterility, follows indirectly), two effects would follow from the surgical removal of the uterus: the elimination of the danger to the whole organism due to the seriously pathological condition of an irreparable uterus, and the termination of the woman's capacity to have children. With at least equal causal immediacy, the surgical operation removes the pathological organ and with it the danger to the whole organism, and also terminates the capacity of the woman to have children. It is absolutely essential, however, that the good effect *directly* intended is the prevention of uterine rupture, and not the foreseen but merely tolerated (hence *indirect*) evil side effect which is the prevention of conception. It is true that the operation produces sterility, but as a foreseen but unintended side effect.[398]

This writer quotes with approval the opinion of Fathers John C. Ford, S.J. and Gerald Kelly, S.J., co-authors of *Contemporary Moral Theology:* ". . . we believe that there is solid intrinsic probability for the opinion that the removal of the damaged uterus is not in itself a direct sterilization . . . The good effect intended is the prevention of uterine rupture, not the prevention of concep-

---

[397] *The Human Body* (cf. note 61), p. 199.
[398] Ford/Kelly, *Contemporary Moral Theology,* II (cf. note 65), pp. 332, 333.

tion."[399] As to the extrinsic probability of this opinion, the fact that a considerable number of theologians share that affirmative opinion provides grounds for following that opinion in particular cases. Since the Holy See has not issued a declaration on this particular application of the Principles of Totality and of the Double Effect, it remains an "open question." Considering the trend in contemporary medical practice with regard to automatic repeat cesarean sections, the surgical procedure in question should be a relatively rare occurrence. The Church expressly rejects any arbitrary "rule of thumb" whereby such a procedure might be justified after "any definite number of cesarean sections" (directive below). It must be admitted that the opinion favoring this procedure could easily be subject to misinterpretation and abuse, and become a veiled excuse for attempting to justify directly-contraceptive surgery.[400]

Serious scandal could result if the Catholic community or the general public were given an overt basis for concluding that the procedure was simply a "backdoor" method of terminating a woman's capacity to have children. In fact, if such an unfavorable impression gained credence and could not be dissipated by a clear explanation of the facts and principles involved, it would constitute a basis for prohibiting the procedure on the basis of scandal.

Directive 22: Hysterectomy is permitted when it is sincerely judged to be a necessary means of removing some serious uterine pathological condition. In these cases, the pathological condition of each patient must be considered individually and care must be taken that a hysterectomy is not performed merely as a contraceptive measure, or as a routine procedure after any definite number of Cesarean sections.

---

[399]*Ibid.*, p. 333. Authors who agree with this opinion include the following: O'Donnell, Thomas J., S.J., *Medicine and Christian Morality* (cf. note 31), pp. 133, 134; Kelly, Gerald, S.J., *Medico-Moral Problems* (cf. note 22), pp. 213–217; Lynch, John, S.J., *Theological Studies,* June, 1957, pp. 230–232; Connery, John, S.J., *Theological Studies,* Dec., 1955, pp. 575, 576. Father Connery compares this case to that of a woman with a non-functioning appendix or gall bladder which would cause no danger unless she became pregnant, and adds: ". . . it would be advisable . . . to have the organ removed before the danger occurred."

[400]This sensitive subject was discussed in chapter I (1.2), and will merit extensive discussion in chapter X (Principle of Material Cooperation).

Directive 15: Cesarean section for the removal of a viable fetus is permitted, even with risk to the life of the mother, when necessary for successful delivery. It is likewise permitted, even with risk for the child, when necessary for the safety of the mother.

1) Caution Required in Analyzing This Procedure

When a hysterectomy is warranted because of the serious pathological condition of the uterus, it would be misleading to say that the procedure is justified because that woman's uterus is "useless." Such reasoning could induce a physician to conclude that a woman whose uterus is not pathological but in effect "useless" (for example, a severely mentally retarded single woman who has advanced arthritis and hence is incapable of attending to her own personal feminine hygiene) would be justified in submitting to a hysterectomy. In terms of the continued potential for contributing to the well-being of the whole organism, the reproductive organs of such a woman still have an important role to play in sustaining a proper sense of womanhood and even of possible motherhood. A quotation from Pope Pius XII is appropriate:

> Man is an ordered unit, one whole, a microcosm, after the fashion of a State whose charter, determined by the end of the whole, subordinates to this end the activity of the parts in the right order of their value and function.[401]

The word "microcosm" is well chosen. The entire organism known as the human body might also be called an "ecosystem" in comparison with the marvellous interdependence and interpenetration among the forces and functions in the world of nature. This ecosystem in the world of nature is threatened by contamination of air and water, by the denuding of marshes and woodlands, by the destruction of soil nutrients, etc. The condition known as "acid rain," for example, even if it portends an irreparable loss of potential oxygenation, does not indicate that nature's air-current system is useless or substantially defective. Likewise, the fact that an arthritic and mentally retarded single woman may not marry and conceive a child provides no basis

---

[401]Address to the *Congress of Psychotherapy and Clinical Psychology*, April 15, 1953; *The Human Body* (cf. note 61), pp. 229, 230.

for characterizing her uterus, or any of her reproductive organs, as useless. In the "cesarean section" case, the surgical removal of the uterus would be justified not on the basis of "uselessness" but because the scarred uterus presents a serious danger to the entire organism.

2) "Uterine Isolation" As a Substitute for Hysterectomy

If the uterus can be removed after repeated cesarean sections because of the danger of rupture, could the procedure be simplified for sound clinical reasons by leaving the uterus "in situ," and simply isolating the uterus from the fallopian tubes? This could be done by a simple surgical separation procedure whereby the tubes are cut or ligated. The clinical reasons for this simple procedure, as compared to the potentially serious surgical removal of the uterus, could include the fact that the simple cutting or ligating of the tubes would obviate the danger (as in a hysterectomy) of adhesions and the possible need of blood transfusions. In some cases, the woman may be so weakened after a difficult cesarean delivery, that proceeding with the hysterectomy at that time would be contraindicated. An additional reason favoring tubal section or ligation could be a psychological one: the woman may be unduly disturbed and depressed by somehow equating the loss of her uterus with the loss of her womanhood.

It seems only reasonable to conclude that in *some* particular cases when hysterectomy could be allowed (as described above), "uterine isolation" could be chosen as an approved substitute. It also follows, however, that the danger of misinterpreting and abusing this simpler substitute procedure would require extreme caution. Obviously, the substitution of tubal ligation for a morally defensible hysterectomy could not be regarded as standard procedure. Father Thomas O'Donnell, S.J. expresses the urgency of caution in the following paragraph:

> The legitimate concept of "uterine isolation" applies *only* to the instance in which hysterectomy is indicated because of dangerous pathology within the uterus itself (which will obviously be mechanical rather than malignant), and in which the isolation of the uterus would be an acceptable clinical substitute for a morally and clinically defensible hysterectomy.[402]

---

[402]*Medicine and Christian Morality* (cf. note 31), p. 134.

> *Preamble, Paragraph 6:* These *Directives* prohibit those procedures which, according to present knowledge, are recognized as clearly wrong. The basic moral absolutes which underlie these *Directives* are not subject to change, although particular applications might be modified as scientific investigation and theological development open up new problems or cast new light on old ones.

Other Applications of the Principle of Totality

The Principle of Totality allows the removal of a damaging organ to be intended *directly*. There is also an evil or unfortunate side effect of such procedures, but it is a *physical* evil, and not a moral one (that is, the risk, pain, resulting physical limitations, etc.). When the damaging organ is a part of the reproductive function of the human body, however, the side effect is a physical and a *moral* evil (a surgical elimination of the capacity to have children). This explains why the Principle of the Double Effect must also be applied. The significance of human reproduction as a prime social good transcends the physical good of the individual; the foreseen side-effect which is the elimination of the capacity to have children cannot be intended, but merely permitted or tolerated (hence, an *indirect* effect). This observation bears repetition.

In the vast panoply of possible medical and surgical procedures, it can be said that generally ("ordinarily") the procedure can be allowed if it is designed to bring about the total good of the patient as a proportionate good—but NOT on the basis of the Principle of Totality alone when the procedure involves the reproductive function. This explains why the word "ordinarily" is used in a brief *Directive* which might be called a brief reminder that the Principle of Totality cannot be used to justify direct sterilization.[403]

> *Directive 6:* Ordinarily the proportionate good that justifies a medical or surgical procedure should be the total good of the patient himself.

---

[403] *Ibid.*, p. 117.

Outside of the many procedures which do involve the human reproductive function (which will be reviewed in the following chapter on the Principle of the Double Effect), therefore, the average medical or surgical procedure is an application of the Principle of Totality—"to assure (the) existence or to avoid, and naturally to repair, grave and lasting damage" to individual parts of the human organism (Pius XII,cf.p.221).

The list gets longer as medical science discovers new treatments and technologies: tonsillectomy, appendectomy, gall-bladder removal, mastectomy, stomach-ulcer surgery, goiter surgery, radiation, chemotherapy, by-pass cardiac surgery, amputations, etc. The intent is not to "cover the field," but to comment on a few procedures which could be subject to controversy as a further illustration of the Principle of Totality.

An appendectomy is called "incidental" when a *healthy* appendix is removed as a precautionary measure in the course of general abdominal surgery. If only slight risk is involved and the patient consents to the "incidental" appendectomy, the very likelihood that the appendix might become seriously inflamed and require a separate operation in the future, would constitute a proportionate reason for removing the appendix. An appendectomy is called "elective" when a *healthy* appendix is removed as a precautionary measure BUT there is no other valid reason for abdominal surgery.

Since the proportion between the risks involved (post operative complications, reactions to anesthesia, etc.) and the anticipated good is out of balance, the general rule would be that such surgery is not justified. An exception would be justified for a person in a military or missionary career, for example, who is being assigned to duty for a protracted period in a part of the world where surgical attention would be unavailable.[404] There is no basis for interpreting the Principle of Totality as referring ONLY to present dangers. In fact, if that military or missionary person had a *past history* of several serious attacks of appendicitis, he or she should feel obligated to "do something about that appendix" before embarking on long foreign service.

Elective tonsillectomy (healthy tonsils, not infected) in these days of "miracle" drugs and antibiotics, is not justified. It is logical to assume that nature's gift of tonsils does contribute to the physical well-being of the individual. If they are infected, they can be treated. If they are diseased, and are not responding to modern methods of treatment, they can be removed.

---

[404]Authors who would allow an appendectomy in such circumstances include the following: Healy, Edwin, S.J., *Medical Ethics* (cf. note 46), pp. 125, 126; O'Donnell, Thomas J., S.J., *Medicine and Christian Morality* (cf. note 31), pp. 73–75; Kelly, Gerald, S.J., *Medico-Moral Problems* (cf. note 22), pp. 252–254; McFadden, Charles, O.S.A., *The Dignity of Life* (cf. note 65), p. 189; Connell, Francis, C.SS.R., *American Eccl. Review* article (cf. note 388), p. 144.

Some authors question the moral validity of routine circumcision of newborns,—that is, when the physician or hospital has a policy of having all newborns circumcised regardless of a clearly identified need. This writer shares the opinion of Father Gerald Kelly, S.J. to the effect that hospitals should adopt a tolerant attitude towards doctors who insist on routine circumcisions. The procedure should not be opposed "as long as it is limited to cases in which circumcision is not actually contraindicated."[405] Before giving or denying permission for the circumcision of their infant, the parents should consider well the arguments which a conscientious physician may offer either for or against the procedure.

In his address to the First Italian Congress of Stomatology on Oct. 24, 1946, Pope Pius XII had words of high praise for "these wonderful sculptors" who "have pooled all the means which the most recent advances have provided" to improve the appearance and function of the human mouth for victims of war, accidents or tumors.[406] Any reasonable efforts to correct or alleviate malfunctions or disfigurements of the body are well within the tenor of the Principle of Totality. It would be unfair and unkind to attribute the desire for such procedures to mere vanity. The variety of such treatments may range from the removal of unsightly moles and blemishes ("birth marks," for example) to the removal or repair of a paralyzed limb or appendage and the substitution of a proper prosthesis.

Caution is required in the search for a physician or plastic surgeon who can back up his or her promises with proven expertise. When liquid silicone came into prominence in the mid 1970's as a means of restoring or forming feminine breasts to proper shape and size, it was found that the injected silicone interfered with blood circulation and with the lymphatic system. Father Charles McFadden, O.S.A. reports on the medical problems which resulted from such injections—as well as from other silicone implants designed both for womens' breasts and for the replacement of mens' testicles.[407] The risks far exceeded the anticipated good results. It would be morally objectionable to entrust such restorative measures to anyone who was not a reputable physician or plastic surgeon . . . or to risk disfigurement by seeking the services of such experts for motives of sheer frivolity (desire for a "new look," contemporary fads, etc.). In all cases of such procedures which are desired for purely esthetic reasons, the need of a due proportion between the validly-

---

[405]*Medico-Moral Problems* (cf. note 22), p. 259. Father Edwin Healy, S.J. in *Medical Ethics* (cf. note 46) presents arguments against the practice of "routine circumcisions," pp. 128, 129.

[406]*The Human Body* (cf. note 61), p. 88.

[407]*The Dignity of Life* (cf. note 65), pp. 191, 192.

anticipated results and the risks involved must be emphasized.

6.3   TOTALITY AND HEALTHY MEMBERS OF THE BODY

Every member of the human race has a right to be identifiable and accepted as a member of one sex or the other. That reasonable statement introduces several crucial questions. What if a person who was born and who developed with definite masculine anatomical structure and characteristics (normal formation of external sexual organs, distribution of fat and body hair, etc.) is nevertheless convinced from deep, abiding psychological needs and desires that he has a right to be "changed into a woman." Sex refers to the anatomical and physiological aspects of human personality; gender refers to the psychological element based on what and how the individual perceives himself or herself to be. Despite the anatomical evidence of the masculine sex, this individual insists on being changed and accepted as a member of the feminine gender.

The Problem of the Transsexual

The transsexual's plight is one of misery and anxiety. Assuming for discussion sake that the individual who is a male by *genotype* or chromosomal sex ("XY" for the male as compared to "XX" for the female), is profoundly anxious over his male *phenotype* (especially the external development as it appears to the observer, from the Greek word "phainein," meaning "to show") and insists on physiological alterations so as to resemble a female. Since such anatomical alterations would involve mutilation of the human body (excision of the testes and penis, and the construction of a vagina through plastic surgery), the predominant view among Catholic moralists is that such physiological alterations could not be justified on the basis of the Principle of Totality.

The reasons for such a moral view of the procedure are multiple. There is no mistaken sex identification as in the cases to be discussed later on in this chapter. There is no question of diseased sexual organs (which might justify their surgical removal for the good of the whole body). The surgery would not change his sex even though he claims to think and feel and react as a female. Such a "reconstructed" individual could never marry a woman, for he would be impotent with regard to the natural functions of the husband in the conjugal act. He could not marry a man, since he remains a member of the male sex. His new life-style would create occasions of sin for himself and his new life partner. He would be a source of grave scandal to others who know the facts.[408] Such an individual would be a mutilated, emasculated man who masquerades as a woman. One author clearly disapproves of such a sex-change procedure even if the individual insists on the surgery purely as a means of relieving the obsessive anxiety and with the intention of living as a celibate.[409]

Some authors have discussed the possibility that the situation in some cases may be one of sexual ambiguity so that it could be permissible to choose the more probable sex and treat the patient accordingly. Father Albert Moraczewski, O.P. would contemplate such a possibility as a last resort in treating the person with this lamentable condition (also known as "gender dysphoria"):

> But before such surgery could gain moral approval from the Church, it would be necessary for the clinical scientist to show that indeed a person's gender, and his or her anatomical sex *can* be discordant. Were an individual to be in that condition, then transsexual surgery might be properly viewed as correcting a defect by altering (as best as one could) the anatomical sex to fit the individual's true gender.[410]

Others list persuasive reasons why such an exceptional case cannot be demonstrated: (1) It has not been demonstrated that the cause of gender dysphoria is biological—the gender ambiguity in question is primarily psychological and should be treated psychotherapeutically; (2) when candidates for surgery are required to undergo psychotherapy in preparation for surgery, many are found to be ambiguous about really wanting it and in the end decide against it; (3) as experience accumulates there is now no solid agreement as to whether it does much good—this type of surgery offers no advantage over psychotherapy; (4) from a theological point of view it is clear that surgery does not really solve these persons' existential problem since it does not enable them to achieve sexual normality so as to be able to enter into a valid Christian marriage or to have children.[411]

---

[408]O'Donnell, Thomas J., S.J., *Medicine and Morality* (cf. note 31), pp. 229–231; Ashley-O'Rourke, *Health Care Ethics* (cf. note 80), pp. 312–316; McFadden, Charles, O.S.A., *The Dignity of Life* (cf. note 65), pp. 38–40; Healy, Edwin, S.J., *Medical Ethics* (cf. note 46), pp. 135, 136.

[409]Ashley, Benedict, O.P. in *Sex and Gender*, Mark F. Schwartz, Sc.D., Albert S. Moraczewski, O.P., Ph.D., James A. Monteleone, MD, editors (St. Louis, Mo: Pope John Center, 1983), p. 43.

[410]*Ibid.*, p. 305.

[411]Ashley-O'Rourke, *Health Care Ethics* (cf. note 80), pp. 313–315. Cf. also "The Transsexual and Marriage" by Msgr. Charles J. Ritty in *Studia Canonica*, Vol. 15, n. 2 (1981), pp. 441–459.

The decision of an appeal case for nullity of marriage before the Sacred Roman Rota (*Coram* Pinto, April 14, 1975) involving a man (age 34 at the time of marriage) who was both a transvestite and a transsexual, was published in the *Canon Law Digest*. The following statement with regard to transsexualism (quoting an Italian expert) is of special significance:

> As regards the *etiology* of the abnormality, 'biological research has not permitted the singling out of any alteration which would point to an organic basis. This is in harmony with the majority of the authors who have endeavored to give biological consistency to the sexual deviations (Vague, Pauly, Benjamin, . . .) . . . Robbe and Girard conclude that psychosexual maturation and orientation are the result more of education and of contacts which the subject has learned to establish with his milieu than the abnormal actions which contribute the elements which the subject ought to integrate into his self image.'[412]

If medical science were to discover some fetal metabolic or hormonal component or some neuro-endocrine influence on man's sexual development which points to discordant anatomical sex, however, it would be possible to contemplate surgical intervention as a "last resort" means of correcting a malfunctioning component of psycho-sexual development. This would be a valid application of the Principle of Totality. From a moral viewpoint, however, such surgical intervention could apply, even in an extreme case of serious excessive anxiety over sexual identity, only to an individual who is determined to live as a celibate. Canonical sources are very clear in stating that transsexuals are perpetually impotent following the "conversion operation."[413]

Transsexuals stand in need of expert psychotherapy and of patient and loving pastoral care. These needs are expressed persuasively in the following quotation:

> The fundamental aim of the therapist as well as of the pastoral counselor in these cases should be to restore the patient's sense of personal self-worth. He or she must be helped to see, as should

---

[412]*Canon Law Digest*, VIII (cf. note 38), p. 757. The decision was negative: "Proof is not had of nullity of marriage in the instance" (p. 768). Cf. also a case involving a transsexual *female* before the Toronto Regional Tribunal, Dec. 23, 1980, as reported in *Studia Canonica*, Vol. 16, n. 2 (1982), pp. 400–411 (especially pp. 408–411) and the article by Msgr. Charles Ritty as listed above (cf. note 411), pp. 441–459.

[413]*Canon Law Digest*, VIII (cf. note 38), p. 763.

homosexuals and those suffering from other sexual problems, that today's culture is grievously mistaken in its exaggerated stress on sexual identity and activity as a primary determinant of human worth. They must be assisted to find interests—spiritual, intellectual and social—which will enable them to escape their preoccupation with their sexual identity and discover their more fundamental value as human persons.[414]

The Problem of Divergent Gender Identity

Dr. James Monteleone, MD, a professor of pediatrics and adolescent medicine at the St. Louis University School of Medicine, calls the birth of an infant with *ambiguous* genitalia "an emergency situation." Time is of the essence. If the decision as to the proper sex of rearing is not determined and acted upon preferably before the infant is taken home from the hospital, the psychological effects on the infant, parents and family members can be deeply disheartening and damaging. Depending upon the complications in each case, facing the challenge may mean the active participation of a team of experts (including a psychiatrist/psychologist), but the situation has the urgency of a "now or probably never" priority. The entire team, together with the parents, should be involved in determining the sex of rearing.[415] Because of the direct relationship of this decision to the life-long well-being of the infant, whatever treatments and medical procedures which may be required are justified on the basis of the Principle of Totality.

As to the biological factor which influences the gender identity, the variety of anatomical differences can range from individuals born with both male and female glands (true hermaphrodites), to individuals born with secondary male characteristics which are superimposed on a genetic female or vice versa, or born with some rudimentary or limited organs of the opposite sex (pseudohermaphrodites), to individuals born with gonads which are composed of a mixture of genetically male and female cells (gynandromorphs). Dr. Monteleone lists the probable causes of ambiguous genitalia as follows: (1) environmental insults ("perhaps viruses, exogenous hormones or other chemicals that affect in utero gonadal development"); (2) sex chromosome aberrations such as Klinefelter and Turner syndromes; (3) birth defects, where ambiguous genitalia are part of an entire syndrome involving several

---

[414]Ashley-O'Rourke, *Health Care Ethics* (cf. note 80), p. 316.
[415]*Sex and Gender* (cf. note 409), pp. 65, 66.

physical abnormalities, and (4) single gene mutations, such as testicular femi-
nization and congenital adrenal hypoplasia.[416]

The subject of ambiguous genitalia and gender identity is too specialized
to be addressed in this chapter. It may suffice to quote an expert such as Dr.
Monteleone to the effect that for the majority of infants at birth, the determination of sex and of sex of rearing is no problem:

> Fortunately the majority of individuals have consistency between
> chromosomal sex, gonadal sex, phenotypic sex, sex of rearing and
> gender identity. For some there may be an error or inconsistency
> in these areas of sex development . . . Sometimes, because of am-
> biguity of the external genitals, genetic sex and gonadal sex are
> difficult to establish without special tests or procedures. In some of
> these cases, the sex of rearing will differ from gonadal and chro-
> mosomal sex.[417]

1) Determining the Sex of Rearing

Once the cause of ambiguous genitalia is determined, it is relatively easy
to decide the optimum sex of rearing, to name the infant, and to perform any
necessary surgery. If the surgery must be done in step stages, it should be
scheduled before the infant is discharged from the hospital and should ideally
be completed in the neonatal period. Dr. Monteleone demonstrates the diagnosis and treatment procedure in his review of four case histories: three *infants*
and one *adult*. According to the chromosomal analysis, all four were normal
46, XY males. As to the sex of rearing, two of the infants were raised as
females, the other (with unhappy consequences) was raised as a male. The
adult chose to assume a male identity.[418]

If an infant has a micropenis, and the diagnosis of that condition is
missed at birth, and the physician does not see him until the age of two or
three when the sex of rearing and gender identity have been established, it
can become a difficult situation. Testosterone therapy may be helpful, but if
there is incomplete penile development, serious thought and consideration
should be given to raising the child as a female. In the words of Dr. Monteleone: "Even the wisest decision will result in some inconvenience and problems." If the child is over 18 months of age when the therapist or physician

---

[416]*Ibid.*, p. 66. Cf. also, same author, *Human Sexuality and Personhood* (St. Louis, Mo.: Pope John
Center, 1981), for a listing and discussion of disorders of sexual development, pp. 71–85.

[417]*Ibid.*, (Sex and Gender), p. 66.

[418]*Sex and Gender* (cf. note 409), pp. 70–75, with photographic illustrations.

enters the case (the age at which the child begins to use language and is establishing gender identity), that child must be dealt with directly and seen on a regular basis until the physician or therapist is confident that the family and child have adjusted adequately to the change in sex rearing. Again, in the words of Dr. Monteleone: "Some feel that a change in sex rearing is feasible until the age of 18 months to about age 3¹/₂ years, but thereafter psychiatric consequences can result. After the age of 5, sex reassignment is rarely possible."[419] An older patient with micropenis may benefit from corrective surgery.

2) The Spectre of Impotence in Cases of Ambiguous Genitalia

The basic directives with regard to impotence are found in the following two canons of the new Code of Canon Law (italics added for emphasis):

> A valid marriage between baptized persons . . . is called ratified and consummated if the parties have performed between themselves *in a human manner* the conjugal act which is *of itself suitable* for the generation of children, to which marriage is ordered by its very nature and by which the spouses *become one flesh* (Canon 1061,1).

> *Antecedent* and *perpetual* impotence to have intercourse, whether on the part of the man or of the woman, which is either *absolute* or *relative*, of its very nature invalidates marriage (Canon 1084,1).

Article 49 of *The Church Today* calls conjugal love *eminently human*, "enriching the expressions of body and mind with a unique dignity;"—and adds that it is perfected (that is, advances to greater perfection) by being "expressed in a manner which is truly human." Undoubtedly this is one of the sources of the phrase *"in a human manner"* in Canon 1061,1, above. An inspiring reflection on this phrase is found in Vol. V of the *Commentary on the Documents of Vatican II*:

> Conjugal love is fully human, personal, total. The whole human being expresses himself or herself in it, with will and heart responsive to the beloved partner in willing self-giving. The bodily element is not considered solely in teleological categories but shares in the personal mode of existence in speech and love. Conjugal love is not regarded one-sidedly as limited to the marital act, but

---

[419]*Ibid.*, pp. 68–70.

as pervading the whole of life. But marital intercourse is a culminating expression of that love and of its continual development.[420]

Such an elevated concept of the "oneness" of marriage casts doubt on the validity of physical conjugal union which is characterized by violence or the "rape" mentality. The great canonist, Gratian, insisted that those who become one in body must become one in mind. He added: "therefore no one who is unwilling should be joined to another" ("ideo nulla invita est copulanda alicui").[421] What an impressive 12th century testimonial to "humano modo!"

Interpretation of Canons 1061,1, and 1084

Impotence means the incapacity for normal sexual intercourse. It is called *antecedent* if this incapacity existed already before marriage; it is called *perpetual* if the condition cannot respond to treatment except through a life-threatening operation. Impotence is *absolute* if it applies to sexual intercourse with all other persons of the opposite sex; it is *relative* if it applies to a particular individual of the opposite sex. Canon 1084,2, specifies further that if the impediment of impotence is doubtful either with regard to the law (the law itself is not clear) or with regard to factual application to this or that individual ("Am I really impotent?"), a marriage is neither to be impeded nor is it to be declared null as long as the doubt persists.

In interpreting the phrase "become one flesh" (Can.1061,1), it is now clear from a decree of the S. Congregation for the Doctrine of the Faith (May 13, 1977) that this does not mean necessarily that the male must be capable of ejaculating semen elaborated in the testicles ("semen verum in testiculis elaboratum"). The discussion of this phrase assumed rather classic dimensions in discussions among canonists and various agencies of the Holy See throughout the years.[422]

This decree of May 13, 1977 does not mean that the doubt as to whether or not "semen elaborated in the testicles" is required for potency is solved;[423]

---

[420](Cf. note 42), p. 237.

[421]*CLSA Commentary* (cf. note 45), p. 745 and footnote 17.

[422]For the background of these discussions, cf. Cappello, Felix M., S.J., *Tractatus Canonico-Moralis de Sacramentis*, Vol. V, *De Matrimonio*, 6th ed. (Rome: Marietti, 1950), nn. 340–389 (pp. 348–388); Roman Rota, "coram Wynen," Oct. 25, 1945, in *Canon Law Digest*, III (cf. note 43), 414–417.

[423]Cappello, *Ibid.*, n. 358,2: "Decisions of the Sacred Roman Congregations by no means constitute an *authentic* declaration, therefore they do not settle the doubt of law."

but it is a definitive declaration in recognizing that the doubt of law exists, and hence those unable to produce semen elaborated in the testicles are not to be considered impotent. The preliminary portion of this decree reads as follows:

> The Sacred Congregation for the Doctrine of the Faith has always held that persons who have undergone vasectomy and other persons in similar conditions must not be prohibited from marriage because certain proof of impotency on their part is not had.

> And now, after having examined that kind of practice and after repeated studies carried out by this Sacred Congregation as well as by the Commission for the Revision of the Code of Canon Law, the Fathers of this S. Congregation, in the plenary assembly held on Wednesday, the 11th of May, 1977, decided that the questions proposed to them must be answered as follows:

This is followed by the "in the *negative*" in response to "whether for conjugal intercourse the ejaculation of semen elaborated in the testicles is necessarily requisite?"[424]

Since that decree of May 13, 1977, the same Congregation for the Doctrine of the Faith received an inquiry with regard to the potency of a man with irremediable bilateral cryptorchidism (both testicles atrophied). The simple reply was: ". . . proceed in accord with the recent decree . . . [of] May 13, 1977."[425] Hence if a man has had a vasectomy, or has lost the function of his testicles through an accident or some disease, he is not to be considered as impotent. The reason is because it is not certain that "semen verum in testiculis elaboratum" is an essential aspect of potency. Cappello states this principle (found in Canon 1084,2) with brevity and clarity: "No one can be deprived of his *certain* right to enter marriage, unless it is *certainly* evident that he is impotent."[426] It still remains to interpret the meaning of the conjugal act as "of itself suitable for the generation of children."

---

[424]*Canon Law Digest,* VIII (cf. note 38), pp. 676, 677. Naturally, this decree was good news to many men who were victims of the legally-imposed sterilization policy of Hitler's Third Reich. Cf. "A Recent Decision of the Holy See Regarding Impotence and Sterility" in the Feb., 1978 issue of *Linacre Quarterly,* by Father Thomas O'Donnell, S.J., pp. 19–21.

[425]*Canon Law Digest,* IX (cf. note 44), pp. 624–627. This was a private response to the Archbishop of Milwaukee, Wis. Cf. also *Canon Law Digest,* VI (cf. note 252), pp. 616–620.

[426]*De Matrimonio* (cf. note 422), n. 379,b (p. 378).

The Minimal Requirements for Sexual Potency

His Eminence, Peter Cardinal Gasparri, and others (before and after him) make a distinction between the *human action* and the *action of nature*. Omitting Gasparri's reference to the ejaculation of true semen (which he considered an essential element), his statement would read as follows: "Human action concludes with the penetration of the penis into the vagina and the effusion of . . . semen therein; then the action of nature begins."[427] Adapting this distinction to contemporary thinking on the subject of impotence, it can be said that both husband and wife can be considered capable of the *human action* "suitable for the generation of children" even though the husband may lack testicles and even though the wife may lack all of her post-vaginal organs (womb, ovaries, fallopian tubes).[428] The fact that children cannot be conceived is viewed as a deficiency in the *action of nature*. The *human action* is accomplished, in the language of Canon 1061,1, in the act whereby, *in a human manner* the spouses *"become one flesh."*[429]

Within these parameters, it is possible to speak of the minimum requirements for human sexual potency. The man is potent if he has a penis of such formation and is capable of sustaining such an erection that he can penetrate and ejaculate into the vagina of the woman he is to marry. A woman must have a vagina which is capable of receiving the male organ. This requirement is fulfilled even though she may have an artificial plastic-surgery vagina—provided that it is constructed of natural, human materials.[430] If she has such a plastic-surgery vagina, however, she has an obligation in charity to inform her intended husband of her lack of a natural, normal vagina.[431] Any priest who learns in the course of premarital instructions that the woman has an

---

[427] *Tractaus Canonicus de Matrimonio,* 9th ed. (Rome: Vatican Press, 1932) Vol. I, n. 509. Cf. also Cappello, Felix M., *De Matrimonio* (cf. note 422), nn. 341, 342 (pp. 348–351); Merkelbach, Benedict Henry, O.P., *Summa Theologiae Moralis,* III (cf. note 250), n. 877.

[428] Cappello, Felix M., S.J., *Ibid.,* nn. 357, 358, lists the following responses on this subject: S. Congregation of the Holy Office, February 3, 1887, July 23, 1890, and July 31, 1895; S. Congregation for the Discipline of the Sacraments, April 2, 1909.

[429] Cappello, *Ibid.,* n. 382 (pp. 380, 381) lists over 30 authors who maintain that the essential element in realizing the consummation of marriage is "ut conjuges fiant una caro" ("that the two partners become one flesh").

[430] *CLSA Commentary* (cf. note 45), p. 765. Cf. also *Canon Law Digest,* VI (cf. note 252), pp. 612–616, and Cappello, *Ibid.,* pp. 363–368.

[431] O'Donnell, Thomas J., S.J., *Medicine and Christian Morality* (cf. note 31), pp. 218–220, discusses this subject of the plastic vagina at length, and mentions that the opinion favoring potency in such cases is shared by Father John C. Ford, S.J., Father Edwin F. Healy, S.J., and by the French theologian, Father P. Tesson, S.J.

artificial plastic-surgery vagina should consult with the bishop of the diocese before agreeing to assist at the marriage.

It is difficult to arrive at a specific answer to the question: "what degree of penetration by the male penis is required in order to render the act 'of itself suitable' for the generation of children?" Father Cappello writes: "Without doubt," the perforation of the vagina or penetration by the masculine member is required. He uses expressions such as "some penetration of the vagina is necessary," and "at least a partial penetration of the vagina is required and suffices."[432] He also mentions a response of the Holy Office of February 12, 1941, which states that it is sufficient if the man penetrates the vagina of the woman to some extent, even though imperfectly ("aliquo saltem modo, etsi imperfecte"), so that he brings about "at least a partial semination into the vagina in a natural manner." The penetration of the entire bulbous tip of the penis into the vagina is not required (a negative response to: "an . . . requiratur, ut glans tota intra vaginam versetur").[433]

The observations in the above paragraph with regard to the absolute "penetration requirement" ("some penetration,"—"at least partial,"—"even though imperfectly") will have to suffice for an understanding of sexual potency. Some sources have speculated as to just how many centimeters of penetration would satisfy the basic requirements;[434] others have inferred that the basic requirements would not be fulfilled if the degree of penetration would not be such as to relieve the concupiscence of both husband and wife.[435] As long as doubt remains regarding such specific aspects of the penetration requirement, whether as to law or as to fact in a particular case, the individuals involved are not to be impeded in their right to marry (Can.1084,2). Positive doubt remains as to the specific extent to which penetration of the vagina

---

[432]*De Matrimonio* (cf. note 422), nn. 342,4 (p. 350), 349,7,1 (360), 382 (p. 380).

[433]*Ibid.*, n. 382,3 (p. 381).

[434]Cf. *Canon Law Digest*, IV (Milwaukee, Wis.: Bruce Publishing Co., 1958), pp. 317–320. This was a private response before the appellate tribunal of Bologna, Italy, in 1954.

[435]Cappello mentions the opinion of authors who would insist that potency must include a penetration which would relieve the concupiscence of both parties: "Potentia enim coeundi includit ut *legitimo et naturali modo concupiscentia* viri et mulieris, per se, sedetur . . ." He states his opinion as follows: "Duo sane requiruntur et sufficiunt: penetratio vaginae per membrum virile et effusio . . . seminis in ea, utraque modo *naturali* facta" (the word *veri* before "seminis" omitted since it would not apply today). *De Matrimonio* (cf. note 422), n. 351,2 (p. 361). The following statement is found among orientations accepted by the Pontifical Commission for the Revision of the Code of Canon Law "which may be considered to constitute an authoritative interpretation of the legislation on masculine and feminine impotence:" "The copula need not be accompanied by complete orgasm or sexual satisfaction on the part of both husband and wife." Cf. *Handbook for Marriage Nullity Cases*, 2nd ed., by Edward Hudson et al. (Ottawa, Canada: St. Paul University, 1976), p. 62, n. 4. The book is listed "for private distribution only."

pertains to the conjugal act, ". . . whereby the spouses become one flesh" (Can.1061,1).[436]

Solving Practical Doubts Regarding Impotence

If the inability to have intercourse clearly existed already before the marriage (antecedent) and cannot be remedied (perpetual), the person involved (man or woman) cannot enter a valid marriage (Can.1084,1). As stated previously, the condition is called *perpetual* if it cannot be remedied "without a probable danger to life."[437] If there are positive reasons, based on qualified medical advice, that the condition may be remedied with the passage of time and/or with medical or surgical treatment, the condition is to be considered *temporary* (impotence uncertain) and the individual cannot be denied his or her *certain* right to marry. If the vagina of the woman is so closed that it cannot be penetrated by the male member in accord with the penetration requirements as outlined by Father Cappello above, and the attending physician judges that remedial surgery would probably endanger the life of the woman, the surgery should be performed *before* marriage.

Due to the lack of specific guidance provided by the discussion above as to the degree of penetration required, and in view of the response of the Holy Office of February 12, 1941, that the penetration of the vagina "to some extent, even though imperfectly" can suffice, every doubtful case should be referred to the bishop of the diocese. If positive doubt remains, the *certain* right to marry should prevail over the *uncertainty* of impotence.

The Liceity of Certain Mechanical Devices for the Husband

Further comment is needed on the statement above that the husband must have "a penis of such formation and capable of such an erection that he can penetrate and ejaculate into the vagina of the woman." This could be of prime importance for individuals who were born with a micropenis and who have been reared as males. The decision as to whether or not such a person is capable of penetrating the vagina "at least to some extent, even though imperfectly" would devolve upon the physician or clinical specialist. If the problem is traced to a structural or organic cause, some patients with inadequate erections can be helped by the administration of human chorionic gonado-

---

[436]For a review of decisions involving potency regarding the vagina, cf. *Canon Law Digest*, VI (cf. note 252), pp. 612–616.

[437]Cappello, Felix M., S.J., *De Matrimonio* (cf. note 422), n. 346,3 (p. 355). This means that the condition might be remedied by *licit* means, without a probable danger to life, or serious risk to salvation ("gravi damno salutis").

tropin (HCG) combined with supportive counseling.[438] The fact remains, however, that the most frequent cause of impotence is traced to psychogenic factors:

> Penile erection depends not only upon structural neuromuscular and vascular components but also to a large degree upon the emotional state of the individual. By far the most frequent cause of impotence is psychogenic factors.[439]

The subject of psychogenic impotence is too involved to be discussed here.[440]

If the cause of impotence is organic, there are limited options for correction of the condition such as a vascular reconstruction or bypass operation to remedy obstruction in the arteries leading to the penis, or recourse to hormonal adjustments, or even a self-injection technique whereby the individual uses a tiny needle to inject drugs directly into the spongy erectile tissue of the penis thus producing a temporary increase in blood flow (not to be attempted without the expert guidance of a physician).[441] Research is also being done on the administration of chemical neurotransmitters (one such chemical messenger is known as vasoactive intestinal peptide) which cause the vascular spaces to widen so as to facilitate the flow of blood to the erectile tissues.[442]

For thousands of men who are concerned about organic impotence, however, relief has been provided by penile prostheses which are surgically implanted completely within the body. One of these is a semirigid rod prosthesis. This device is made of two silicone rubber rods which are surgically inserted into the shaft of the penis. Although this device remains firm after it is implanted, it is flexible and can be bent so that the penis is close to the body for concealment when the individual is not engaged in sexual intercourse.[443] The more satisfactory and more expensive device (total cost may amount to sev-

---

[438]Amelar-Dubin-Walsh, *Male Infertility* (cf. note 86), p. 206.

[439]*Ibid.*, p. 205.

[440]For a brief survey of this question, cf. Dr. Carlo Rizzo in *Dictionary of Moral Theology* (cf. note 346), pp. 608, 609, and 816, 817. Cf. also Niedermeyer, Dr. Albert, *Compendium of Pastoral Theology* (cf. note 89), pp. 123–126.

[441]Cf. the *Mayo Clinic Health Letter* (Mayo Clinic, Rochester, Mn.), Medical Essay entitled "Impotence in America," May, 1986, pp. 6, 7.

[442]*Ibid.*, p. 8. Cf. also the December, 1985, issue of the same publication.

[443]This device would seem to be the most questionable of the prostheses mentioned in this chapter as facilitating adequately the conjugal act. Since the device is always in place, and semirigid, it is difficult to understand how it could activate neuromuscular components to bring about any type of an ejaculation of natural fluids. Even more questionable are external splints, sometimes called "coital training devices," which are mentioned by Amelar-Dubin-Walsh in *Male Infertility* (cf. note 86). They are applied to the limp penis to give it an outer skeleton of support, but "are largely unsatisfactory both to the patient and to his sexual partner" (p. 208).

eral thousand dollars) is the *inflatable prosthesis* of the more complex type. It consists of three parts: a balloon-shaped reservoir which is filled with fluid and placed beneath the lower abdominal muscles, two artificial cylinders inserted into the two natural cylinders of the penis (which normally fill with blood to cause an erection), and a pump which is placed in the scrotal sac (which contains the testes). All of the parts are connected by tubing, and the prosthesis is implanted through a small incision near the penis (only a short hospital stay required).[444]

This more complex type of implanted inflatable prosthesis is described in a medical journal as follows:

> The inflatable prosthesis is designed to produce an erection whenever the patient desires. It neither contributes to nor detracts from the capability of the patient to experience an orgasm. The prosthesis does enable the patient to penetrate the vagina and, if he was capable of it before becoming impotent, to ejaculate and impregnate a woman.[445]

There is also a less complex type of implanted inflatable prosthesis which is less costly. It is also less satisfactory due to the fact that the erection it produces is not as firm as the one produced by the more complex version described above. The *less complex* type is contained entirely within the penis (two silicone-encased cylinders, each with its own small pump and fluid reservoir). The small pumps for each cylinder are located near the tip of the penis and the reservoirs on the opposite end. There are no implantings in the lower abdominal muscles and in the scrotal sac with connecting tubing as in the more complex installation.[446] Presumably, however, the quotation from the medical journal above would apply to both types of inflatable prostheses.

The moral principles involved in the use of such devices as listed above (including surgical, chemical and self-injection techniques) have not been discussed widely among Catholic theologians. The following observations are presented in an effort to stimulate such discussions, and subject (as always) to correction or rejection by Church authorities.

The following basic principles must be kept in mind: (1) the essentials for the male's capacity for sexual intercourse must include a sustained erection, penetration of the vagina, and ejaculation into the vagina; (2) if it is *certain*

---

[444]*Mayo Clinic Health Letter,* May, 1986, pp. 7, 8.

[445]"Erectile Impotence Treated With an Implantable, Inflatable Prosthesis," by F. Brantley Scott, MD, et al., *Journal of the American Medical Association,* June 15, 1979, p. 2612.

[446]*Mayo Clinic Health Letter,* May, 1986, p. 7.

that the male's inability with regard to any one of these three aspects of intercourse existed before the marriage (antecedent impotence) and cannot be remedied (perpetual impotence), he cannot enter a valid marriage contract (Can.1084,1); (3) if there is a positive doubt, whether of law or of fact, with regard to either of the two principles mentioned above, the individual cannot be impeded from entering marriage for as long as that doubt persists (Can.1084,2); (4) the Church does not necessarily forbid the use of certain artificial means designed solely to facilitate the natural act or to achieve the attainment of the natural act of intercourse normally performed (Pope Pius XII, cf. chapter II, p.42).

In applying these principles to the situation of a young man who is impotent from birth and who had never married (hence "antecedent"), the answer as to whether or not he could enter marriage would depend upon whether or not the physical or psychic impotence could be remedied. As an illustration of the requirement that the male must be capable of *having and of sustaining* an erection and of ejaculation, an actual case cited by Cardinal Gasparri, will be helpful. After his marriage to Julia, Caius noted the same problem which he had experienced before marriage. According to Julia, Caius had difficulty in achieving an erection. Whenever he was successful in that effort, however, it was not a proper erection ("formalis erectio") but rather a moderate erection ("modica") which disappeared immediately and was followed by the emission of some type of liquid. Furthermore, he had a small and flaccid penis, small testicles, and lacked a proper manifestation of the heat of passion ("calor"). The marriage was declared invalid on the grounds of impotence. The declaration was confirmed by a higher congregation of the Holy See. Three years later, however, Caius had overcome his inability to sustain an erection, and was allowed to contract marriage with another woman.[447]

The problem which Caius experienced in his first marriage could have been due to *relative* impotence (as opposed to *absolute* impotence) because of a temporary disease or illness, or because of a strong dislike or aversion to his first wife. Another possibility could be that his condition was remedied by medical treatment or professional counseling. Although this case involved a married man, one might consider the possibility of a single man who was diagnosed as congenitally impotent and was capable of only a moderate erection (small penis and testicles, absence of a passionate approach to intercourse), and who became capable of sustaining an erection with the installation of an implanted, inflatable prosthesis.

In such a case, the implanted, inflatable prosthesis would be, in effect, an artificial means of "facilitating the natural act," and of "achieving the attain-

---

[447] *Tractatus Canonicus de Matrimonio,* Vol. I, 9th ed. (cf. note 427). nn. 520 and 548.

ment of the natural act of intercourse normally performed" (cf. principles above). Presuming that the individual was also capable of ejaculating some type of natural fluid, there would be no reason to question his right to marry. He would be obligated, however, to inform his future spouse of his condition well in advance of the date of marriage.

If an individual lacks even the minimal capacity for erection and ejaculation as in the case cited by Cardinal Gasparri above, he remains incapable of entering a valid marriage contract for as long as the condition fails to respond to medical, psychological or psychiatric treatments. In such a case, the implanted penile prosthesis would not be a measure which facilitated some degree of natural capacity for human intercourse, but rather a pathetic mechanical *substitute* for the absence of sexual potency. This would be a violation of Catholic moral standards. There is also the possibility that such an unfortunate individual might be tempted to compensate for his lack of sexual prowess by using the implanted device to engage in grossly immoral practices.

In some cases, the masculine opening of the urethra is not at the tip of the penis but rather on the underside (hypospadias) or in some other area of the penis. If such a condition precludes the possibility of ejaculating into the vagina, and the condition does not respond to corrective measures, the impediment of impotence exists. If the position of the abnormal opening is such that it can be covered by a perforated condom so that the ejaculation can be directed to the perforated opening and hence enter the vagina, there should be no moral objection to having recourse to such a *facilitating* device. Upon the recommendation of the physician, the "silastic" type of condom (also known as a seminal pouch, cf. chapter II, pp.52,53) might well be used for that purpose. The claim is that such a device prevents the spillage of the ejaculate if properly used (cf.note 93). Depending upon the actual location of the urethral opening, the physician is best qualified to decide whether or not the device could be effective in facilitating ejaculation into the vagina, and also in advising the patient as to the best location for the perforation.

In the event that a man becomes impotent after marriage due to an accident, illness or disease, there should be no moral objection to the implanting of an inflatable prosthesis providing that there are no reasonable and available alternatives (counseling, hormonal or chemical treatments, medical or surgical measures, etc.). Such impotence cannot be characterized as either antecedent or perpetual. It is known rather as *subsequent* impotence, and has no effect on the validity of the marriage.[448] Likewise it has no effect on the liceity of continued sexual union. The Pontifical Commission for the Revision of the Code of Canon Law has accepted an interpretation of legislation on

---

[448]*CLSA Commentary* (cf. note 45), p. 766.

impotence which states that conjugal union "need not be accompanied by complete orgasm or sexual satisfaction on the part of both husband and wife."[449]

A word of caution is in order regarding a decision to submit to the implantation of an inflatable prosthesis. The physical and psychological risks involved (possible depression, danger of infection in view of the man's age, general state of health, and personal hygiene habits, etc.) may well outweigh the reasonably anticipated benefits. Extensive psychological counseling may be required so that personal expectations do not exceed realistic benefits.

In the treatment of *antecedent* impotence, there is little that can be done for a male who is born without a penis and is reared as a male. Unless the art of plastic surgery or phalloplasty (but from natural human tissues and materials) advances to the point of fashioning existing neuromuscular and vascular tissues into functioning erectile and ejaculatory components, the patient would have nothing more than a facsimile or replica of a true penis. He would remain impotent and incapable of entering a valid marriage contract.[450]

The *female* form of impotence known as *vaginismus* is often of psychosomatic origin. This type of *functional* impotence is described as a spasm of the sphincter muscle of the vagina with extreme sensibility of the adjacent parts. This condition makes penetration of the vagina painfully difficult or impossible. Since this condition usually responds to medical and/or surgical treatment (if of anatomical origin) or to psychological counseling (if of psychosomatic origin), it ordinarily is not perpetual, and hence does not constitute the impediment of impotence.[451]

Unnecessary Surgery

The contraceptive pill held first place among the various means of avoiding pregnancies for many years. As of late December, 1984, however, the U.S. Center of Health Statistics authorized the media to announce to the American public the startling news: "the pill has been superceded by male and female sterilizations."[452] These surgical procedures for contraceptive purposes,

---

[449]Cf. note 435.

[450]Ritty, Msgr. Charles J., "The Transsexual and Marriage," in *Studia Canonica*, Vol. 15, n. 2 (1981), p. 459, note 41.

[451]O'Donnell, Thomas, S.J., *Medicine and Catholic Morality* (cf. note 3), p. 218. Among the orientations accepted by the Pontifical Commission for the Revision of the Code of Canon Law (cf. note 435) was one stating that "it is not yet decided whether functional impotence constitutes a diriment impediment of impotence." *Ibid. (Handbook for Marriage Nullity Cases)*, p. 62, n. 14.

[452]*Time*, December 17, 1984, p. 79.

whether by excision or ligation of reproductive organs, are violations of the Principle of Totality because of the lack of a proportionate reason. In fact, on the basis of the Principle of the Double Effect (which is also involved), there can be no adequate justifying reason because of the presence of very reasonable and available alternatives (among them, Natural Family Planning). From a Catholic moral viewpoint, this is a prime example of unnecessary surgery. It is not a "classic" type of unnecessary surgery, however. In the classic sense, the patient neither wants nor needs the surgery.

As mentioned previously, and reported in the Jan. 28th, 1985 issue of *Time* magazine, the price tag for physician orders for additional procedures and diagnostic tests which really are not necessary, adds anywhere from $15 billion to $40 billion to the national health-care cost. The fact that this "defensive" tendency may be due in large part to the physician's fear of malpractice prosecution cannot justify such a flagrant abuse of the law of justice and of charity. Accepting a fee for such professional practices compounds the injustice and the evil. If the patient is put into a life-threatening condition because of such unnecessary ministrations, the physician cannot evade responsibility in conscience for the added suffering, expense and inconvenience. The Code of Medical Ethics of the American Medical Association states in section 4: "Physicians . . . should expose, without hesitation, illegal or unethical conduct of fellow members of the profession." If the members of the medical profession are unwilling or unable to observe that section of the code, they cannot merit the trust and confidence mentioned in section 1 of the same code: "Physicians should merit the confidence of patients entrusted to their care, rendering to each a full measure of service and devotion."[453]

Physicians are not infallible. With even the best will and highest of intentions, a physician may make an error in judgment which subjects a patient to a procedure which, in hindsight, was not medically indicated. He must also be aware of the danger of looking for short cuts, when the only proper treatment for a patient is a more complicated procedure. A severe crushed-hand injury sustained in an industrial accident, for example, can be treated by surgical amputation, or by the far more tedious diagnostic and surgical procedure of repairing the bones, nerves, tendons, arteries, etc., in several operations if required so as to restore the use of the hand. Unless it is an emergency situation where time permits no delay (danger of gangrene and loss of the entire arm, etc.), the physician is bound in conscience to propose the procedure which is in the best interests of the patient regardless of the expertise involved.

With regard to surgical vasectomy and tubal ligations (or cutting), it

---

[453]"Codes of Medical Ethics" in *Health Matrix*, Summer, 1984, pp. 43–48.

must be stressed that these immoral methods of sterilization are not devoid of danger. Even though the vasectomy of the male is a rather simple procedure (sometimes called "bandaid surgery"), there can be some danger of thrombosis and embolism. Even the mere ligation of the "vasa deferentia" can have what is called a "Steinach effect," which can condition an increase in sexual libido because the patient now feels "sexually safe." This can dispose a man to marital infidelity, domestic discord and even separation and divorce. Authors also speak of profound sexual neuroses and imaginative ills which can afflict some types of men when they have been rendered sexually safe.[454]

For a woman who has her fallopian tubes ligated or severed as a contraceptive measure, the procedure itself is more complicated since it usually involves laparotomy (opening of the abdomen) and anesthesia. The psychological dangers associated with vasectomy for men apply also to women who can now feel sexually safe. Neuroses can also arise from the depressing realization that she has lost her capacity to conceive and nurture new life. Sometimes the procedure involves severing the fallopian tubes and then burying the distal ends in the folds of the broad ligament, in the hope that the capacity to conceive another child might be restored at some future date. With the advent of microsurgery and laser technology today, the re-joining of the fallopian tubes and of the vasa deferentia (for males) is within the realm of possibility more frequently than in the past.

> *Directive 33:* Unnecessary procedures, whether diagnostic or therapeutic, are morally objectionable. A procedure is unnecessary when no proportionate reason justifies it. *A fortiori,* any procedure that is contra-indicated by sound medical standards is unnecessary.

---

[454]Niedermeyer, Dr. Albert, *Compendium of Pastoral Medicine* (cf. note 89), p. 268. Cf. also Healy, Edwin, S.J., *Medical Ethics* (cf. note 46), p. 177.

CHAPTER VII

The Principle of the Double Effect

In the depths of his conscience, man detects a law which he does not impose upon himself, but which holds him to obedience. Always summoning him to love good and avoid evil, the voice of conscience can when necessary speak to his heart more specifically: do this, shun that. For man has in his heart a law written by God. To obey it is the very dignity of man; according to it he will be judged (*The Church Today*, n.16).

PRINCIPLE: AN ACTION, GOOD IN ITSELF, WHICH HAS TWO EFFECTS, AN INTENDED AND OTHERWISE NOT REASONABLY ATTAINABLE GOOD EFFECT, AND A FORESEEN BUT MERELY PERMITTED CONCOMITANT EVIL EFFECT, MAY LICITLY BE PLACED, PROVIDED THERE IS A DUE PROPORTION BETWEEN THE INTENDED GOOD AND THE PERMITTED EVIL (from *Medicine and Christian Morality*, by Father Thomas J. O'Donnell, S.J., p.29).

The two most general and universal precepts of the natural law, accepted by fair-minded people of all times and nations, are: "Do good," and "Avoid evil." The latter ("Avoid evil") is a negative precept, and like all negative precepts, obligates always and everywhere. Due to the many life situations in which foreseen but unintended evil effects are associated with doing good, however, the question is bound to arise: "Does the obligation to avoid evil oblige one to abstain from a good action, in order to prevent a foreseen but merely permitted concomitant evil?"

It is important to emphasize that both effects of a double-effect action are to be considered in their moral implications. Even though the evil effect cannot be willed directly, it is foreseen as something that would be morally wrong if willed directly either as an end or as a means to an end. Father Thomas O'Donnell, S.J. explains this moral-viewpoint aspect as follows:

> Here we must distinguish carefully between moral and physical evil. We are speaking of an evil effect in the moral order only. The evil effect is that which, if directly willed, would be morally evil.
>
> For example, contrast the amputation of a gangrenous leg with the death of a non-viable fetus. In the former case the loss of the leg is a physically, but not morally, evil effect. The leg, as a part of the whole body, is subordinated to the good of the whole. In this case the amputation, although a physical evil, is not a moral evil, if directly willed.
>
> In the latter case, however, granted a cancer of the cervix with a non-viable fetus in situ, the surgeon intends the removal of dangerously diseased tissue. He foresees that the result of his attaining this good effect will be fetal death. He does not seek, intend, or directly will fetal death, but merely foresees it. If he directly willed fetal death, his action would be morally evil.[455]

If the Principle of the Double Effect were denied or rejected, the possibilities for doing good would be limited drastically. The moral responsibility of the individual for foreseen and unwelcome side effects which are recognized as evil if willed directly can be obviated by excluding them as a direct object of the human will—by tolerating them as inevitable but merely permitted side effects of a good action. Jesus said as much when he responded to St. Peter's question regarding moral evil by saying:

> Do you not see that . . . what comes out of the mouth originates in the mind? . . . From the mind stem evil designs—murder,

---

adulterous conduct, fornication, stealing, false witness, blasphemy. These are things that make a man impure" (Matthew, 15: 17-20).

If the object of a human action is intrinsically evil, however (to be discussed presently), it cannot be justified in any circumstances or even for the highest of motives (for example, blasphemy). In such cases, there is no way of alienating the one who performs the action from direct responsibility for the evil action. The basic principle, "the end does not justify the means," is based on St. Paul's response to possible confused and misleading concepts of the Christians of Rome:

> Or why may we not do evil that good may come of it? This is the very thing that some slanderously accuse us of teaching; but they will get what they deserve (Romans, 3:8).

"Do good" is a positive precept. Like all positive precepts, it does not obligate in every possible situation of doing good. The reason is simply because there is a limit to the good that can or should be done. Even the most highly motivated individual is not obligated to spring into action every time he or she sees the opportunity of doing good. To be expected to do good in all possible situations would constitute a crushing and insupportable burden. This is not to deny or to minimize, however, the common teaching of theologians that there are many situations in life when the individual is obligated to do all that is reasonably within his or her power to do so as to foresee and prevent the emergence of evil consequences. Among the many examples that could be mentioned there is the common obligation to make choices and decisions so as to avoid occasions of sin; the obligation of parents and teachers to protect those under their care from bad companions; the obligation of civil officials and administrators to uphold justice in the discharge of their duties; the obligation of all citizens (based on the virtue of charity) to yell out a warning to others who may be unaware of approaching danger, etc.[456]

7.1 Explanation of the Principle of the Double Effect

There are many situations in everyday life when an action results in more than one effect with moral implications—that is, effects which the agent per-

---

[456]Merkelbach, Henry, O.P., *Summa Theologiae Moralis,* vol. I (cf. note 151), nn. 60-63 and 172, pp. 67-70 and 164, 165.

ceives as either good or evil. Some actions have two good effects from a moral viewpoint. If a woman forgives an unfriendly neighbor who spread lies about her, there is the good effect of an example of Christian forgiveness, and the good effect of turning an enemy into a friend. Other actions have two evil effects from a moral viewpoint. If a man stops at his favorite tavern and imbibes to the point of drunkenness after a hard day at the office, there is the evil effect of drunkenness, and the foreseen evil effect of serious domestic trouble when he gets home that night. Many human actions have a good effect and an evil effect as perceived by the agent in their moral implications. The good effect is intended and can be willed directly. The evil effect, although foreseen in its moral implications, is not willed directly, but merely permitted or tolerated. For example, a judge acquits an innocent man. There is the good effect of the triumph of justice, and there is the evil effect of incurring the bitter criticism of the opposition. Without the judge's good action, the evil effect would not have materialized. He cannot be held responsible, however, for the foreseen but merely permitted evil effect.

The Principle of the Double Effect validates "doing good" regardless of foreseen but unintended evil effects (perceived in their moral implications) provided that, all things considered, the intended good effect is of such merit that its omission would be, in the judgment of prudent individuals, too high a price to pay for preventing the concomitant evil effect. It should also be noted that in the example above, the judge was under an obligation to render a just decision by virtue of his position as a public, civil official. By virtue of his position, he was obligated to render a just decision in behalf of the common good. The principle would not validate the actions of imprudent "do gooders" who thoughtlessly launch out into performing ill-conceived good deeds without regard for possible evil consequences.[457]

The Five Conditions Involved in the Principle of the Double Effect

The last half of this chapter will focus on the application of the Principle of the Double Effect to medical situations. For illustration purposes, it may be well to use the example mentioned in the writings of St. Thomas Aquinas—the breaking-and-entering thief who was mortally wounded by the vigilant master of the house. Although St. Thomas does not furnish details, it will be presumed that the master of the house was caught by surprise, and had reasons to fear that his life was in danger (dangerous and armed prowlers had

---

[457]Public officials are obligated to perform their duties for the common good, as St. Thomas Aquinas points out in his *Summa Theologiae* (cf. note 168), II-II, Q.64, art.3, corp.

wounded home owners in similar incidents in the area, etc.). Other details will also be presented as imaginary.

The following conditions are quoted from the statement of the Principle of the Double Effect as found at the beginning of this chapter:

(1) "An action, good in itself (or at least indifferent) which has two effects . . ."

This refers to the action itself, considered independently of its effects. The surprised and terrified master of the house grabbed the first heavy object he could find (a large solid-glass paperweight), hid behind the door, and administered a direct blow to the head of the intruder as he entered. The action of striking someone with a blunt object is in itself indifferent from a moral viewpoint. It could be perceived as good or as evil depending on the circumstances.

Many actions are good in themselves (for example, praising God, helping a neighbor), while others, considered in the abstract and apart from concrete circumstances, are said to be indifferent as in the example above. Common human actions such as walking, eating, running, etc., are indifferent from a moral viewpoint. The moral evaluation would depend on the circumstances surrounding the action (for example, walking down the street fully unclothed) and the intention of the one who performs the action (for example, running away from the scene of a serious accident so as "not to be involved"). Furthermore, both actions which are good in themselves or indifferent from a moral viewpoint can be evil because the person who performs them has no right or authority to do so. These might be called reserved actions. Thus a person who is not a duly elected or appointed judge or magistrate has no right to hand down decisions in a civil court.

Other human actions are evil with regard to the very substance of the action. These actions are called morally evil in themselves ("in se") or intrinsically evil. As mentioned previously, if such actions are performed with due knowledge and deliberation, they are morally evil in all circumstances regardless of the high purpose or intention of the one who performs them. Classic examples of such actions are blasphemy, perjury, masturbation, killing of the innocent, etc. The morality of such actions is called absolute or "exceptionless" ("we may not do evil that good may come of it," or "the end does not justify the means").

When considering the morality of a human act in a concrete situation, attention must be given to three considerations: the objective nature or substance of the action, the circumstances under which it is performed, and the purpose or intention of the one performing the action. The classical teaching is that the act must be good on all three counts ("bonum ex integra causa"). If it departs from this standard of moral goodness on only one count (objectively evil, sinful circumstances, evil purpose or intention), it is an evil action ("malum ex quolibet effectu"). If a young man gives an expensive gift to his girl friend in proper circumstances (brings it to her apartment on the evening of her birthday) but with the purpose or intention of overwhelming her with a sense of gratitude so that she will consent to his lustful desires, the action is evil regardless of the propriety of the object of the action and the circumstances.

(2) The good effect: "An intended and otherwise not reasonably attained good effect . . ."

The good effect must be the only effect which is the *direct* object of the human will. Hence it is called the "direct voluntary." There is no reason to believe that the master of the house, in this particular case, had any reasonable alternative. There was no time to call for help or to run for safety without the danger of being detected and assaulted by the intruder. The good effect of his defensive action was his protection from possible serious harm. If that good effect could have been obtained in some other way, equally attainable and effective, without causing the evil effect (physical harm to the intruder), he would have been obligated to choose that other way.

(3) The evil effect: "And a foreseen but merely permitted side effect . . ."

Since St. Thomas mentions that the thief was mortally wounded, the scenario may be sketched to include the calling of the police, and their discovery that the blow on the head actually caused the death of the intruder. In the words of St. Thomas: "Inasmuch as an action of this type is intended to protect one's own life, it is not illicit: since it is natural for anyone to protect life itself to the extent possible."[458] It can be presumed that the frightened master of the house foresaw the possibility, at least in a confused manner, that the blow on the head might bring about the death of the intruder. The action, however, was a moderate type of violence which was required in the situation.[459] The master of the house did not intend to bring about the death of the

---

[458]*Ibid.*, art. 7, corp.

[459]*Ibid.*, St. Thomas quotes a legal guideline: "vim vi repellere licet cum moderamine inculpatae tutelae." It would be illicit, however, to use more violence than required ("majori violentia quam oportet"). *Ibid.*, corp.

intruder, but merely permitted it as a possible *indirect* consequence of his action. Again, in the words of St. Thomas: "Moral actions are reckoned ("recipiunt speciem") according to what is intended, and not according to what is beyond the intention ("praeter intentionem"), since that is not an intended consequence ("per accidens").[460]

(4) No relationship of causality: The evil effect is "a merely permitted concomitant effect . . ."

The evil effect must not cause the good effect. In other words, the good effect must not be realized through the evil effect. If such a relationship of causality between the two effects is present, the evil effect is *directly* intended either as an end or as the means to the contemplated end. In the example provided by St. Thomas (self-defense against the unjust intruder), the action of the master of the house against the intruder did not refer to the protection of the life of the master of the house as a means to an end, nor as an end in itself, but as a consequence due to the *necessity of the end*—his intention to save his own life ("ex hoc quod intenditur conservatio propriae vitae").[461] It is not essential that the two effects (good and evil) must proceed from the same action with split-second simultaneity, but that the agent must not intend the evil effect *directly* even as a means to realizing the good effect. Sometimes this condition is expressed by saying that the good effect must be at least equally immediate with the evil effect. Father Francis Connell, C.SS.R. notes, however, that ". . . this immediacy refers to the order of *causality,* not the order of *time.* In the order of time the bad effect may preceed the good effect."[462]

(5) Proportionate reason: "Provided there is a due proportion between the intended good and the permitted evil effect."

There must be a proportionate reason for permitting the foreseen evil to occur. The good to be realized must compensate for the evil which is permitted or tolerated. Disregard for this imperative would amount to causing injury to others without necessity contrary to Christian standards of justice and charity.

"Proportionate" means that if the evil effect is slight, a slight reason would suffice for performing the action; if the evil effect is serious, only a serious reason would justify the action. The difficulty of determining the

---

[460]*Ibid.*, corp.
[461]*Ibid.*, corp.
[462]*Outlines of Moral Theology* (Milwaukee, Wis.: Bruce Publishing Co., 1953), p. 23, n. 3.

exact proportion that is due between the intended good and the permitted evil should not be minimized. It depends not only on a proper spirit of justice and charity, but also on a strong sense of human prudence. Father Gerald Kelly, S.J. provided a practical guideline when he wrote: "In practice, this means that there must be a sort of balance between the total good and the total evil produced by an action." He also noted that the difficulty of estimating the due-proportion element is so great in some cases, ". . . that even the most eminent theologians may disagree in their solution."[463]

In the case under discussion, the need of protecting life itself provided the master of the house with a proportionate reason for his violent defensive action. As an illustration of the connection between this condition (proportionate reason) and condition (2) above, however, the scenario might be changed to involve apprehension and fear in the neighborhood due not to the criminal behavior of dangerous and desperate adult thieves, but to the miscreant behavior of young boys of the poverty-stricken section of the area. Presuming that the master of the house is in fairly-robust health, he would not be justified in resorting to the violent type of self-defense as mentioned above (armed with a heavy blunt object) unless he had reasons to fear that the boys were armed with dangerous weapons (knives, guns, etc.). The reason is because the master of the house then has an alternative method or means of protecting himself and his property without afflicting serious injuries; as soon as he sees that the culprit entering the door is a young boy, he could overpower him by his superior physical strength.

The virtue of charity might inspire the master of the house to deal kindly with the young culprit (after overpowering the boy) by not turning him over to the law, or taking an interest in the poverty condition of the boy's family, but the virtue of charity would not obligate him to do so unless he were obligated in some way to provide for the welfare of the young boy (for example, if it happened to be his own grandson).[464]

An Evaluation of the Principle of the Double Effect

The Principle of the Double Effect is valid and defensible as a reliable guideline for doing good and avoiding evil. If individuals had to abstain from performing good actions because of foreseen evil side effects, not only would much good remain unattempted and undone in the world, but many would be tempted to use that prospect of evil side effects as an excuse to pass up

---

[463]*Medico-Moral Problems* (cf. note 22), p. 14.

[464]St. Thomas Aquinas, *Summa Theologiae* (cf. note 168), II-II, Q.64, art.7, corp. and footnote 11.

opportunities of doing good and even to shirk their duties in their personal, social and professional lives. Meanwhile, the forces of evil are advancing with diabolical ingenuity. The words of a great writer come to mind: "All that is needed for the triumph of evil, is that good people do nothing."

It is a simple principle, and yet difficult of application in complicated cases. Father Gerald Kelly, S.J. points out that conscientious people often use the Principle of the Double Effect without knowing the conditions listed above:

> The aviator who bombs an important military target, foreseeing but not desiring the deaths of some civilians, is, perhaps unwittingly, applying the principle. The student who must read a treatise on sex, foreseeing but not desiring temptations against chastity, is also using the principle, although he too may have no training in its use. And all of us, whether we realize it or not, are following the same principle when we perform some good and necessary action, realizing that, despite our best intentions, some others will misunderstand and will be led to rash judgments and criticisms. The deaths of the civilians, the sexual temptations, and the harsh thoughts and criticisms are all simply unavoidable and unwanted by-products of actions that are good in themselves and of sufficient importance to be performed despite the evil effects that accompany them.[465]

It is also clear that complications can arise to make the application of this principle difficult. A rather common pastoral problem might illustrate how complications can combine to make definite action difficult. Mr. and Mrs. Gin, parents of four small children, have been in to see the pastor, separately and together, over the past four months regarding serious marital problems. Mr. Gin, unemployed, is given to drink when he feels depressed (has "sworn off" many times) and has vented his anger and depression again and again by beating his wife—often in front of the children. Drunk or sober, however, Mr. Gin is always kind to the children. His parents, veritable pillars of the parish, have said to the pastor: "If you allow that couple to break up and separate, we are through with this parish." Is there an alternative to separation, like insisting on Alcoholics Anonymous for Mr. Gin yet another time (tried it and dropped out twice before)? Could professional counseling be attempted yet another time (Mrs. Gin broke it off last time,—"they ask too many personal

---

[465]*Medico-Moral Problems* (cf. note 22), p. 15.

questions"?). The pastor asks himself: "Am I exaggerating the risks of a separation?—Am I really thinking of the welfare of the children who need their father? Do I have a proportionate reason for giving up in my efforts to reconcile this couple? Should I try getting the police to intervene? Will a civil separation lead to divorce—will it drive Mr. Gin to become a chronic alcoholic?"

The Principle of the Double Effect often is abused, especially by individuals with the mentality of "It worked in that case, why can't it work in this case." It is often misunderstood by individuals who have not been trained to make distinctions. Some professionals seem to think for example, that "merely permitting foreseen evil side effects" is the same as "intending such side effects as a means to an end,"—which is an unfair appraisal of the principle. The *President's Commission* reveals such a mentality in the following quotation:

> The commission makes use of many of the moral considerations found in this doctrine (referred to as "doctrine of double effect"), but endorses the conclusion that people are equally responsible for all of the foreseeable effects of their actions, thereby having no need for a policy that separates "means" from "merely foreseen consequences".[466]

Evidence of the abuse of the principle will be presented in the discussion of the problem of proportionalism.

7.2 THE PROBLEM OF PROPORTIONALISM

The following commentary on a passage of Vatican II's document, *The Church Today* (n.16) provides a fitting introduction to the subject of proportionalism:

> The fathers [of Vatican II] were obviously anxious . . . not to allow an ethics of conscience to be transformed into the domination of subjectivism, and not to canonize a limitless situation ethics under the guise of conscience. On the contrary, the conciliar text implies that obedience to conscience means an end to subjectivism, a turning aside from blind arbitrariness, and produces

---

[466]*Deciding to Forego Life-Sustaining Treatment,* President's Commission (cf. note 215), p. 80, note 110.

conformity with the objective norms of moral action. Conscience is made the principle of objectivity, in the conviction that careful attention to its claim discloses the fundamental common values of human existence.[467]

Father Peter Knauer, S.J., who might be called the "Father of Proportionalism," formulated the question: "How does man recognize whether an act is morally good?" First he considered the possibility that good might be determined in relation to man's last end, which is God, but he rejected that approach as "pious" and "abstract." He then considered the possibility that good might be determined by a human act's "correspondence to human nature" [on which, in large part, "conformity with objective norms of moral action" is based], but found that standard "ambiguous." He then answered his question by saying (writing in 1965):

> The most exact is the third definition, according to which the morally good is "the simply good." By "good" is here meant nothing other than the physical goodness of any reality whatsoever, that goodness by which something becomes desirable in any sense, according to the axiom *ens et bonum convertuntur* ["being and good are one and the same," our translation]. What is "simply" good, and therefore morally good, is such a value, if it is willed in such a way that the physical evil possibly associated with it remains objectively beyond the intention of the person willing. The good alone, that is, "the simply good," determines the intention.[468]

Obviously this "good" is not the "good in itself" mentioned in the first condition of the Principle of the Double Effect as explained in the first section of this chapter (requirement "that the action be good in itself"). Thus "saying your prayers" or "helping your neighbor" or "disciplining your child" are actions good in themselves because they are in conformity with the virtues of religion, charity and parental love respectively. Father Knauer rules out such norms because they are simply physical acts. He insists that they can be considered as moral acts only when viewed in their entirety, encompassing all of the circumstances associated with the placing of the act: "Moral good

---

[467]*Commentary on the Documents of Vatican II,* vol. V (cf. note 42), p. 135.

[468]"The Hermeneutic Function of the Principle of the Double Effect," in *Readings in Moral Theology, No. I,* ed. by Charles E. Curran and Richard A. McCormick, S.J. (New York, N.Y.: Paulist Press, 1979), p. 2.

consists in the best possible realization of any particular value envisaged in its entirety."[469] What is the determinant which makes an act morally good or evil? It is the "commensurate reason" (which he also calls the "proportionate reason,"—hence, "proportionalism"): "The commensurate reason occupies the same area as what is directly willed and alone determines the entire moral content of the act. *If the reason of an act is commensurate, it alone determines the finis operis, so that the act is morally good.*"[470]

His thought is illustrated in his discussion of telling a lie—which to him, in itself, is a physical evil (later called a "pre-moral evil"):

> A lie consists in telling what is false without commensurate reason and therefore directly or formally causes the error of another . . . If such behavior were permitted, then trust in its existential entirety would be impossible; . . . But it is something entirely different if, in order to preserve a secret, a false answer is given to an indiscreet question. Then the case is parallel with self-defense; the error of the other is not directly willed. Morally, the answer has the meaning that I will not give away my secret. That the questioner is deceived is an evil which is rightly accepted in exchange for preservation of the secret.[471]

If other acts traditionally regarded even as intrinsically evil are substituted for lying (blasphemy, perjury, masturbation, direct sterilization, killing of the innocent, etc.), a commensurate reason or a combination of commensurate reasons could "determine the finis operis, so that the act is morally good."

The Basic Tenets of the Theory of Proportionalism

Father Servais Pinckaers, O.P. rightly calls proportionalism a "transition from a morality centered on the relationship of the act to its *object* conferring on it a moral quality in itself, independent of the *subject's* finality, to a morality centered on the *subject's* finality which becomes constructive of the *object itself* by means of a proportionate reason" (Emphasis added). This amounts to an interpretation of the Principle of the Double Effect as "no longer starting from its first condition and from the principle that one cannot do that which is evil in itself to attain a good, but starting from its last condition, proportionate reason, which serves henceforth to determine what is good or evil."

---

[469]*Ibid.*, p. 17.
[470]*Ibid.*, p. 11.
[471]*Ibid.*, p. 24.

257

He adds: "We are therefore participating in a sort of revolution within post-Tridentine Catholic morality."[472] It is a discordant rejection of *objectivism* in favor of *subjectivism* in determining the morality of human acts.

Traditional theology does not deny that a *moral judgment* cannot be made if one looks only at the object of the act, independently of the circumstances surrounding the act and the end intended. A person cannot judge that sexual intercourse is morally wrong unless he is aware of the circumstance that the two parties involved are not married; he cannot judge that a man is a thief for secretly taking the lawnmower of another unless he knows that the culprit intends to keep it as his very own; he cannot judge that a woman is guilty of sterilization unless he knows that she has contraception in mind. Such moral judgments cannot be made without knowing the circumstances and the end or intention of the person who performs the action; but there is no hesitancy in calling premarital intercourse, stealing, and direct sterilization objectively immoral.

In contrast, the proportionalists pass over the *objective* aspects of human acts and concentrate on *subjective* aspects. They seek to assemble as many favorable circumstances as possible in order to evaluate an action as morally good. This leads to an "IF" or "appendage type" of moral standards: stealing is wrong IF there is no proportionate reason; premarital sex is morally good IF there is a proportionate reason; contraception is wrong IF there is no proportionate reason. Otherwise, such human acts, in themselves, involve merely physical or pre-moral evil.

It was always admitted that there are physical evils which are not, in themselves, moral evils—for instance, illness, death, surgical mutilation, etc. The proportionalists group together all such physical evils which are a part of the human condition, along with the propensity of human nature to fail in achieving satisfaction in human endeavors, and call them *ontic* evils or disvalues. Louis Janssens defines ontic evil as "any lack of perfection at which we aim, any lack of fulfillment which frustrates our natural urges and makes us suffer. It is essentially the natural consequence of our limitation."[473] In applying this concept to the use of contraceptives, he states that contraception can be justified if these means do not obstruct the partners in the expression of conjugal love, and if they keep birth control within the limits of responsible parenthood.[474] Strange to say, the statement infers that "no obstruction in

---

[472]"The Question of Intrinsically Evil Acts and 'Proportionalism'," in *The Question of Intrinsically Evil Acts,* mimeography publication (Washington, D.C.: U.S. Catholic Conference, 1984), 2nd section, pp. 11, 12. This second section has separate pagination.

[473]*Readings in Moral Theology,* vol. I (cf. note 468), p. 60.

[474]*Ibid.,* pp. 72, 73.

conjugal love," and "respecting the limits of responsible parenthood" are morally good norms. Otherwise, to quote again the words of Knauer, how could such circumstantial aspects "determine the finis operis, so that the act is morally good?" They seem to be approved as a means to an end; and morality consists precisely in the relationship of a means to an end.

What is the attitude of the proportionalists regarding objective norms based on Holy Scripture, on declarations from the Holy See and on the natural law? They are not rejected outright, but are rationalized into benign oblivion as standards of determining right from wrong. Father Joseph Fuchs, S.J. grants such norms a certain "pedagogical" importance:

> The moral task of the Christian is not to fulfill "norms" but to "humanize" (Christianize) each of man's concrete realities, understood as a divine call. Norms of moral behavior should "help" to bring this about rightly, "objectively." The true significance of these norms consists in this "pedagogical" service—not in a universal validity that could compromise objectivity. Accordingly, the function of the norms is then "only" pedagogical.[475]

He considers norms based on the Holy Scriptures: "God's speaking in human mode signifies that the moral imperatives appearing in Holy Scripture should not be interpreted as direct divine "dictates" . . . Holy Scripture was never meant to be a handbook on morality: consequently it may not be so used."[476] He explores the validity of the "norms of the ecclesial community" and comments on such "non-definitive authoritative orientations of the Church" as follows: ". . . a certain "presumption" of truth must be granted them. Yet one may not see in such instances any conclusive legislation or doctrinal laying down of an ethical norm, the validity of which would be guaranteed by the Holy Spirit."[477]

With regard to the natural moral law as a source of moral norms, Father Fuchs betrays his predilection for "recta ratio" (right reason). He insists that reason is the only reality of the natural order which can provide a basis for or affirm any moral laws. Speaking of "recta ratio" he says: "The human is in it, that which is humanly right. Whatever is not recta ratio is necessarily non-

---

[475]*Ibid.*, pp. 130, 131, article entitled "The Absoluteness of Moral Terms." The author must be thinking of mankind before original sin when he writes that in the future, there will be less detailed and fewer behavioral norms, but rather "fundamental principles, a deepened insight into human and Christian values and a heightened sense of responsibility."

[476]*Ibid.*, p. 97.

[477]*Ibid.*, p. 105.

human, not worthy of man, antithetic to a steadily advancing "humanization." "[478] When applying this concept to the natural moral law, he insists that "nature is not understood as human, unless it is thought of as a *personal* nature," and that man is "essentially person-reason." To think of man in any other way is to consider him "infrapersonally." His commentary on the natural law as a source of moral norms follows:

> In any case, nature, considered infrapersonally, cannot be the norm of moral behavior. Rather man is essentially person and has to understand himself therefore as a person—"in a human nature"—and achieve self-realization according to this self-understanding. Self-realization entails that he himself must discover the available possibilities for his action and his development and determine on the basis of his present understanding of himself which of these possibilities are "right," "reasonable," "human" (in the full and positive sense of these words), and so contributive to "human progress." In this way he arrives simultaneously at the moral judgment of a concrete situation and the affirmation of moral norms.[479]

What the proportionalists are saying is that the norms based on Holy Scripture, Church pronouncements, as well as those based on the natural moral law are not necessarily exceptionless. In a given case, such norms can be brushed aside if there is a proper balance of good and evil effects of a contemplated human action, and a proportionate reason for performing an act which is contrary to such norms. The statements presented above make this switch from guidance by objective standards to guidance by subjective standards abundantly clear.

An Evaluation of Proportionalism

There is no record in Church sources of any specific condemnation of proportionalism. The following passage from Vatican II's *The Church Today* might be considered as an inferred disapproval of the theory of proportionalism (objective vs subjective):

> Hence the more that a correct conscience holds sway, the more persons and groups turn aside from blind choice and strive to be

---

[478]*Ibid.*, p. 111.
[479]*Ibid.*, pp. 108, 109.

guided by objective norms of morality. Conscience frequently errs from invincible ignorance without losing its dignity. The same cannot be said of a man who cares but little for truth and goodness, or of a conscience which by degrees grows practically sightless as a result of habitual sin.[480]

The situation might be likened to any human endeavor which attempts to operate by circumventing established rules and regulations; for instance, the football coach who might say to his NFL team: "Forget about the rules. Be competitive, and be honest and fair. If anyone violates this directive, he had better have a proportionate reason." The following observations are submitted as reflections on the dangers inherent in the theory and practice of proportionalism.

a) Terminology—the Focus on Ontic Good and Evil

Distinguished authors have singled out the concept of ontic values and disvalues as the basic error of proportionalism as considered from a philosophic viewpoint.[481] The consequences of such a concept are even more damaging from a pastoral viewpoint. *Moral* good reflects concerns about spiritual motivation, the search for true happiness, the pursuit of virtue, conforming to gospel standards and values, etc. *Ontic* good reflects preoccupation with "down to earth" humanistic and existential concerns such as health, life, pursuit of progress, etc. To say that this represents a basic change of perspective from the spiritual to the material would be unfair. Proportionalists do not advocate the exclusion of spiritual values. It can be said, however, that the reprimand of the Lord Jesus to St. Peter (who tried to dissuade Jesus from loyalty to His Father's will) would have some application to preoccupation with ontic concerns: "You are trying to make me trip and fall. You are not judging by God's standards but by man's" (Matthew, 16:23).

This drastic shift of emphasis—this reversal of the frame of reference (from the objective to the subjective imperative)—implies a downgrading of concepts of moral good. It is no longer a matter of potential right and wrong, but merely of "values" and "disvalues." Again, to quote Father Knauer:

---

[480] *The Documents of Vatican II,* Walter M. Abbott, S.J., ed. (cf. note 50), p. 214. The opening quotation of the chapter is from this article 16 of *The Church Today.*

[481] Ashley/O'Rourke, *Health Care Ethics* (cf. note 80), pp. 160–162. Cf. also Connery, John, S.J., "Catholic Ethics: Has the Norm for Rule-Making Changed?," in *Theological Studies,* June, 1981, pp. 232–250. Father Connery refers to proportionalism as aiming at the "demoralization of all the good and evil that is found in human acts." p. 247.

"moral good consists in the best possible realization of any particular value envisaged in its entirety" (cf.p.257). Is the ontic value of preserving health on the same level as the gospel value of responding to the needs of your neighbor? Would a "value" which happens to correspond to an objective norm for a non-proportionalist be given prior consideration by a proportionalist (that is, because it is based on conformity with virtue, or with the natural moral law)? Father Servais Pinckaers, O.P. comments on this alienation of moral norms from their sources as follows:

> The consequences of the separation established by the "proportionalists" between the virtues and the concrete norms is to render the virtues inoperative in behavior as well as in morality. The moralist will be able to elaborate morality and perform his work of deciding norms and cases without really having need of the virtues, not even of charity.[482]

b) The Effective Circumvention of Authority

Even against the background of the vagaries of "personalism" following Vatican II, and the controversy over Pope Paul VI's encyclical letter on birth control ("Humanae Vitae") during the same turbulent period, there is no justification for outright disregard for the authority of the Holy Scriptures as reflected in Church teaching and of the authority of papal pronouncements. To say that the Holy Scriptures may not be used as a source of moral standards because the bible is historically and culturally conditioned to the extent that it is an unreliable guide for moral behavior, deserves the response: "what is freely asserted (without foundation) can be freely denied" ("quod gratis asseritur, gratis negatur"). To say that papal pronouncements should not be accepted as a valid "laying down of ethical norm(s)" amounts to questioning the validity of the doctrine of the magisterium of the Church. One proportionalist may have touched the very core of the problem (autonomy vs authority) when he wrote: "Our ability to resolve which action we want to effect at a certain moment is an expression of our autonomy, of our self-determination."[483]

In their glorification of "right reason," the advocates of proportionalism should reflect that the *"right"* in "right reason" should imply a preferential regard for moral norms as based on Holy Scripture, authoritative Church

---

[482] *The Question of Intrinsically Evil Acts* (cf. note 472), p. 39.

[483] Janssens, Louis, "Ontic Evil and Moral Evil," in *Readings in Moral Theology,* I (cf. note 468), p. 61.

pronouncements, pursuit of virtue, etc. It cannot be denied that accepting and respecting the voice of authority is difficult for mankind today as it was for our first parents who were tempted to reject authority and to "be like gods who know what is good and what is bad" (Genesis, 3:5). The "spirit of the age" is one of intolerance for authority on just about every level of life. Yet, Our Savior won for all human individuals the grace to overcome that primordial revolutionary tendency (even if some reject that grace), and to be encouraged in that effort by the words of St. Paul to the Romans (12:2):

> Do not conform yourselves to this age but be transformed by the renewal of your mind, so that you may judge what is God's will, what is good, pleasing and perfect.

c) The Tendency to be Motivated by "Utility"

The term "consequentialism" refers to a system which is based on the same internal logic as proportionalism. In both systems, moral judgment depends on a proportionate reason, with a view to the end or purpose of the action. The difference is that the former stresses a balancing of the good and evil *consequences,* while proportionalism stresses a balancing of the good and evil *circumstances* of an action. The proportionate reason refers to all of the good expected of a particular action. Since both systems are teleological (from the Greek "telos," meaning "end"), they are designed to judge and interpret following the relationship between the means and the end. As Father Pinckaers, O.P. says, such a system "inevitably approximates utilitarianism, for the useful is defined precisely by the correspondence of the means to the end . . . towards the submission of every moral value to the consideration of the useful as its foundation."[484]

Without obligatory objective moral norms to set the parameters, that tendency to seek the "useful" would be amplified. Again, quoting Father Knauer:

> In ethics, only the obligation to seek the best possible solutions in their total existential entirety is unchangeable. The best solutions cannot be determined in advance as in a catalogue; they must be developed within the dynamic of the affirmative obligation that there be development.[485]

---

[484] *The Question of Intrinsically Evil Acts* (cf. note 472), p. 17.
[485] *Readings in Moral Theology,* I (cf. note 468), p. 10.

The subject of utilitarianism is too complicated to be discussed here. Suffice it to say that the type referred to here is what is known as "utilitarianism of the norm," or "restricted" utilitarianism" as distinguished from "utilitarianism of the act" or "extreme" utilitarianism." Utilitarianism of the norm admits, as criteria of actions, certain norms of universal significance which nevertheless must have been previously justified on the utilitarian level. This could be compared to a process of testing over a long period to show that certain behavior is always good, or always evil and harmful. Such a process tends to bring about a certain relativity of moral reality and the admission of certain exceptions to every law.[486]

d) Tendency to Permissiveness in Moral Behavior

Undoubtedly the application of the theory of proportionalism has led to permissiveness in moral standards over the past twenty years. This is demonstrated by the opinions of advocates of this theory as mentioned earlier in this discussion of proportionalism (for example, with regard to lying and contraception). As Father John Connery, S.J. has pointed out: "Some authors have shown surprising facility in uncovering proportionate reasons, particularly in the area of sex. These authors have used proportionalism more as an exception-making tool than as a metaethical explanation of moral norms and principles."[487] If such instances are due not to the system of proportionalism itself (as some advocates of the system claim), but to the abuse of the system, it must be admitted that proportionalism is vulnerable to abuse in practice. To the extent that it is abused, more and more of the devout and loyal faithful (not to mention critics not of the Catholic faith) are perplexed and confused by the ingenuity of fellow-members of the Church in justifying behavior which is contrary to the teachings of the magisterium.

If the Church did adopt proportionalism as its basic norm, it does not follow that the Church would necessarily change the basic objective moral norms as taught and practiced in the past. Father John Connery, S.J. stresses this important observation as follows: "(The Church) might continue to condemn without exception adultery, abortion, etc. What would change is that instead of claiming that these acts are morally wrong in themselves, it would simply say that they are morally wrong because there is no proportionate reason to justify them. It could do this even though it held the theoretical position that a proportionate reason would justify them."[488] In proportionalist

---

[486]Pinckaers, Servais, O.P., *The Question of Intrinsically Evil Acts* (cf. note 472), pp. 18, 19.

[487]"The Teleology of Proportionate Reason" in *Theological Studies,* Sept., 1983, p. 495.

[488]*Theological Studies* (cf. note 481), June, 1981, p. 245.

language, the Church would be saying that all actions which are performed without a proportionate reason are "intrinsically evil." This position is stated clearly by Father Knauer, S.J.:

> What is intrinsically an evil act is brought about when no commensurate reason can justify the permission or causing of the extrinsic evil, that is, any given premoral physical evil or injury. This is a thesis which has special significance for contemporary ethics. It says that "morally evil" and "intrinsically evil" are synonymous expressions.[489]

If a proportionalist mentality ever does flourish in the Church with official approval, however, it is very likely that procedures now forbidden in our Catholic hospitals such as direct sterilizations (vasectomies, tubal ligations), masturbation, artificial insemination by husband, will be allowed with increasing frequency—to the detriment of morals and human dignity and the consternation of the faithful.

The following directives apply to the traditional understanding of the Principle of the Double Effect as based on the observance of *objective* norms of morality (vs the *subjective* orientation of the theory of proportionalism). The application of directive 13 (below) will be illustrated throughout the rest of this chapter.

Directive 5: Any procedure potentially harmful to the patient is morally justified only insofar as it is designed to produce a proportionate good.

Directive 26: Therapeutic procedures which are likely to be dangerous are morally justifiable for proportionate reasons.

Directive 13: Operations, treatments, and medications, which do not directly intend termination of pregnancy but which have as their purpose the cure of a proportionately serious pathological condition of the mother, are permitted when they cannot be safely postponed until the fetus is viable, even though they may or will result in the death of the fetus. If the fetus is not certainly dead, it should be baptized.

---

[489]*Readings in Moral Theology,* I (cf. note 468), p. 7.

7.3   APPLYING THE PRINCIPLE OF THE DOUBLE EFFECT

The practical application of the *Principle of the Double Effect* in cases of *indirect* sterilization was discussed in chapter III. It can also be applied to rare instances when procedures which are *indirectly* abortive can be warranted. The Church's viewpoint with regard to abortive procedures differs considerably from the medical viewpoint. Physicians generally define abortion as the "delivery or loss of the products of conception before the 20th week of gestation . . . delivery between 20 and 28 weeks is considered premature birth."[490] The Church's definition of abortion is stated in *Directive 12* as "the directly intended termination of pregnancy before viability . . . [including] the interval between conception and implantation of the embryo."

Physicians speak of *induced* abortions whereby the life of the nonviable fetus is attacked *directly* by one or more of the three major methods of terminating a pregnancy: either by the instrumental evacuation of the uterus, by stimulation of uterine contractions, or by surgical procedures. If these are performed in order to save the life or health of the mother, they call them *therapeutic* abortions. The Church rejects that phrase (therapeutic), and considers all *direct* attacks on fetal life, including intrauterine devices and contraceptive medications which may prevent implantation, as crimes against the inviolability of human life.

As indicated above, the distinction between *direct* abortion and *indirect* abortion is essential to an understanding of the Church's teaching on abortion. A *direct* abortion is one which is intended either as an end in itself or as a means to an end. It is a direct attack on the life of the nonviable fetus which is intended to terminate the pregnancy. An *indirect* abortion is the foreseen but merely permitted uterine evacuation of a nonviable fetus which is the side-effect of a procedure which is directed toward some good end and legitimate purpose.[491] The surgical removal of a cancerous uterus to save the life of the pregnant mother, for example, involves the unintended side effect of terminating the pregnancy.

Since the medical concept of an *induced* abortion (as mentioned above) is associated with the *direct* termination of pregnancy by artificial means, the medical concept of a *spontaneous* abortion (which occurs without any external intervention) might be compared to what theologians call an *indirect* abortion. It is a "natural" (as opposed to "artificial means") process. In like manner, even though artificial means are used in an approved procedure which involves the side effect of terminating the pregnancy (for example, the surgical

---

[490] *The Merck Manual* (cf. note 56), p. 1723.
[491] O'Donnell, Thomas, S.J., *Medicine and Moral Theology* (cf. note 31), p. 140.

removal of a cancerous uterus), that foreseen but unintended side effect is an *indirect* abortion which could be described as "the spontaneous result of an artificially produced condition in the mother." Father Thomas O'Donnell, S.J. explains this helpful observation as follows:

> Even though the uterine evacuation of indirect abortion is the result of some artificial procedure, in the moral order this artificial procedure has no direct connection with the uterine evacuation."[492]

It should be noted in passing that women who are in danger of a *spontaneous* abortion (due to natural causes) have a moral obligation to follow the physician's orders in taking reasonable precautions to safeguard the new life within the womb. If the physician diagnoses a *threatened* abortion (which is defined as any bleeding or cramping during the first 20 weeks of pregnancy), his orders may involve additional bed rest, the definite curtailment of "on your feet" activities, and even a reduction of days or hours of employment outside of the home. If the danger advances to that of an *imminent* abortion (also known as an *impending* abortion), the physician will prescribe conservative management so as to contain the impending threat of abortion. If an expectant mother in such a situation cannot check in as a hospital patient, she must cancel all activities outside of the home. Furthermore, a reliable adult should be with her in the home or at least be conveniently "on call" so as to be able to provide transportation to the hospital when needed. The woman who faces the greater danger of an *inevitable* abortion is subject to pain and bleeding caused usually by the rupture of the membranes and the dilation of the cervix. The pain can be characterized as intolerable; to all indications, the expulsion of the fetus cannot be prevented. A pregnant woman who is not a hospital patient at the onset of such pain and bleeding must be rushed to the hospital without delay.

1) Ectopic Gestation—"Out of Place" Pregnancies

The first trimester is the period when 85% of spontaneous abortions (miscarriages) occur. It might be said that this is nature's way of preventing the birth of malformed infants. Statistics indicate that in 60% of spontaneous abortions, the fetus is either absent or grossly malformed. In another 25% to 60% of spontaneous abortions, the fetus is found to have chromosomal abnormalities which limit drastically the proper development of the infant.[493]

---

[492]*Ibid.*, p. 141.
[493]*The Merck Manual* (cf. note 56), p. 1723.

A considerable number of spontaneous abortions result from a type of abnormal pregnancy which is known as ectopic (from the Greek word for "out of place"). This means that the implantation has occurred outside of the endrometrium and endometrial cavity of the uterus; that is, in the cervix, fallopian tube, ovary, or in the abdominal or pelvic cavity. Ectopic pregnancies in the U.S.A. have increased from 17,800 in 1970 to 42,400 in 1978 (from 4.5 per 1000 reported pregnancies to 9.4 per 1000). There is greater risk for non-white women as compared to white women.[494] The most common ectopic site of implantation is in some portion of the fallopian tube (ampullar, isthmic, interstitial). Usually these pregnancies rupture into the lumen of the tube as early as the 6th week and are carried out through the fimbriated distal end of the tube and deposited in the peritoneal cavity. These are known as tubal abortions.[495]

In other cases (the subject of discussion here), the embryo remains in the tube, but the tube has been so traumatized and weakened by the "boring in" action in the nidation (nest-making) process, that it presents a serious threat to the life of the mother. This "boring in" process leads to the perforation of the inner layers of the tube; resultant gradual hemorrhaging can result in rapid hemorrhaging, hypotension or shock. At about the 6th or 8th week of pregnancy, the woman may experience a sudden lower abdominal pain, followed by fainting. Usually this indicates that the tube has ruptured.[496] Modern medical understanding of this condition today makes it very clear that the serious threat to the mother is due not to the developing fetus, but to the diseased and weakened condition of the fallopian tube. Hence the physician does not have to wait until the tube has ruptured before responding to the threat to the mother's life by appropriate surgical action.[497]

Surgical Removal of the Fallopian Tube (Salpingectomy)

As soon as the physician has sufficient evidence to make the diagnosis that the tubal pregnancy has advanced to the stage which constitutes a serious

---

[494]Rubin, George L., "Ectopic Pregnancy in the United States 1970 Through 1978" in *The Journal of the American Medical Association*, April 1, 1983, p. 1727.

[495]O'Donnell, Thomas, S.J., *Medicine and Christian Morality* (cf. note 31), p. 198. Cf. also McFadden, Charles J., O.S.A., *Medical Ethics* (cf. note 17), p. 215.

[496]*The Merck Manual* (cf. note 56), p. 1725.

[497]For the listing of the pronouncements of the Holy See on this subject and interpretation thereof, cf. *Canon Law Digest*, III (cf. note 43), pp. 669, 670; Kelly, Gerald, S.J., *Medico-Manual Problems* (cf. note 22), pp. 107–110; Davis, Henry J., S.J., *Moral and Pastoral Theology*, II (New York, N.Y.: Sheed and Ward, 1943), pp. 174–186.

threat to the life of the mother, he can and should tie off the arteries which supply blood to the tube, and then remove the tube surgically. Some medical authorities debate the propriety, in particular cases, of removing only the traumatized section of the tube, and leaving the tube in situ after repair. This would not be morally objectionable. The objection to this procedure is that it could predispose the woman to future ectopic pregnancies.

Before initiating the surgical procedure, the physician must be assured of three conditions: (a) That the tube is presumed to be damaged and dangerously affected to such an extent as to warrant the surgery. The procedure would be immoral if the physician said to himself: "practically every ectopic pregnancy in time threatens the life of the mother; so I will anticipate that serious and foreseen pathological condition and perform the surgery before the onset of that serious danger." (b) The procedure is not just a separation of the embryo or fetus from its site within the womb. If the physician decided to save the mother by slitting open the tube and removing the embryo, or by terminating its life by radiation or by using drugs, it would be a *direct abortion* (cf. forthcoming discussion of salpingotomy). (c) That the procedure cannot be postponed without notably increasing the danger to the mother.

Presuming that the pregnancy has not advanced to a stage approaching viability, the procedure outlined above would fulfill all the conditions required for the application of the Principle of the Double Effect. First, the excision of the tube in itself is an indifferent action. Medical opinion is overwhelming in saying that it is not the embryo that makes the procedure necessary, but the diseased and disintegrated condition of the fallopian tube. There is no reasonable alternative to removing this serious threat to the mother's life. The evil side effect (death of the embryo) is not willed or intended, but merely permitted. The good effect does not emerge through the evil side effect—the mother's life is saved not through the death of the embryo but by the excision of the tube. Saving the life of the mother constitutes a proportionate reason which is sufficient to compensate for the loss of the life of the embryo.

It should be apparent that each individual case of tubal pregnancy must be judged on its own merits. This critical guideline is emphasized by a sobering statistic: between 1914 and 1959, there were ten cases of advanced tubal pregnancy wherein both mother and infant survived. Seven of the infants went to full term.[498] In a recent survey of specialists in obstetrics and gynecology on the subject of ectopic pregnancies, 47% of the physicians who responded to the survey (32 in number) felt that there would be a 50% chance of finding a living embryo in an *unruptured* fallopian tube—thanks to the ear-

---

[498]O'Donnell, Thomas, S.J., *Medicine and Christian Morality* (cf. note 31), p. 199.

lier diagnoses of ectopic pregnancy made today.[499] Among the available modern methods of early diagnosis, special mention might be made of laparoscopy ("visualization" of in internal organs through an opening in the abdominal wall), testing of HCG levels (the hormone known as Human Chorionic Gonadotropin) and ultrasonography (whereby the conceptus can be "seen" especially after the 7th week).

Several authors have speculated as to what could be done if the surgeon discovers a tubal pregnancy in the course of an abdominal operation (appendectomy, for example). Father Edwin Healy, S.J. would allow the excision of the tube "if to wait would necessitate performing another grave operation later on." Father Charles McFadden, O.S.A. would allow the excision in some cases if the physician "judges the tube to be in a pathological condition," and if based on the sound judgment that "the woman would be incapable of sustaining another operation within a few weeks."[500] Other authors view the problem sympathetically, but are reluctant to answer in the affirmative.[501] Authors Healy and McFadden would allow the excision of the tube even *outside* of the situation of undergoing some additional type of abdominal surgery, if her condition with the tubal pregnancy requires close observation and she simply would not or could not return for additional surgery if required later on (e.g., lacks financial resources, lives too far away from the hospital, etc.).[502]

The present writer would approve of the excision of the fallopian tube in both situations provided that modern methods of early diagnosis yield positive indications that the woman may be in a pathological condition—not simply presumed, but based on *some* positive evidence. The fact that she might have to submit to another operation in the near future while recuperating from the other operation (case n.1) or that lack of observation would increase the danger to her life (case n.2) increases the compensating qualities of the proportionate reason for allowing the procedure. Moralists mention that in situations such as outlined above, a physician is justified in solving a *positive* doubt (as to the serious nature of her condition) in favor of the woman. In these

---

[499]"Physicians' Reactions in Ectopic Pregnancy Survey" in *Ethics and Medics,* May, 1984, pp. 3, 4. It should be noted that many of the respondents recognized other causes of death besides the rupture of the tubes. This survey was conducted by Father Donald McCarthy, Ph.D. of the staff of the Pope John Center (author of the article).

[500]McFadden, Charles, O.S.A., *Medical Ethics* (cf. note 17), p. 225; Healy, Edwin, S.J., *Medical Ethics* (cf. note 46), p. 224.

[501]Bender, Louis, O.P. in *Dictionary of Moral Theology* (cf. note 346), p. 509; Davis, Henry, S.J., *Moral and Pastoral Theology,* II (cf. note 497), pp. 181, 182.

[502]Healy, Edwin, S.J., *Medical Ethics* (cf. note 46), p. 224; McFadden, Charles, O.S.A., *Medical Ethics* (cf. note 17), pp. 224, 225.

situations, as in so many other sensitive and complicated moral-medical dilemmas, the moralist must admit the extent to which the ultimate decision must be left up to expert medical opinion and expertise.

In the rare case when the tubal pregnancy has advanced to the stage approaching viability, special consideration must be given to the possibility of relying on expectant treatment (postponing any proposal to excise the tube) in the *reasonable* hope of a successful delivery of the infant. If the situation is such that the danger to the mother significantly outweighs the chances of the survival of the infant, the proximity to successful delivery of a viable infant must be considered. If the infant is very close to safe delivery, the condition of the mother would have to be almost equivalent to certain death before the excision of the tube could be permitted.[503]

Father Thomas O'Donnell, S.J. considers the rare possibility that after the tubal rupture, the maternal connections may remain and the embryo might continue to develop between the layers of the broad ligament or in the peritoneal cavity. In that event, "a large thin placenta may become attached to the proximate internal organs, drawing all or part of its blood supply from the viscera." Every effort must be made to allow such a secondary abdominal pregnancy to advance to viability. If dangerous hemorrhaging developed, however, and the fetus was nonviable, the physician would be allowed to intervene surgically to control the bleeding. Any direct attack on the fetus, of course, would be immoral.[504]

The Rare Possibility of Transferring the Embryo by Salpingotomy

Salpingotomy (as distinguished from "salpingectomy," or removal of the tube) refers to the surgical procedure of leaving the fallopian tube intact, but removing the embryo from the tube. If this is done (presuming the presence of a serious pathological condition which threatens the life of the mother) but with the intention of transplanting that new life in the uterine cavity of the mother, and there is solid clinical evidence that provides genuine hope for the survival of the embryo without adding significantly to the danger for the mother, the procedure (in theory) could be morally acceptable.

Whether or not such a procedure could be warranted in practice, however, is quite another matter. In February of 1984, an eight-question survey was sent to 157 obstetricians in an effort to assess the medical feasibility of salvaging the embryo from an unruptured tube for transfer to the uterus of the mother. The responses of the 69 obstetricians who cooperated in the sur-

---

[503]*Ibid.* (McFadden), p. 226.
[504]*Medicine and Christian Morality* (cf. note 31), pp. 199, 200.

vey (44%) might be summarized as follows: 32 of the obstetricians (47%) felt that there was a better than 50% chance of finding a living embryo in an unruptured fallopian tube; 19 of the obstetricians (29%) allowed a better than 50% chance of successfully removing the embryo from the tube with sac intact; 70% of the obstetricians felt that the chances of successfully transferring the embryo in an intact sac to the uterus of the mother were 5% or less. The majority of the obstetricians (88%) felt that an ectopic embryo would not survive to viability in 95% of the cases whether the tube is ruptured or unruptured.[505]

The survey of obstetricians was followed by a survey of 15 Catholic ethicists from throughout the nation as reported in the September, 1984 issue of *Ethics and Medics*. The author of the survey concluded: "Most of the eleven other ethicists whom we consulted [that is, 11 of the 15] would not consider the action a direct killing and would permit it in some circumstances," — subject, of course, to official Church approval. The prevailing intention behind such a procedure would have to be removed from any objective to tamper with the reproductive process for experimental purposes. The prevailing intention would have to be to save the life of the embryo against terrific odds with some clinically-established hope of a successful outcome. Some slight hope of eventual success might be gleaned from contemporary efforts at embryo transfer (also known as S.E.T. or Surrogate Embryo Transfer), which would not be immoral if no surrogate is involved so that the embryo is the mother's own conceptus. The author of the survey properly concludes: "But clearly this delicate subject deserves further study."[506]

The question of the removal of the embryo by salpingotomy not for transfer to the uterine cavity (as above), but precisely as a means of saving the tube for a future pregnancy, was also proposed in the survey of Catholic ethicists as referred to above. In this survey, the problem was stated as follows:

> Our problem is one of analysis of whether salpingotomy should be ruled out by the moral norm against direct killing of the innocent . . . if the death of the embryo cannot be determined, can salpingotomy be ethically justified for a woman who wants to

---

[505]"Physicians' Reactions in Ectopic Pregnancy Survey" by Father Donald McCarthy, Ph.D. of the staff of the Pope John Center in *Ethics and Medics*, May, 1984, pp. 3, 4.

[506]"Ethicists' Reactions to Ectopic Pregnancy Survey" by Father Donald McCarthy, Ph.D. in *Ethics and Medics*, September, 1984, pp. 2-4. This printed report did not list the ethicists or quote their actual opinions. Such information is filed, along with the responses of both the obstetricians and the ethicists, at the main office of the Pope John Center, Braintree, Ma.

preserve her fertility [that is, preserve the tube for a future pregnancy].[507]

Eight of the respondents indicated approval of the proposal that the ectopic embryo could be removed along with its surrounding tissue to correct the pathological condition, and that the physician's effort must be to preserve the fertility of the mother and to remove but not kill the embryo. Five of the other respondents (including this writer) expressed sincere convictions that "salpingotomy [in this context] should be considered direct killing and cannot be ethically justified in Catholic teaching." One of them drew a comparison between such procedures and "classical abortions" as follows:

> The demonstration of the salpingotomy thesis seems to me to depend on showing how we *can* "shell out" of the tube but *can't* do classical abortions; or how the *finis operis* of the two procedures differ essentially, so that one is not the other, irrespective of the *finis operantis* ("motive"). Unless that can be clearly shown, it seems to me to be very clear that approval of salpingotomy opens the way for any therapeutic abortions done for sufficiently serious reasons.[508]

The two remaining respondents took a position which was closer to the opinions of the *five* ethnicists (against salpingotomy as described in the "statement of the problem"), than to the opinions of the *eight* ethnicists as above. One of them insisted that salpingotomy as described was direct abortion, but that it was not *direct killing*. The other admitted that ". . . the directives hold that salpingotomies are direct abortions."[509]

A passing reference might be made to other rare types of ectopic pregnancies. If the implantation of the fertilized ovum occurs within the ovary, there is a possibility that the pregnancy may go to full term. Surgical intervention could not be justified as long as there remains some real hope of delivering a viable fetus. Surgical intervention would be allowed if rupture occurs, or if the riddled and traumatized ovary must be removed because it presents a serious threat to the life of the mother. If the fertilized ovum is implanted in the cervix, the temptation to remove the fetus as a source of future trouble must be resisted. If the life of the mother is in serious danger from profuse bleeding, rupture of the amniotic sac, or perforations of the

---

[507] *Ibid.* (*Ethics and Medics* article and Pope John Center files).
[508] *Ibid.*
[509] *Ibid.*

cervical wall, however, a hysterectomy could be permitted. This is yet another application of the Principle of the Double Effect.

> *Directive 16:* In extrauterine pregnancy, the dangerously af-
> fected part of the mother (e.g., cervix, ovary or fallopian
> tube) may be removed, even though fetal death is foreseen,
> provided that: a. the affected part is presumed already to be
> so damaged and dangerously affected as to warrant its re-
> moval, and that b. the operation is not just a separation of
> the embryo or fetus from its site within the part (which
> would be a direct abortion from a uterine appendage); and
> that c. the operation cannot be postponed without notably
> increasing the danger to the mother.

2) Placenta Praevia—Abnormal Implantation

"Placenta praevia" is the Latin term for the condition caused by the implantation of the placenta (Latin word for "cake") of the pregnancy over or near the internal mouth of the cervix. It may cover the mouth of the cervix (called "low implantation"). The word "praevia" is well chosen, for it means literally "in front of the passageway." This condition occurs about once in every 200 pregnancies; usually in a woman in her first pregnancy or in patients with abnormalities of the uterus such as fibroids, that inhibit normal implantation.[510] The onset of the symptoms of this condition (sudden, painless, scant or profuse bleeding) is noted in late pregnancy when the lower uterine segment begins to thin and lengthen. Frequently it is difficult to distinguish this condition from "abruptio placentae" (separation of the placenta from the uterine wall). The need of vaginal examination in order to identify the condition can be obviated by the use of ultrasound (which can locate the placenta).

Since the uterus is some 40 times larger at term than in its non-pregnant state, the placenta appears to "migrate" as the pregnancy develops and is carried upward on the uterine wall. Hence if a low-lying placenta is noted in an early ultrasound scan, no further diagnostic or therapeutic precautions are undertaken unless bleeding is noted. If the placenta is covering the mouth of the uterus completely, the patient is put on pelvic rest with a full explanation

---

[510]Wynn, Ralph M., MD, *Obstetrics and Gynecology,* 3rd ed. (Philadelphia, Pa.: Lea and Febiger, 1983), p. 126. Cf. also *The Merck Manual* (cf. note 56), pp. 1729, 1730.

of the problem. This emphasizes the importance of confirmation of the diagnosis of placenta praevia prior to operative delivery.[511] If massive bleeding occurs and the fetus is viable or near term, the patient must be transferred to an operating room which is prepared for either immediate cesarean section or vaginal delivery. Blood must also be available for replacement as needed.

Since the fetus usually is close to term, it is easy to understand why the dilation of the cervix and the contractions of the upper segment of the uterus would present a danger of some detachment of the placenta. A viable fetus may be removed whenever there are sound reasons for a medical judgment that the procedure is in the best interests of the mother and of the infant. If the fetus is nonviable however, and bleeding is not severe, expectant treatment and vigilance can lead to control of the bleeding. If the bleeding becomes severe, the solution proposed in some medical books, "Empty the uterus" (bring about an abortion), is absolutely forbidden. This would be the elimination of the danger to the mother by terminating the life of the fetus in a direct manner,—a direct attack on a nonviable fetus. In rare cases, the placenta may be only partially separated from the uterine wall. If the separation is *complete,* however, a nonviable fetus may be removed after the complete separation of the placenta from the uterine wall has been verified. Father McFadden justifies this conclusion as based on "the fact that the fetus dies within ten minutes of a complete separation of the placenta." He adds: "Consequent emptying of the uterus therefore involves only an already-deceased fetus."[512]

3) Abruptio Placentae—Detachment of a Normal Implantation

The condition known as "placenta praevia" and the condition known as "abruptio placentae" (detachment of the placenta) are the two most common sources of serious third-trimester bleeding. The latter occurs in about 1% of all pregnancies.[513] In the premature detachment of a normally-implanted placenta (abruptio placentae), the danger to both mother and infant cannot be minimized. In the bleeding which signals the onset of placental separation, the blood may pass behind the membranes and though the cervix (external hemorrhage), or may be retained behind the placenta (concealed hemor-

---

[511]Queenan, John t., MD and Warsof, Steven L., MD in *Management of High-Risk Pregnancy,* 2nd ed., John T. Queenan, MD, ed. (cf. note 189), p. 224.

[512]*Medical Ethics* (cf. note 17), p. 203. Cf. also O'Donnell, Thomas, S.J., *Medicine and Christian Morality* (cf. note 31), p. 192; Healy, Edwin, S.J., *Medical Ethics* (cf. note 46), pp. 239, 240. The separation can be considered as complete even though some strands of tissue may still adhere to the uterine wall.

[513]Wynn, Ralph M., MD, *Obstetrics and Gynecology* (cf. note 510), p. 128.

rhage). Depending upon the degree of separation and blood loss, the symptoms in severe cases can include vaginal bleeding, a tender and tightly contracted uterus, evidence of fetal cardiac distress or death, and maternal shock. It may also lead to both renal failure and the degeneration of the outer layer of the kidneys (renal cortical necrosis).[514] Again, ultrasonography can be very helpful in providing evidence that the problem is *abruptio placentae* and not *placenta praevia*.

If the pregnancy is not near term, and the fetal heart tones are normal, cases of mild bleeding can be managed by bed rest and observation in the hospital. Fortunately abruptio placentae usually occurs near term or near the onset of labor when the fetus is *viable*. If the bleeding continues or grows more severe, and the physician judges that premature delivery of the viable fetus is in the best interests of both mother and infant, induction of labor would be permissible. If the uterine activity is insufficient for vaginal delivery, some obstetricians feel that an adequate trial with oxytocin in order to promote vaginal delivery should be preferred to the more risky and expensive route of cesarean delivery.[515] The operating room should be prepared as to staff and equipment, however, for both vaginal and cesarean delivery.

If the fetus is *nonviable* and the bleeding endangers the life of the mother, it is morally permissible to try to control the bleeding by drug therapy or by the use of tampons even though it is foreseen that this might result in premature labor from such procedures. In extreme cases, it may even be necessary to perform a hysterectomy. All such measures would not be intended to expel the fetus but to control the bleeding. In keeping with the Principle of the Double Effect, the evil effect, the threat to the life of the fetus, is foreseen but merely permitted.

It is also permissible to remove the nonviable fetus whenever *complete* separation of the placenta has occurred. The reason is because the fetus is without its life-source and will be dead within minutes. Father Healy, S.J. would extend this permission also to a situation where an insignificant portion of the placenta may still adhere to the uterine wall. He remarks appropriately that such an insignificant attachment no longer serves as a source of life for the fetus, and concludes: "The abruptio is such that the nonviable fetus cannot possibly be saved. At present, it is bleeding to death. In such circumstances the complete deathblow has already been struck and the fetus may and should be delivered at once in order to administer baptism."[516]

---

[514]Lindheimer, Marshall D., MD, and Katz, Adrian I., MD in *Management of High-Risk Pregnancy* (cf. note 189), p. 323.

[515]Quilligan, Edward J., MD in *Management of High-Risk Pregnancy* (cf. note 189), pp. 596, 597.

[516]Healy, Edwin, S.J., *Medical Ethics* (cf. note 46), p. 240.

Hemorrhaging can become a serious threat in all stages of implantation and gestation. In the premature detachment of a *normally* implanted placenta (abruptio placentae) it is known as an "accidental" hemorrhage; in the detachment of an *abnormally* implanted placenta (placenta praevia) it is known as an "unavoidable" hemorrhage. Other situations can present the danger of accidental hemorrhage. The first line of defense is conservative and expectant treatment; bed rest, transfusion, drug therapy, etc. The physician must select the treatment which is best designed to protect the lives of both mother and fetus in the given situation. It is never permissible to choose a treatment which would *directly* terminate the life of the fetus or uproot it from its life line (site of implantation). If the treatment of choice has to be a measure or technique (such as drug therapy) which directly controls the hemorrhage but indirectly endangers the life of the fetus or indirectly threatens to destroy its life line within the womb, the situation calls for the careful application of the Principle of the Double Effect. The choice of such measures or techniques is justified only if a given situation has reached a critical stage. If there is another measure or technique which does not have a concomitant evil side effect (or has a less serious evil side effect), and which is reasonable and available in the situation, that should be the measure or technique of choice.

The concept of "viability" was discussed in the chapter on the Principle of the Right to Life. It is a relative term, depending not only on the number of weeks of gestation, the anatomical and functional development of the fetus, the weight and length of the fetus, the race of the parents, etc., but also on the medical facilities and expertise available in the area. Leading hospitals in the nation are inclined to define viability of the fetus (all things considered) as beginning "at about 24 weeks."

Directive 14: Regarding the treatment of hemorrhage during pregnancy and before the fetus is viable: Procedures that are designed to empty the uterus of a living fetus still effectively attached to the mother are not permitted; procedures designed to stop hemorrhage (as distinguished from those designed to expel the living and attached fetus) are permitted insofar as necessary, even if fetal death is inevitably a side effect.

---

4) Hyperemesis Gravidarum—Pernicious Vomiting

Many pregnant women with "morning sickness" may claim that they are vomiting everything they have ingested. Yet, they continue to gain weight and are not dehydrated. Such women are not victims of "hyperemesis gravidarum" (literally: "excessive vomiting of pregnant women") in the strict sense of the phrase. Authors admit that the specific cause of this "nervous form" of vomiting and nausea in pregnancy is not known, but that in the majority of cases, it can be traced to a psychogenic origin. In some cases the cause can be traced to a physical factor such as liver disease, a kidney infection, pancreatitis, intestinal obstruction, or to GI tract lesions or intracranial lesions.

The pregnant woman does not have the condition known as hyperemesis gravidarum unless starvation (weight loss), dehydration, and acidosis are added to the vomiting syndrome. If the condition does not respond to treatment, some medical manuals urge termination of pregnancy (abortion) especially if hemorrhagic retinitis appears. One manual recommends the following: "Even in the absence of developing retinitis, termination of the pregnancy should be considered in the rare cases that it does not respond to therapy (as evidenced by continued weight loss, jaundice, and increasing pulse rate)."[517]

This is a good illustration of a case which cannot justify the application of the Principle of the Double Effect. Clearly the evil effect (expelling the fetus) is directly willed, and is the direct means of bringing about the good effect (eliminating the threat to the mother). Since this condition usually occurs during the early months of pregnancy, there is still hope of relying on psychotherapy and expectant treatment until the fetus is viable. If the condition occurs as late as the 6th month, however, and the fetus is viable, there is no moral objection to a premature delivery by means of induced labor.

Medical experts agree that the occurrence of hyperemesis gravidarum as late as the 6th month of pregnancy would be rare indeed. As long as over 45 years ago, however, medical science provided the proper management of this condition in the earlier months of pregnancy with only an occasional maternal death. Both Father Charles McFadden, O.S.A., and Father Thomas O'Donnell, S.J., mention the record of the Margaret Hague Maternity Hospital of Jersey City, N.J. (Catholic) in treating 299 cases of hyperemesis gravidarum over a ten year period (1930's and early 1940's) with no maternal deaths and only one therapeutic abortion.[518] Father McFadden compares the overall obstetrical record of that hospital to the record of a prestigious American non-Catholic hospital. The latter recorded 1,903 deliveries between 1941 and 1942 including 55 therapeutic abortions; the Margaret Hague Maternity

---

[517] *The Merck Manual* (cf. note 56), p. 1727.

[518] McFadden, Charles, O.S.A., *Medical Ethics* (cf. note 17), p. 188. Cf. also O'Donnell, Thomas, S.J., *Medicine and Christian Morality* (cf. note 31), p. 167.

Hospital of Jersey City, N.J. recorded 67,000 deliveries in the 13-year period, 1931–1942, with only 4 therapeutic abortions.[519] This illustrates the extent to which the abortion mentality influences medical and surgical practice.

Medical research and obstetrical practice have advanced dramatically since the 1940's. With maximum use of contemporary aids in the management of high-risk pregnancies, loss of life either for mother or infant in hyperemesis gravidarum cases (as in so many other obstetrical challenges) should be unheard of in the annals of modern medical practice.

5) Eclampsia—Pregnancy-induced Hypertension

Eclampsia (from the Greek word "to flash forth") and its forerunner preeclampsia have been called the "engima of obstetric practice and research." The reason for such a statement is that so little is known about the basic cause or etiology of this affliction.[520] Other terms for preeclampsia/eclampsia which convey a more realistic concept of the condition are "acute hypertension" or "pregnancy-induced hypertension." Preeclampsia develops in about 6% of pregnant woman,—especially in women who are pregnant for the first time, or in women who have pre-existing hypertension, albumin in the urine, and edema (fluid retention). The condition may be diagnosed as *mild* preeclampsia, *severe* preeclampsia, or eclampsia. The latter stage (eclampsia) is marked by convulsive seizures. The mortality rate for eclampsia indicates the serious and challenging nature of the affliction. The rates are 1% to 17% for the mother, and 10% to 35% for the infant.[521]

Obstetricians insist that preeclampsia/eclampsia *should* be preventable even in its severest forms. The incidence can be reduced by exemplary prenatal care, and by identifying those women who have a statistical probability of developing that condition. Dr. Frederick Zuspan, Chairman of the Department of Obstetrics and Gynecology of the Ohio State University College of Medicine (Columbus), writes as follows:

> The time has come for obstetricians to individualize prenatal visits and not to set predetermined interval times. Early on, high-risk patients should be seen at least every two weeks, and more often late in pregnancy. If the patient fails to keep her appoint-

---

[519]*Ibid.* (McFadden), pp. 188, 189.

[520]Dilts, Preston V., Jr., MD, and Sibai, Baha M., MD in *Management of High-Risk Pregnancy* (cf. note 189), p. 477.

[521]Zuspan, Frederick P., MD, "Acute Hypertension," in *Management of High-Risk Pregnancy* (cf. note 189), pp. 405–408.

ment, as many primigravidas do, she must be contacted and reminded again of the importance of prenatal care. The woman undergoing her first term pregnancy should be considered a potential high-risk patient since 6% of patients in this group will develop acute hypertension.[522]

Since the specific causative factor remains unknown, however, the possibilities of prevention are necessarily limited.

Since this condition normally does not occur until late in pregnancy when the fetus is viable, labor may be induced as to time and method which is best calculated to save the lives of both mother and child. In the rare instances when eclampsia does develop before the fetus is viable, contemporary medicine cannot advance any moral justification for bringing about the termination of the pregnancy. Hence the Principle of the Double Effect cannot be used to justify medical intervention before the fetus is viable. Such intervention would amount to a direct abortion. The specific objectives of treatment of this serious condition should be to prevent convulsions, to deliver a live infant, and to prevent postpartum complications for both mother and child.[523]

6) Erythroblastosis Fetalis—The Rh Factor

The Rh factor, an element in human red blood corpuscles, gets its name from the Rhesus monkey, in whose red corpuscles a similar element was discovered. Persons with this element in their blood are known as *Rh positive;* those without it are *Rh negative.* If Rh positive blood finds its way into the blood stream of an Rh negative person, the latter developes what is called a sensitivity to Rh positive blood. This sensitization is not harmful to the Rh negative person except in two possible situations: if this sensitized Rh negative person receives Rh positive blood again after sensitivity develops, and if an Rh negative pregnant woman is sensitized by her Rh positive fetus. This event can occur when the mother of the fetus is an Rh negative, and the father is an Rh positive. In the U.S.A., 85% of whites are Rh positive, and about 13% of marriages among whites result in the pairing of an Rh positive man and an Rh negative woman. Only one out of 27 children born of these couples will have the serious disease of the newborn known as erythroblastosis fetalis (hemolytic anemia of the fetus).[524]

---

[522]*Ibid.,* p. 405.

[523]*Ibid.,* This author concludes that with proper treatment, "fetal loss should not exceed 10% and maternal deaths should seldom occur" (p. 410).

[524]*The Merck Manual* (cf. note 56), p. 1730.

How does the fetus become a victim of this disease? The red blood cells (erythrocytes) of the Rh positive fetus enter the mother's circulation system usually at the time of delivery, but occasionally earlier in pregnancy through breaks in the placenta.[525] This stimulates maternal antibody production against the Rh factor. Rh-negative individuals have no Rh antigen on the surface of their erythrocytes. When they are exposed to the antigen, they may become immunized. Although an exposure to even slight amounts of Rh-positive blood may immunize the Rh-negative individual, the general rule is that a clinically significant immunization requires two exposures to Rh antigen. The Rh-negative individual then developes antibodies, some of which can cross the placenta and become responsible for coating the Rh-postive *fetal* erythrocytes (red blood cells) and causing their destruction (hemolysis). If this process is extensive, it can cause hydrops fetalis (gross edema with severe anemia) and intrauterine death. This is known as *erythroblastosis fetalis.* If the hemolytic process is milder, the fetus may compensate by increasing the production of erythrocytes (red blood cells).[526]

Usually, however, the immunization which sets up the dangerous invasion of antibodies is not caused by the crossing over of erythrocytes or of white cells from fetal into maternal circulation, but rather by the large transfer of erythrocytes from the fetus to the mother at the time of delivery. Since most immunizations occur at delivery, a full-term pregnancy carries a substantial risk of immunization. The antibodies appear either postpartum or following exposure to the Rh antigen in the next pregnancy. The incidence of Rh immunization has been cut sharply by the administration of Rh immune globulin within 72 hours of birth. In an attempt to eliminate the immunization which may have occurred through transplacental hemorrhage (crossing over of erythrocytes or of white cells from fetal into maternal circulation during pregnancy) in the third trimester (1% to 2% of Rh cases), a proper dose of Rh immune globulin is administered at 28 weeks' gestation.[527]

Amniocentesis is used to determine the need of intrauterine transfusions. A careful analysis of the amniotic fluid can detect signs of fetal deterioration. If the antibody standard (titer) is just at the critical level and the patient has not had an infant with erythroblastosis fetalis, the initial amniocentesis may be done between 28 and 29 weeks' gestation. If the titer or history suggests that the disease may be more severe, the amniocentesis may have to be done as early as 23 weeks' gestation. Transfusion is indicated only if the fetus would

---

[525]Wynn, Ralph M., MD, *Obstetrics and Gynecology* (cf. note 510), p. 144.

[526]Queenan, John T., MD, "Rh and Other Blood Group Immunizations," in *Management of High-Risk Pregnancy* (cf. note 189), pp. 505, 506.

[527]*Ibid.,* pp. 506, 507.

die before it can safely be delivered. The life of a severely affected fetus can be saved by instilling Rh-negative, irradiated, washed, packed erythrocytes into the fetal peritoneal cavity. Since they are Rh-negative, they will not be destroyed. Dr. John T. Queenan, MD, Chairman of the Department of Obstetrics and Gynecology at the Georgetown University School of Medicine, describes one large cooperative study of the success rate of intrauterine transfusions as follows:

> A total of 1,097 transfusions were done on 607 immunized, Rh-negative patients with 614 fetuses. The procedure saved 206 (34%) of the fetuses. This is a significant gain when you consider that the procedure was not done unless the fetus would otherwise have died in utero at a stage too early for extrauterine survival. With improved technique, some investigators have achieved survival rates of 70% to 75%. The use of real-time ultrasound not only avoids radiation exposure to the patient, fetus, and clinicians but also allows for monitoring the fetal heart rate during injection of the blood.

He also states that intravascular transfusion by fetoscope (directly into the umbilical vein) "has been shown to be successful."[528]

Ultrasound scanning and amniocentesis provide reliable means of determining and monitoring the condition of the fetus especially with regard to the fetal heart size (congestive heart failure is a possibility) and the progression of the accumulation of serous fluid in the abdominal cavity (known as "ascites"). It is a question of balancing the risks of extrauterine life due to prematurity with the hostile intrauterine environment. Usually an Rh-immunized mother should be delivered by 38 weeks. If the analysis of the amniotic fluid indicates the advisability of an earlier delivery, careful clinical judgment is required. Dr. John Queenan states that generally a vaginal delivery can be accomplished from 36 weeks onward, but the fetus must have electronic heart rate monitoring during labor. He adds that if delivery is to be done between 34 and 35 weeks' gestation, it could be either vaginal or abdominal, depending on the condition of the cervix. "For all earlier deliveries," he continues, "cesarean section seems more prudent."[529] Provided that the infant is viable, there is no moral objection to inducing labor before term if the physician judges this to be in the best interests of mother and infant.

---

[528]*Ibid.*, p. 512.
[529]*Ibid.*, pp. 512–515. Quotation on p. 515.

Unless the mother was sensitized by a blood transfusion prior to her first pregnancy, the fetus of that first pregnancy usually is not affected. The risks of sensitization increase, however, with each subsequent pregnancy. In women who have developed Rh sensitization, the second pregnancy often produces a mildly affected infant. Succeeding pregnancies produce more seriously affected infants until, at the third, fourth, or fifth pregnancy, the fetus may die in the womb. The survival rate is higher today than in the past. Just three decades ago, 50% of the Rh-immunized mothers lost their babies. Today, with proper diagnostic and therapeutic management, perinatal mortality should be 5% to 6%.[530] Needless to say, the Rh factor even in high-risk situations would never justify recourse to directly-sterilizing procedures. With proper consultation and spiritual guidance, however, a couple that is at high risk as evidenced by former pregnancies could be justified in resorting to Natural Family Planning. The fact that one partner of a proposed marriage is Rh positive and the other Rh negative should in no way affect their right to marry. Charity would require, however, that both parties have a mutual knowledge and understanding of the situation.

The Principle of the Double Effect could be applied if amniocentesis and ultrasonography indicate that a particular infant simply cannot survive until viability. This would justify the use of any reasonable and available procedure, even though it is of a risky and aggressive nature, in order to *bring the infant through to viability*. The direct intention would be to save (and baptize) the endangered infant.

7) Hydatidiform Mole—A Trophoblastic Disease

The hydatidiform mole (from "hydatis," the Greek word for "a drop of water") often is noted soon after conception by a rapid increase in the size of the uterus. Other symptoms are vaginal bleeding, lack of fetal movement, severe nausea and vomiting, and the passage of typical grapelike tissue. Good-Kelly mention three characteristics of this formation as proliferation (rapid growth), degeneration (of the chorionic villi) and edema (fluid retention), and add: "the three result in the formation of small cystic bodies which cluster together to give the whole mass the appearance of large bunches of grapes." It is their opinion that this begins in the very early days of pregnancy, and "progresses so rapidly that the fetus is quickly destroyed."[531]

Contemporary methods of diagnosis can be used to identify this condition. In a normally-progressing pregnancy, a well-formed sac should be seen

---

[530]*Ibid.*, p. 519.

[531]Good-Kelly, *Marriage, Morals and Medical Ethics* (cf. note 79), p. 106.

after 5¹/₂ weeks of gestation, embryonic echoes by 7 weeks, and fetal heartbeat and fetal movements can be detected by ultrasound by the 8th week of gestation. A molar gestation is easily diagnosed, as the uterus will be completely filled with high-density echoes rather than the expected fetus and amniotic fluid.[532] Other modern means of diagnosis are electrocardiography to determine whether or not there is a fetal heartbeat, x-ray to detect any evidence of skeletal formation, and testing of human chorionic gonadotropin (HCG) levels. Since there is the slightest possibility that the formation might include a human conceptus, Good-Kelly recommend an additional precaution as follows:

> When we see a case of hydatidiform mole, we always have another obstetrician see the patient with us and if he agrees in the diagnosis we then consult a clergyman, appraising him of all the facts and asking him to decide on the licitness of operating the patient.[533]

That possibility of including a human conceptus envisons two possible situations: (1) that the presence of a living fetus cannot be ruled out by clear and definite evidence to the contrary, and (2) that there is definite evidence that a surviving *twin pregnancy* may be present together with the hydatidiform mole. In the former case, the induced delivery of the presumed fetus, living and inviable, would amount to a direct abortion. If the mole is definitely diagnosed as a dead fetus or as incompatible with the presence of a living fetus, dilation and curettage, hysterotomy or even hysterectomy are morally acceptable and indicated, according to the medical indication. In the latter case (suspected evidence of a surviving *twin pregnancy*), Father Thomas O'Donnell, S.J. prescribes the proper procedure as follows:

> In such a case surgical interference would have to await the viability of the surviving fetus as long as the maternal life was not in imminent danger from the presence of the mole. If the maternal danger became imminent one could, under the principle of the double effect, institute procedures for the removal of the mole,

---

[532]Queenan, John T., MD, and Warsof, Steven L, MD, "Ultrasonography," in *Management of High-Risk Pregnancy* (cf. note 189), p. 222.

[533]*Marriage, Morals and Medical Ethics* (cf. note 79), p. 109.

even though the surviving fetus would then perish . . . several cases of this type have been reported in the periodical literature.[534]

The danger to the mother can rate as very serious in a minority of cases. Although 80% of hydatidiform moles are benign, complications of such a condition can include intrauterine infection and septicemia, hemorrhage, toxemia of pregnancy, and even the development of cancer of the chorion of the placenta. The latter is a highly malignant carcinoma which may spread early and widely by way of the venous and lymphatic systems. As soon as a diagnosis is made which definitely rules out the presence of a living fetus, efforts to save the life of the mother by dilation and curettage or by other surgical procedures (not excluding hysterectomy if warranted) are morally permissible.

8) The Anencephalic Fetus

Somewhat similar to the treatment of a hydatidiform mole pregnancy is the treatment of an *anencephalic* pregnancy (from the Greek "an" which means "no," and the Greek word "enkephalos" which means "brain"). In both cases, the proper procedure depends on whether or not the conceptus represents human life. In both cases, the removal of the conceptus would be a direct abortion unless there is incontrovertible clinical evidence, in each particular case, either that the fetus is dead, or that the conceptus is not a human individual.

The term "anencephaly" covers a wide rage of conditions extending from the loss primarily of only the cortex of the brain down to the total absence of a brain including the absence of even a brain stem. If clinical evidence clearly indicates the absence even of a brain stem, it is logical to conclude that the conceptus is not a human being. The reason is because the human brain, including the brain stem, is an essential component for the functioning of a unified human being and the root of all potentiality for rationality. If there is evidence of some brain tissue, including especially the brain stem which is necessary for basic vital functions such as respiration and proper cardiac activity, the prevailing presumption must be that the fetus is a human individual.

The question as to just when the spiritual soul is infused into a human

---

[534]*Medicine and Christian Morality* (cf. note 31), p. 176. The following statement is found in *Williams Obstetrics,* 16th ed., by Jack A. Pritchard, MD, and Paul C. MacDonald, MD (New York, N.Y.: Appleton-Crofts, 1980), p. 561: "Jones and Lauersen (1975) identified and described hydatidiform mole with a coexistent fetus 8 times in 175,000 pregnancies."

individual was discussed in chapter III (cf.3.5). The fact remains that a human conceptus is of human origin and destiny from the moment of conception ("incipiently human," cf.p.96), unless there is overpowering evidence to the contrary. Contemporary medical facilities for testing and monitoring a pregnancy such as ultrasonography, amniocentesis, chorionic villus sampling, human chorionic gonadotrophin levels (HCG), etc., can help the obstetrician in arriving at the proper diagnosis especially if used in combination. A recent text on obstetrics refers to a survey which was designed to detect neural tube defects in 1,271 high-risk patients, for example, and reported as follows: "There were 26 anencephalics; 100% were detected."[535] The dependability of these contemporary facilities would depend upon how far the pregnancy has advanced, the age and condition of the mother, etc., and the phrase "in combination" is important. Ultrasonography can detect fetal heartbeat and fetal movements by the 8th week of gestation; amniocentesis can be done after 14 weeks of gestation and can be used effectively in combination with ultrasonography, etc.

If there is any positive doubt after delivery as to whether or not the infant is a true anencephalic (that is, lacking even a brain stem), conditional baptism should be administered. As long as that positive doubt persists, however, there would be no moral obligation to use aggressive measures or extraordinary means to maintain the fragile life of the infant. Since the infant can be said to be "born dying," the use of aggressive measures would only prolong the dying process. If there is clinical evidence that the infant is undoubtedly anencephalic (lacking even a brain stem), there would be no moral obligation to administer nutrition, hydration or medication.

9) Radiation Therapy

In applying the Principle of the Double Effect to radiation therapy, two aspects in particular merit special attention: (1) is there a reasonable and available alternative procedure which is effective but presents less dangers of unfavorable side effects, and (2) if radiation is the only answer to the problem at hand, is there a proportionate reason for resorting to radiation therapy despite the involved risks and dangers?

Significant advances in pharmacology and chemotherapy should provide a response to the first question in most cases. If radiation is the procedure of

---

[535]Queenan, John T., MD, "Maternal Serum a-Fetoprotein Screening," in *Management of High-Risk Pregnancy* (cf. note 189), p. 58.

choice, however, the proportionate reason would have to be based on an adequate consideration of the dangers or risks associated with radiation. There is a general agreement on some aspects of the use of radiation such as the cumulative effects of radiation exposure, the special sensitivity of certain tissues to radiation exposure (lymphoid cells, gonads, etc.), the delayed effects of radiation, etc. Some obstetricians call x-irradiation the "agent with the best-defined responsibility for chromosomal damage," and add: "In the past few years, increasing evidence has shown that exposure of women and men to ionizing radiation can lead to nondisjunction in the offspring and/or increase the incidence of spontaneous abortion."[536] The possibility of an increased number of genetically-defective infants due to the uncontrolled use of radiation imposes a moral obligation to "limit radiation exposure to that which is absolutely necessary for valid diagnostic or therapeutic purposes, and to strictly control occupational exposure."[537]

If radiation is contemplated by the physician during pregnancy, he is obligated to take all due precautions so as not to subject the fetus to needless radiation. If such precautions are taken, and the life of a pregnant woman with an advanced metastatic cancer of the uterus can be saved only by resorting to radiation therapy, he may proceed with such therapy even though the life of the fetus might be endangered. If the fetus is near viability, however, and the radiation therapy can be postponed without endangering the life of the mother, he is obligated to postpone the radiation therapy until after the mother has been delivered by vaginal delivery or by cesarean section. If the fetus is not near viability, and the condition of the mother requires prompt action, the physician might decide to do a radical hysterectomy instead of proceeding with the radiation therapy. In that event, presuming that both procedures are indicated as equally effective, the hysterectomy should be the preferred choice. The reason is based on the spiritual welfare of the infant: the infant probably would be a still-living subject of baptism as soon as the uterus has been excised.

Directive 25: Radiation therapy of the mother's reproductive organs is permitted during pregnancy only when necessary to suppress a dangerous pathological condition.

---

[536]Fabricant, Jill D., Ph.D., Boué, Joëlle, MD., Boué, André, MD., "Cytogenic Abnormalities in Spontaneous Abortions," in *Management of High-Risk Pregnancy* (cf. note 189), p. 69.

[537]*The Merck Manual* (cf. note 56), pp. 2131, 2132. Quotation on p. 2132.

10) Hysterectomy in the Presence of Pregnancy

It is encouraging to know that the medical world has decreased significantly the reasons often alleged for what abortionists call "therapeutic abortions." The following observations are found in *The Merck Manual* (1982) with page numbers indicated. With regard to cardiac disease: "Cardiac disease in pregnancy fortunately is becoming uncommon today, mainly because of the marked decline in rheumatic heart disease in the USA" (1735); and "Most patients with congenital heart disease who are asymptomatic are not under an increased hazard during pregnancy" (1736). With regard to hypertension: "About 75% of patients with hypertension will have no difficulty with pregnancy; the other 25% will have to be delivered early to avoid abruptio placentae or unexplained intrauterine death"(1737). With regard to malignancies: "Malignancy of any kind is generally treated as if the patient were not pregnant. Malignancies of the upper abdomen, lung, or extremities are fortunately uncommon in pregnancy and should be treated as usual"(1741); "Carcinoma of the cervix is becoming less common, since cytologic smears allow early diagnosis of the preinvasive form;" "Hodgkin's disease is not so rapidly fatal, and cure is possible. If Hodgkin's disease is confined above the diaphragm, a pregnant patient may receive appropriate irradiation therapy with shielding of the abdomen" (1742).

Unfortunately there are still many pathological conditions of a pregnant mother which are considered "medical indications" for inducing a nonviable fetus, including some situations in the categories listed above. The fetus possesses the same right to life that belongs to any other human being. It is never permitted to perform an operation or procedure if the *direct* purpose is to save the life of the mother by killing or ejecting a nonviable fetus. The stimulating challenge for the contemporary obstetrician is to use the marvels of medical technology to save both mother and child.

There is a vast difference, however, between *causing* the death of a fetus, and *permitting* the death of a fetus for a sufficiently compensating reason. As noted in this chapter (application of the Principle of the Double Effect), such a permitted or tolerated (and unintended) side effect could be justified in advanced cases of "placenta praevia" and of "abruptio placentae" (after a complete separation of the placenta from the uterine wall), but would not be justified in conditions known as "hyperemesis gravidarum," "eclampsia," and the Rh factor. If a pregnant woman is found to have cancer of the cervix, and the physician judges that the cancer will spread beyond the confines of the underlying uterine wall within one or two months (when the fetus still will be nonviable), he is justified in resorting to radiation therapy or a radical hysterectomy even though, as an indirect and unintended effect, the fetus will die.

If the mother who is pregnant with a nonviable fetus has an inoperable cancer of the reproductive organs (*nothing* can be done to save her life), however, the physician's chief concern must be the best interests of the fetus. Since it is impossible to save the life of the mother, the Principle of the Double Effect cannot be applied. The physician must wait until the fetus is viable using radiation to retard the growth of the cancer only to the extent that it does not have serious effects for the fetus-and deliver the fetus by cesarean section at the opportune time.

If while pregnant, a woman suffers a severe appendicitis attack, or a gall-bladder attack, etc., and surgery simply cannot be postponed until the fetus is viable without endangering the life of the mother, the surgery is permissible even though the death of the fetus is foreseen but not intended. The unfortunate death of the fetus would be an *indirect* consequence of the procedure. The presumption is that the physician would have no other alternative in his effort to postpone the surgery until the child is viable. Proceeding with the surgery could well lead to premature labor and the loss of the nonviable infant. If this is the only solution in saving the life of the mother, it would be allowed as an application of the Principle of the Double Effect.[538]

> *Directive 17:* Hysterectomy, in the presence of pregnancy and even before viability, is permitted when directed to the removal of a dangerous pathological condition of the uterus of such serious nature that the operation cannot be safely postponed until the fetus is viable.

11) Induced Labor

The Church looks upon the artificial induction of labor *before* viability (that is, before the fetus is capable of extrauterine life) as direct abortion. In medical circles, such a procedure often is recommended "when contraception or sterilization is not used or fails." The reasons for abortive procedures are listed as either medical (therapeutic) or non-medical.[539] The choice of one of the three major methods of "evacuating the uterus" (vaginal instrumental evacuation, stimulation of uterine contractions, major surgery) depends upon the stage of development of the fetus. Such abortive procedures must not be confused with the theological concept of induced labor. In the theological

---

[538]Healy, Edwin F., S.J., *Medical Ethics* (cf. note 46), p. 232.
[539]*The Merck Manual* (cf. note 56), p. 1706.

concept (and indeed, the proper clinical concept) induced labor is described as the initiation of the birth process by artificial or mechanical means *after* a reliable judgment as to the *viability* of the fetus. The procedure is permissible provided that there is a proportionate reason in view of the risks involved in each particular case. In other words, it is warranted premature delivery.

While some obstetricians consider eclampsia or pregnancy-induced hypertension to be the "enigma of obstetric practice and research" (cf.p.279), others might join Dr. Tom Barden, Chairman of the Department of Obstetrics and Gynecology, University of Cincinnati College of Medicine, in his appraisal of premature birth:

> Premature birth remains the most perplexing problem of modern obstetrics, with its parthogenesis usually obscure, the propriety of certain forms of treatment unclear, and the result of drug therapy far less than ideal. It is the major contributing factor to approximately two-thirds of neonatal deaths in the United States. The incidence of premature birth in the United Sates has remained relatively stable in recent years, at about 5.5% when defined as birth before 37 weeks' gestation, or at 7.5% when defined as birth weight less than 2,500 g.[540]

The good news is that risk factors to premature birth can be recognized early in pregnancy and decreased by appropriate treatment. This imposes an obligation not only on the observant and dedicated obstetrician, but also on a couple with a record of a previous low-birth-weight infant:

> The oxytocic action of prostaglandin, the large quantity of prostaglandin in male seminal fluid, and the possible role of prostaglandin in female orgasm suggest the potential danger of coitus in such patients [that is, with a record of the previous delivery of a low-birth-weight infant]. They should also be advised to stop smoking because of its well-established dose-dependent effect on reduced birth weight.[541]

Medical indications for inducing labor before full term have been mentioned previously in this chapter. The discussion of the management of a true anencephalic pregnancy, for example, could include the possibility of an ear-

---

[540]*Management of High-Risk Pregnancy* (cf. note 189), p. 535.
[541]*Ibid.*, p. 537.

lier delivery because the mother is subject to serious psychiatric repercussions over the anguish of carrying a seriously handicapped infant. There could be other situations involving a viable normal pregnancy (infant not handicapped) where a high-strung or hypertensive mother is so overwrought by fear and anxiety that the physician judges that a slight advance in delivery is the only alternative in the effort to sedate her fears and anxieties. The final judgment rests with the physician or obstetrician; based on prenatal care and monitoring, he or she is presumed to know the patient. Provided that the risks for the infant are minimal, and that all due precautions are observed, there could be rare exceptions to the general rule of "wait until full term."

It must be admitted, however, that the inclination to allow such rare exceptions could pave the way for "elective interventions:" for example, an earlier delivery so that the baby might be born on the couple's wedding anniversary, or so that the baby might be born before the wealthy visiting father-in-law's scheduled departure, or so as not to delay the obstetrician's departure for a vacation or a medical convention, etc. Such excuses, considered in the absence of a valid medical indication, cannot constitute a proportionate reason for an earlier delivery. Dr. Barden proposes a prudential guideline for obstetricians as follows:

> Finally, the obstetrician must avoid premature births from elective interventions by induction of labor or cesarean section until the fetus is mature. Even now, neonatal intensive care units report that significant numbers of premature infants with life-threatening respiratory distress have been delivered by elective intervention.[542]

In the interests of the intrauterine development of the infant, the conscientious obstetrician will delay the premature delivery as long as possible.

Solutions to problems of induced labor are to be sought in the application of the Principle of the Double Effect. The application is not valid, however, if there is a reasonable and available alternative to induced delivery. In view of the formidable arsenal of aids and equipment which are at the disposal of the contemporary obstetrician (ultrasonography, amniocentesis, fetoscopy, antibiotics, monitoring devices, etc.), such alternatives should be possible on an ascending scale. A list of proportionately serious reasons for performing a premature delivery could include the following: unless the birth process is hastened, the infant will die in the womb without baptism; a delay would

---

[542]*Ibid.*, pp. 537, 538.

present a more serious danger to the mother as compared to the danger of premature delivery for the infant; the mother is in imminent danger of death and delay in hastening the birth process could mean the death of the viable infant as well. In the last case (mother in imminent danger of death), the delivery should be delayed as long as is reasonably possible so as not to shorten appreciably the life of the mother. If hastening the birth is necessary to save the mother's life, premature delivery would be allowed even if the infant is only *probably viable* provided that there is a basis for genuine hope of saving the infant's life. The obstetrician actually would be doing his best to save both mother and infant.[543]

One reason for premature delivery as advanced in former years was based on the danger of normal delivery due to the narrow dimensions of the woman's pelvis. The solution to such a situation today would be delivery by cesarean section.

Another emergency situation involving a nonviable fetus would be an early spontaneous abortion when the uterine contractions of labor are completely beyond control. Abortion is inevitable. The physician is concerned about the baptism of the fetus while still alive, and uses hand pressure on the woman's abdomen so as to hasten delivery. The physician is not causing the death of the fetus. He is merely bringing the fetus from a situation where it cannot be baptized to a position where baptism is possible. The cause of death is attributed to the uncontrollable contractions of labor.[544]

The possibility of a secondary abdominal pregnancy must also be considered. After the rupture of the fallopian tube in a tubal pregnancy, for example, the maternal connections may remain, and the fetus could continue to develop between the layers of the broad ligament or in the peritoneal cavity. If the mother is doing well, the pregnancy should be allowed to continue as long as possible beyond viability. If serious complications arise, however, and the fetus is *viable,* the physician may prepare at once to open the abdomen and deliver the fetus.[545] If the fetus is nonviable, however, the physician would not be allowed to intervene and deliver the fetus unless the mother developed a serious pathological condition such as severe and uncontrollable hemorrhaging at the placental site of the secondary abdominal pregnancy. This would be an application of the Principle of the Double Effect. The surgical intervention

---

[543]Healy, Edwin, S.J., *Medical Ethics* (cf. note 46), p. 245. In borderline cases of viability, the conscientious obstetrician or physician should seek verification of his own judgment through consultation with one or more specialists in obstetrics. Cf. McFadden, Charles, *Medical Ethics* (cf. note 17), p. 211.

[544]Healy, Edwin, S.J., *Medical Ethics* (cf. note 46), p. 235.

[545]*Ibid.*, pp. 245, 246. Cf. also Kelly, Gerald, S.J., *Medico-Moral Problems* (cf. note 22), pp. 113, 114; O'Donnell, Thomas, S.J., *Medicine and Christian Morality* (cf. note 31), pp. 199, 200.

required to save the life of the mother could not be by way of a *direct* attack on the life of the fetus. In this case it would be an unintended side-effect of a life-saving intervention.[546]

In addition to repeated condemnations of direct abortion, the Holy See has issued several directives which would apply to induced premature deliveries. They might be summarized as two responses on the immorality of craniotomy (Nov. 28, 1872, and May 28, 1884), and two responses on the evil of directly aborting an infant in order to save the life of the mother or of the infant (August 19, 1889, and July 24, 1895). Another response of the Holy Office under date of May 4, 1898, states that acceleration of birth for just reasons and without harm to the life of the fetus is licit, with special mention of the situation "when the mother would otherwise perish." Finally, a response of the Holy Office under date of March 5, 1902, concerns the immorality of extracting an immature ectopic fetus. [547]

Directive 23: For a proportionate reason, labor may be induced after the fetus is viable.

---

12) Premature Rupture of the Amniotic Membranes

In their discussion of the very-low-birth-weight infants, Moore and Resnik state that the majority of such infants beyond 28 weeks' gestation can now survive, and predict that 80% of such babies born in the 1980's "can have productive futures with few or no neurologic disabilities."[548] Realizing that prediction, however, depends upon closely coordinated obstetric and neonatal care during labor, birth, and early neonatal life. A delay of even 7 days in delivery improves chances of survival dramatically; a fetus at 26 to 30 weeks' gestation gains 100 to 150 grams per week.

One of the serious complications of late pregnancy is brought about by the premature rupture of the amniotic membranes. This occurs in as many as 38% of very-low-birth-weight infants, and leads to serious risks including

---

[546]Father Kelly refers to a report on two cases of full-term abdominal pregnancies. One was delivered alive and well. The other apparently would have been saved if the diagnosis had been made in time. *Ibid.* (cf. note above), p. 114.

[547]*Canon Law Digest,* III (cf. note 43), p. 669.

[548]Moore, Thomas R., MD, and Resnik, Robert, MD in *Management of High-Risk Pregnancy* (cf. note 189), p. 545.

fetal sepsis or chorioamnionitis and preterm labor. The situation is explained as follows:

> Generally, because risk of prematurity exceeds risk of sepsis in pregnancies complicated by premature rupture of membranes, a conservative, expectant approach is warranted. Respiratory distress syndrome accounts for 50% to 70% of perinatal deaths, whereas neonatal infection is associated with only 10% to 20%. In comparing two groups of patients with premature rupture of membranes and very-low-birth weight infants, Graham and associates encountered no chorioamnionitis or fetal sepsis in the expectantly managed group. Perinatal mortality, intraventricular hemorrhage, and respiratory distress were 55% to 60% higher in the group delivered early.[549]

In theory, it should be possible to diagnose the destructive infection known as chorioamnionitis in advance and to identify fetuses who will become infected and deliver them before the infection becomes established. In practice, however, there seems to be no test which will predict chorioamnionitis in a consistent manner. Moore and Resnik propose the following guideline in the management of very-low-birth-weight (VLBW) pregnancies:

> Therefore, base your decision to deliver the VLBW fetus, when you suspect sepsis, on such traditional clinical criteria as maternal fever and uterine tenderness, fetal distress on fetal heart rate (FHR) monitoring, or herpes simplex lesions or positive herpes culture . . . On balance, such fetuses will benefit from expectant management through both interval weight gain and continued lung maturation. For the minority of fetuses who develop sepsis in utero, aggressive treatment with antibiotics and expeditious delivery are likely to provide the best outcome.[550]

The 1983 edition of *Obstetrics and Gynecology* by Ralph M. Wynn, MD defines the rupture of the membranes as premature when it occurs more than one hour before the onset of labor. The aggressive management of this condition includes delivery within 24 hours of the rupture of the membranes. The

---

[549]*Ibid.*, p. 548.
[550]*Ibid.*, p. 549.

preferred method of delivery is induction by the administration of oxytocin if there are no contraindications to this drug.[551] It is generally agreed, however, that this drug must be administered cautiously and in doses sufficient to stimulate strong, normal labor.

When sepsis or chorioamnionitis infection occurs after the rupture of the amniotic membranes, the lives of both infant and mother are in danger. If the mother survives, she may have to become reconciled to sterility for life. Fortunately, the rupture of membranes usually occurs late in the second trimester or in the early third trimester when the infant is viable or close to viability. If rupture occurs when the infant is alive and viable, but is not followed by the complete loss of the amniotic fluid nor by the chorioamnionitis infection, careful and continuous monitoring of the pregnancy can lead to a successful delivery. The situation calls for cautious expectant management of the pregnancy. Likewise there is no moral problem if the infant is judged to be dead within the womb by reliable medical standards. The mother then is to be delivered as expeditiously as possible.

The obstetrician encounters a very challenging situation, however, when the infant is alive but nonviable (not able to live outside of the womb), and the rupture of the amniotic membranes is accompanied by the loss of amniotic fluid and the chorioamnionitis infection. In most cases, Mother Nature provides the solution by bringing about the spontaneous expulsion of the infant. If the live but nonviable infant remains attached to the womb, however, the deadly infection cannot be controlled by any known drug or medical treatment. The standard treatment in such cases is to protect both infant and mother from the damaging effects of chorioamnionitis by inducing delivery through the administration of oxytocin. The 1986 edition of the *Physician's Desk Reference* makes it very clear that the drug was designed, when used "ante partum," as a means of initiating or improving uterine contractions "where it is desirable and considered suitable for reasons of fetal or maternal concern, in order to achieve early vaginal delivery."[552]

The situation is similar to the treatment of hemorrhage during pregnancy and before the fetus is viable when, in the words of *Directive 14* (cf.p.277) "Procedures that are designed to empty the uterus of a living fetus still effectively attached to the mother are not permitted." Unless it is also a clear case of a complete "abruptio placentae," it is evident that the fetus is still effectively attached to the mother. Distinguished moralists stipulate that a direct attack is made on the life of the fetus not only if the fetus is expelled from the amniotic sac, but also if a positive effort is made to separate the fetus from the

---

[551]*Obstetrics and Gynecology* (cf. note 510), p. 124.
[552]*Physicians' Desk Reference* (cf. note 67), p. 1966.

placental connection or "mooring" which is the essential lifeline of the fetus:

> It also should be noted that the specific moral malice of direct abortion does not wait upon the actual removal of the pre-viable infant from the uterus, but is identified in the separation from the uterus of the essential life support system of the fetus (the placenta), just as the specific moral malice of embryotomy is the dismembering of the fetus within the uterus.[553]

A comparison might be made between separating an infant from his or her life source either by induction from the amniotic sac or by separation of the placenta from the uterine wall, and separating an electric lamp from its light source either by removing the bulb or disconnecting the electric plug from the wall receptacle. In both cases, it is a direct effort to render the source of life (or light) powerless. If the drug oxytocin could be viewed medically as a means of controlling the chorioamnionitis infection with the foreseen but unintended initiation of uterine contractions and labor as a possible side effect, the Principle of the Double Effect could be applied, provided, of course, that no equally effective treatment is available to safeguard the lives of the infant and/or mother. In such circumstances, the risk of the foreseen but unintended separation of the placenta from the uterine wall could be justified in the intended objective of saving human lives by controlling the virulent infection. As stated above, however, oxytocin cannot be viewed as having a direct effect of controlling the infection when used as an ante-partum treatment.[554]

There are situations in which the Principle of the Double Effect could be applied to save the life of a woman who is pregnant with a living but non-viable fetus whereby the loss of the fetus would be an *indirect* consequence of a medical intervention. One possible situation (which would NOT involve the use of oxytocin): the scenario could be that the onset of the chorioamnionitis infection is so invasive and virulent (following the rupture of the amniotic sac) that it leads to the rupture of the uterus itself. This might occur because the

---

[553]O'Donnell, Thomas, S.J., *The Medical-Moral Newsletter,* Dec., 1983, p. 37.

[554]In *Medico-Moral Problems* (cf. note 22), pp. 87–89, Father Gerald Kelly, S.J. discusses the use of "ergot" (a drug which stimulates uterine contractions) in the case of a woman who is in imminent danger of death due to excessive hemorrhaging. The fetus is still alive but cannot be saved. Providing that no other alternative to save the fetus is available, he would allow the use of *ergot* in view of the fact that "independently of the presence or absense of a fetus, ergot has an effect on hemorrhage." Father O'Donnell, S.J. expresses the same opinion in *Medicine and Christian Morality* (cf. note 31), pp. 197, 198. The problem under discussion here, however, is not the control of hemorrhaging, but the control of the chorioamnionitis infection.

uterus is in a weakened condition due to a previous cesarean section, or due to scar tissue which had formed as a result of an injury in a previous pregnancy.[555] Depending upon the location and size of the rupture, the obstetrician may judge that the woman is in such a serious, pathological condition, that a hysterectomy is the only means of saving the life of the mother (cf. *Directive 17*, p. 289).

Another situation (which would involve the use of oxytocin) is more problematical, since it would involve the prudential judgment of the obstetrician with regard to the relative nature of viability. Even hospitals with the most advanced obstetric and gynecological equipment and neonatal facilities would hesitate to consider anything much less than 24 weeks of gestation as basis for a judgment of viability in a particular case. Father Thomas O'Donnell outlines the possibilities and the parameters of the use of oxytocin in such a situation as follows:

> Even though the vital uterine environment is itself rapidly becoming potentially lethal for the baby as well as for the mother, the only morally acceptable removal of the baby would be into an environment which would offer at least as good, or preferably better, chances of survival for at least as long a time, or longer, than the baby could be expected to survive in the infected uterus. If the available intensive neonatal care is judged to be incapable of prolonging the extrauterine life of the baby for any considerable length of time, it seems clear that the emptying of the uterus, even to avert serious danger for the mother, would simply be a direct abortion which the fact that the infant is going to die anyhow would neither justify or change . . .
>
> It should be carefully noted that even if the judgment is proposed that the baby delivered would not be in any worse situation than it is in the uterus, this would have to be a conclusion of clinical objectivity rather than a personal value judgment of the physician. The personal value judgment of the physician could take the form, "if the uterus is not emptied both will die," whereas the only acceptable clinically objective judgment would have to be, "if we do empty the uterus both mother and baby will live longer."[556]

---

[555] *Marriage, Morals and Medical Ethics*, by Frederick L. Good, MD, LL.D., and Rev. Otis F. Kelly, MD (cf. note 79), pp. 93, 94.

[556] *The Medical-Moral Newsletter*, Dec., 1983, p. 39.

In applying the Principle of the Double Effect in these circumstances, the use of oxytocin could be justified so as to induce delivery of the at-least-marginally viable infant in an attempt to save the lives of both infant and mother, but with the foreseen but unintended side-effect of risking the ability of the viable infant to survive outside of the womb. It would be up to the obstetrician to judge, in view of the advanced extensive neonatal care and monitoring facilities of the hospital and his own professional skill and patience, whether or not the infant would have that at-least-equal chance of extrauterine survival as described in the quotation above. It should be less difficult to make such a favorable judgment in particular cases, if and when medical science and technology brightens the prospects for premature infants with improved incubators or the long-awaited artificial placenta.

Since nature usually provides the solution to chorioamnionitis infections by initiating spontaneous labor contractions and the eventual delivery of the infant, some obstetricians may be inclined to justify the use of oxytocin when such contractions are not spontaneous, by saying that they are simply "assisting nature in the labor process." Such an argument is both unwarranted and invalid. One might imagine the possibility of applying the same defective logic to patients who are in imminent danger of death so as to justify medical interventions to "assist nature in the dying process." If such reasoning were to prevail with regard to a difficult and threatening birth process, the next step might well be to justify the artificial induction of labor (infant non-viable) immediately following a major premature rupture of the membranes even without the complication of the chorioamnionitis infection.[557] This could be characterized as "slippery slope" medical practice (one "rare exception" justifies another).

A recent article on neonatal sepsis states that the major disease-producing microorganisms (pathogens) in neonatal sepsis have changed over the years. The authors add: "Now, the most common bacterial pathogens are Group B streptococci and *Escherichia coli*."[558] The observations above would apply to any

---

[557]In *Health and Medicine in the Catholic Tradition* (cf. note 206), Father Richard McCormick, S.J. refers to the Catholic Church's rejection of abortion "in the vast majority of instances" (Guideline 15, p. 12), but questions the propriety of applying the word "abortion" to the "instance of rupture of the membranes." His position is stated as follows: "If nature has started a process (with extremely low fetal survival expectation and rather high incidence of serious maternal infection in attempting to bring the fetus to term), does human completion of this process deserve the rejection implied in the term "abortion"? I raise these as questions for those concerned to protect fetal life but not to expand the protection deductively in a way harmful to the overall health of the position." p. 135.

[558]"Neonatal Sepsis," by David A. Driggers, MD, et al. (4 others), in *AFP* (Academy of Family Practice), August, 1985, pp. 129–134. Cf. p. 129.

other serious bacterial infections ante-partum (besides chorioamnionitis) which are accompanied by a premature rupture of the membranes. It is only proper to add that some authors would permit the removal of the fetus in cases when "both a spontaneous abortion and a probably lethal uterine infection are inevitable" not on the basis of providing an at-least-equal chance of extrauterine survival for the fetus as described above, but on the basis that the uterus is "*substantially useless* to the fetus".[559] Since the life-sustaining placental connections are still intact, however, this writer cannot share that opinion. Again, to quote *Directive 14* of the *Catholic Hospital Directives*: "Procedures that are designed to empty the uterus of a living fetus *still effectively attached to the mother* are not permitted" (emphasis added). Furthermore, the argument based on the "uselessness of the uterus" (cf.chapter VI,pp.223,224) is inaccurate and misleading.

---

[559]Cf. "May a Catholic Hospital Allow Drugs that Accelerate Abortion?" in *Health Progress*, Dec., 1984, pp. 48–50. The author was a member of the staff of the Pope John Center. Cf. also the opinion of Father Richard McCormick, S.J. in footnote 557.

CHAPTER VIII

Principle of the Common Good

No era will ever succeed in destroying the unity of the human family, for it consists of men who are all equal by virtue of their human dignity. Hence there will always be an imperative need—born of man's very nature—to promote in sufficient measure the universal common good; the good, that is, of the whole human family (Pope John XXIII, *Pacem in Terris*, April 11, 1963, n.132).[560]

PRINCIPLE: INDIVIDUALS, FAMILIES, AND VARIOUS GROUPS WHICH COMPOSE THE CIVIC COMMUNITY ARE AWARE OF THEIR OWN INSUFFICIENCY IN THE MATTER OF ESTABLISHING A FULLY HUMAN CONDITION OF LIFE. THEY SEE THE NEED OF THAT WIDER COMMUNITY IN WHICH EACH WOULD DAILY CONTRIBUTE HIS ENERGIES TOWARD THE EVER BETTER ATTAINMENT OF THE COMMON GOOD . . . NOW, THE COMMON GOOD EMBRACES THE SUM OF THOSE CONDITIONS OF SOCIAL LIFE BY WHICH INDIVIDUALS, FAMILIES, AND GROUPS CAN ACHIEVE THEIR OWN FULFILLMENT IN A RELATIVELY THOROUGH AND READY WAY (*The Church Today*, n. 74).

---

[560]*The Papal Encyclicals, 1968–1981* (Wilmington, Del.: McGrath Publishing Co., 1981), p. 121.

The footnotes to articles 74 and 75 of Vatican's II's *The Church Today* indicate the extent to which the concept of the common good is based on Pope John XXIII's two encyclicals, *Mater et Magistra* and *Pacem in Terris*. The term "common good" can be understood in two senses: as a value in itself, and as a means to an end. The term is used here primarily in the second sense—as a relative value and a means to an end. In the words of the *Commentary on the Documents of Vatican II*, the common good is described as follows: ". . . it is the sum of all the general presuppositions or conditions which the individual cannot provide for himself and which must be already available for him if he is to develop in a fully human way, at all, or without too much difficulty."[561] It was Pope John XXIII who shifted the concept of the common good from the Aristotelian emphasis on "the good of the state," to the good of the whole of humanity.

A discussion of the extent to which the common good is superior to the good of the individual must include due consideration of both *objective* and *subjective* factors. *Subjectively,* a person who has been blessed with an abundance of material possessions or educational advantages has a greater obligation to contribute to the common good: "More will be asked of a man to whom more has been entrusted" (Luke,12:48). *Objectively* considered, several situations might be mentioned for illustration purposes. When two sets of good are not of the same order, any conflict between them should be settled in favor of the higher order; for example, the spiritual good of an individual or group vs the demands of *material* progress. Another objective consideration is that a private good may be of such a nature as to justify the sacrifice of some portion of the common good; for example, a young man's exemption from military service in wartime because of the number of dependents on the home front. Furthermore, a good of a lower order but of high urgency may justify putting off a higher good of a less urgent nature; for example, a young man interrupts his studies for the priesthood for reasons of health.

Of special importance from the viewpoint of motivation is the distinction between voluntary and imposed sacrifice for the common good. A highly motivated individual may licitly sacrifice his or her own personal good for a common good in so many circumstances when society would have no right to impose or demand such a sacrifice; for example, donating a kidney to a victim of renal failure. In the highest form, such voluntary sacrifices can be motivated by the love of God: "Whatsoever you do for one of my least brothers . . ." (Matthew,25:40).

In the application of the priorities of the Principle of the Common Good to the healing ministry, three imperatives come to mind: fidelity to Catholic

---

[561]*Commentary on the Documents of Vatican II, Vol. V* (cf. note 42), p. 318.

ideals and values (8.1), building on community of concerns (8.2), and promoting the common good (8.3).

8.1   THE COMMON GOOD—IDEALS AND REALITIES

Pope John XXIII's inspiring vision of advancing the common good based on the equality of all humankind "by virtue of their human dignity" (opening quotation of this chapter) emphasizes a Christian ideal which is somewhat similar to the ideal enunciated in Lincoln's Gettysburg address in the phrase "One Nation under God." In the real world, however, there are numerous insurmountable divisions. Of particular importance in the discussion of the pursuit of the common good in the mission of healing, there is the reality of conflict with non-Catholic views on the morality of medical issues. In most cases, the Catholic health facility exists side by side with other medical facilities which are not committed to Catholic concepts of right and wrong. On many issues, the Catholic health facility administrators can form a common cause with their counterparts of other medical facilities. This is a matter of some civic urgency in view of the fact that not only Catholics but also individuals and groups of other religious denominations (or of no religious denomination) lend financial support to the healing ministry of Catholic health facilities (fund drives, hospital committee memberships, etc.). This is true especially if the Catholic health facility is the only health facility in the community. Yet, the temptation to compromise on moral principles must be resisted.

In those communities where the Catholic health facility is the only one conveniently available to all members of the community, a special "ecumenical vision" requires due consideration of the divergent convictions of the non-Catholic citizens on moral-medical matters. The very concept of "regional morality" as advanced by some authors has overtones of compromise. Tempering the publication of procedures which cannot be offered in a Catholic health facility is one thing; making unwarranted exceptions regarding the forbidden procedures, however, is another, and must be avoided as a matter of principle.

There can be regional circumstances and pressures which justify a more frequent application of the *Principle of Material Cooperation*. This is not regional *morality* but rather regional *reality*. The issue will be discussed and illustrated at length in chapter X. Collaboration to the degree possible is one thing; compromise is akin to abdication of principles. An appropriate answer to those who say that Catholics in hospital practice are imposing Catholic morality on others, is the following statement of Archbishop Pilarczyk of Cincinnati:

> Catholic health care exists primarily as a witness to the Church's
> reality, as a witness to Church teaching, as a witness to the love of
> Christ for his people in the context of sickness and wellness. If we
> believe that certain procedures or practices are in disaccord with
> the law of the Gospel and with the law of the love of Christ for his
> people, to cooperate in such procedures or practices is to give
> counterwitness to the love of Christ . . . If others come to us and
> want us to do things that we believe are contrary to the Gospel law
> of Christ, they ask us to be false to our reason for being . . . it is
> not inappropriate for a Catholic hospital to be true to its con-
> science. It is not imposing anything on anybody.[562]

Progress in advancing the common good will not be made by denying the
difficulty presented by the situation outlined above, or by denying the common sense of inadequacy in meeting the challenge,—but rather by continued
dedication to Catholic values and ideals. Fair-minded individuals and groups
of other religious persuasions will understand—and even admire Catholic
hospital authorities for "standing up for their convictions." It is only when
Catholic values and ideals are made secure in a spirit of loyalty and dedication that Catholic efforts in pursuit of the common good can be effectively
extended and reciprocated (collaboration, consultation) on the basis of "no-
blesse oblige."

When dedicated sisters and brothers came to America in the early 19th
century to pioneer in establishing Catholic health facilities at great personal
sacrifice and expense, they were motivated both by Christian humanism and
by apostolic ideals. The humanistic motive was manifested by their concern
for extending the healing mission to the poor; the apostolic motive was manifested by their desire to use their presence and ministrations as a means to
witness to the ethical and spiritual aspects of health care in accordance with
Catholic values. Although contemporary circumstances make it difficult for
Catholic health facilities to emphasize concern for the poor, their Catholic
identity is compromised if the apostolic motivation is allowed to pass into
oblivion: ". . . unless a Catholic hospital gets its vitality from its own religious
faith and system of values, it will become more hurtful than healing, a scan-

---

[562]The response of the Archbishop of Cincinnati, Most Rev. Daniel E. Pilarczyk, to this
question as found in *Ethics Committees: A Challenge for Catholic Health Care* (cf. note 226), pp. 22, 23.

dal, rather than a witness of Christ's presence in a suffering world".[563] Loyalty and dedication to Gospel values and the teachings of the Catholic church must continue as the distinctive, identifying mark of every Catholic health facility in the present and future as in the past. Any feelings of "insufficiency" in this regard can be calmed by recalling the words of the Divine Healer: "For man it is impossible, but for God, all things are possible" (Matthew, 19:26).

> *Preamble, paragraph 3:* A Catholic-sponsored health facility, its board of trustees, and administration face today a serious difficulty as, with community support, the Catholic health facility exists side by side with other medical facilities not committed to the same moral code, or stands alone as the one facility serving the community. However, the health facility identified as Catholic exists today and serves the community in a large part because of the past dedication and sacrifice of countless individuals whose lives have been inspired by the Gospel and the teachings of the Catholic Church.

8.2   BUILDING ON COMMUNITY OF CONCERNS

The Second Vatican Council focused particular attention on the need of consultation as a means of advancing the common good. This is reflected in the new Code of Canon Law (English edition as published by the Canon Law Society of America). The index provides 25 entries under the heading of "consultation/counsel." This listing involves approximately 60 canons of the code. It is significant that the word "council" is defined as "an assembly of persons called together for consultation, deliberation, or discussion;" and the advice resulting from such an assembly is known as "counsel" (from the Latin "consulere,"—to consult). The propriety of consultation is urged in situations as diverse as a bishop consulting with his auxiliary bishop (Can.407), or with a pastor preliminary to appointing an associate pastor (Can.547), or with religious superiors with regard to apostolic works (Can.678), to consultative assemblies such as the presbyteral council (Can.495) and parish pastoral councils (Can.536).

---

[563] Ashley-O'Rourke, *Health Care Ethics* (cf. note 80), p. 140.

Without doubt, the concept of individuals and groups "contributing their energies" as sources of consultation and advice is a powerful means of building and sustaining a sense of community. Unfortunately the true value of consultation was weakened or clouded for over a decade since Vatican II with a misplaced emphasis on decision-making . . . as if authorities with decision-making responsibilities were to be sidetracked or circumvented by their advisors. Actually the inherent value of consultation is to enable decision-makers to fulfill their responsibilities with increased knowledge, foresight and prudence. The new Code of Canon Law is saying that consultors are urged to advise; decision-makers are obligated to listen and to take advantage of this rich source of communal counsel in fulfilling their duties.[564]

Within the scope of the mission of healing, the following areas of pursuing the common good through consultation and common deliberation are in line with the *Ethical and Religious Directives for Catholic Health Facilities*.

The Role of Ethics Committees

The subject of ethics committees was introduced in chapter three with a brief review of the U.S. government's intervention in behalf of such consultative groups in advancing and protecting the best interests of the health facility patient. Whereas only 1% of non-Catholic hospitals in the nation had ethics committees or similar groups as of late 1983, 41% of Catholic hospitals claimed to have such committees as of the same date. This favorable statistic can be attributed to the unique identity of Catholic hospitals, "represented through their commitment to the Church and their sponsoring congregations' charisms."[565] The motivation behind the ethics committees in non-Catholic hospitals was not oriented to patient welfare to any significant degree. Some were organized primarily to protect the hospital from malpractice suits, or to facilitate the reduction of costs in life-support cases. Another potential weakness was due to the fact that such committees often were dominated by physicians and other health professionals whose primary concern was not uniformly ethical.[566]

By virtue of having been exposed to the potential and advantages of an ethics committee over a longer period of time, Catholic health facilities per-

---

[564]Cf. article on parish councils by Msgr. Orville Griese in *Homiletic and Pastoral Review*, January, 1985, pp. 47–53.

[565]"Ethics Committees and Ethicists in Catholic Hospitals" by Sr. Joan Kalchbrenner, RHSJ, et al., in *Hospital Progress*, Sept., 1983, p. 47.

[566]"Are Ethics Committees Alive and Well?" by Judith Randall in *The Hastings Center Report*, Dec., 1983, pp. 10–12.

sonnel should be in a position to exercise leadership in the growing ethics-committee movement. In addressing the question of the purpose of such committees, it may be helpful to compare Catholic thinking with non-Catholic thinking on the subject. The *American Society of Law and Medicine* proposes three functions of such a committee which are jurisdictional in nature: 1) to review a case to confirm a physician's diagnosis or prognosis; 2) to review decisions made by physicians or surrogates about specific treatment, and 3) to make decisions about suitable treatment for incompetent patients.[567] Such "jurisdictional" functions are inappropriate for an ethics committee. The first two are concerns which are the prime responsibility of professional physicians who must make "on the spot" judgments based on medical evidence. "Second guessing" physicians by a committee after-the-fact could also lend undue consideration to cost control to the detriment of the patient. The 3rd function (decision making) is the responsibility of the competent patient or the family members of the incompetent patient, or of the administrator, based on adequate expert medical evidence and advice. Furthermore, intrusion into the field of decision-making on the part of ethics committees could also induce those who have that responsibility to "cop out" in the discharge of their duties.

Three other functions listed by the same source—functions which are educational in nature—are highly recommended as right and proper for ethics committees: 1) to provide education programs on how to identify and solve ethical issues; 2) to *recommend* (not "make") policies to be followed in certain difficult situations ("do-not-resuscitate" policy, "irreversible coma" policy, etc.); 3) to serve as consultants to physicians, patients, family members of patients, administrators. Based on 1982 data from a survey conducted by the Catholic Health Association, ethics committees in Catholic hospitals favored the three functions above as follows: 1) educational programming, 56%; 2) policy recommending, 79%; 3) consultation (advisory), 84%. Policy-*making* received a low rating of 17%; decision-making received a 19% rating.[568] In a 1984 publication on Catholic ethics committees, 6 models for such committees for hospitals repeatedly list functions such as education and study, recommend or confirm policy, consult and advise. Significantly, there is no mention of policy-*making* or of *decision*-making.[569]

---

[567]"Ethics Committees in Hospitals" by Kevin D. O'Rourke, O.P. in *Parameters 83* (quarterly, St. Louis University Medical Center), Vol. 8, n. 3, p. 19. Cf. also *Deciding To Forego Life-Sustaining Treatment* (cf. note 215), pp. 160, 161.

[568]Kalchbrenner, Sr. Joan, RHSJ, et al. article in *Hospital Progress* (cf. note 565), p. 49.

[569]*Ethics Committees: A Challenge for Catholic Health Care* (cf. note 226), pp. 113-123.

1) Ethics Committees: Purpose and Membership

The purpose of an ethics (or "moral-medical") committee in a Catholic hospital should be to assist the trustees and administration of the hospital as well as the professional staff in fulfilling their responsibilities in attending to the "total good of the patient, which includes his higher spiritual as well as his bodily welfare" (Preamble, paragraph 2). Since the hospital is committed to the observance of the *Ethical and Religious Directives for Catholic Health Facilities,* the work of the committee members is best described as a *sharing in* "the responsibility to reflect in (hospital) policies and practices the moral teachings of the Church, under the guidance of the local bishop" (preamble, paragraph 4), and a *submission to* "the teaching authority of the Church in the person of the local bishop, who has the ultimate authority for teaching Catholic doctrine" (preamble, last paragraph). Briefly stated, the purpose is to share in the responsibility for establishing and maintaining the Catholic identity of the hospital. This explains why some authors favor "Catholic Identity Committee" as a name for such an assembly of consultants.

Undoubtedly the greatest need is for adequate and effective consultation. In order to guarantee *adequate* consultation, the membership should be interdisciplinary so as to make the assembly a rich "sharing of knowledge" entity. In order to guarantee *effective* consultation, education and educational programming must be made function number one—as a means to an end. In a discussion of "Committee Formation and Function" at the headquarters of the Catholic Health Association in Sept., 1983, each of the experienced panelists stressed education as the primary purpose of their committees. The report continues:

> The entire workshop group, through written responses, also validated education as the principal purpose of institutional committees. The continued development of new medical technology, with its attendant ethical challenges, suggests the continued dominance of this purpose well into the 1990's. It was also generally agreed that educational activities must first be undertaken within the committee itself and then extended to staff, personnel, patients, family, and even the public, particularly legislators.[570]

The report continues with practical suggestions for educational endeavors (recommended as first function of ethics committees) and policy-

---

[570]*Ibid.*, p. 86.

recommending activities (recommended second function).[571] Such a "university of learning" on moral-medical issues is bound to produce rich dividends in the consultation potential of the committee (recommended third function).

As to organization for *adequate* consultation, the purpose of the committee is defeated if representation on the committee is too heavy in any one discipline. In any ethical or moral problem, whether it concerns an individual patient or a policy, there will be a limited number of options open. These options will be medical, moral, administrative, social and legal. In order to define and evaluate these options, the committee should represent these professions. Due to the ecumenical nature of the population served by most Catholic hospitals, at least one member should be a non-Catholic who shares the hospital's commitment to Catholic ideals and values. Each member should be fully competent in his or her own field. A special effort should be made to select members who are willing and able to take the time required for effective service, and who are willing to learn and able to tolerate ambiguity and conflict.

The recommendation is that, depending upon the size of the hospital, the membership be limited to not less than 7 and not more than 15 members. The following composition of an ethics committee is suggested for a 400-bed Catholic hospital—representation consisting of:

Administration 1	Religious Community (sponsor) 1
Board of Trustees 1	Non-Catholic staff member 1
Medical staff 2	Lawyer (NOT the hospital attorney). .1
Pastoral Care Dept. 1	Business community representative. . .1
Priest (theologian). 1	Nursing staff (1 of intensive care) 2
Social worker. 1	

Consultation with in-house staff members should be encouraged. Several non-staff members might be designated as consultants (for example, a psychiatrist, the bishop's representative for hospital matters, etc.) to attend particular sessions as required.

Ethics committee members are appointed by the administrator or by the board of trustees. A three-year term of service is suggested, with the proviso that when first organized, one-third of the membership be appointed for 2 years and one-third for 1 year. With this proviso, approximately one-third of the members will be replaced each year. It is also recommended that the head of the medical staff be asked to designate the two medical-staff members. Some ethics committee members elect their own officers: Chairperson, Vice-

---

[571] *Ibid.*, pp. 85, 86. For a practical listing of concerns for committee consideration, cf. Ashley-O'Rourke, *Health Care Ethics* (cf. note 80), pp. 143–145.

chairperson and Executive Secretary (for a one-year term, eligible for a second one-year term). Others suggest that the officers be appointed by the administrator or by the board of trustees.

2) Activities of an Ethics Committee

The very purpose of an ethics committee (education/policy recommendation/consultation) would suggest two standing committees chosen from within the membership of the ethics committee. The first is the "Education Committee" (some prefer the term "values committee") which would be in charge of planning and promoting of ventures such as workshops, panel discussions, etc., for hospital personnel, staff members, community groups and even the general public. A good subtitle for such a group could be the "let your light shine" committee; because its potential in expanding awareness of medical-moral situations and possible solutions would make it a significant vehicle of public relations in the hospital's mission of healing. A second standing committee is the "Appropriate Care Committee" which would be available for consultation in emergency problem cases. There is no reason why such a standing committee could not serve also as the "Infant Care Review Committee" as stressed by the Federal Department of Health and Human Services in the wake of the "Baby Doe" publicity in 1984. The federal agency proposed such a committee to review specific decisions to withdraw or withhold medical care, and to monitor periodically the hospital's actual practices in the treatment of handicapped infants (cf. chapter III, p.115). Hopefully such a role could be pursued without invading the "jurisdictional" field, and without casting aspersions on members of the medical staff. The overall purpose should be to profit by past experiences.

It is recommended that the members of the standing committees be chosen by the chairperson of the ethics committee, and that the vice-chairperson be designated to chair one of the standing committees. In all of the activities of the ethics committee, the obligation to respect confidentiality whenever particular cases are brought up for discussion, must be kept in mind.

Catholic hospitals also have social concerns: personnel relations, adequate compensation for employees, response to the needs of the poor, retirement benefits, union activities, etc., which indicate a need for a special "Social Concerns" committee.[572] If all of these concerns are added to the province of the ethics committee, however, the effectiveness of the committee in moral-medical matters will be compromised. The increased membership

---

[572]"Corporate Conscience: Governance and Management" by Sr. Mary Roch Rocklage, RSM in *Ethics Committees: A Challenge for Catholic Health Care* (cf. note 226), pp. 69–77.

required (adding experts on labor relations, insurance, finance, etc.) and the added burden on individual members (so many disciplines to be mastered) will make it difficult to persuade qualified individuals to serve on the committee. If the ethics committee is expanded and given responsibility for such a variety of concerns, the first function to be curtailed would be the most important one—the educational function. Medical-moral concerns are too crucial for the Catholic identity of the hospital to be "watered down" with social, managerial and financial responsibilities.

Many bishops have assigned a qualified priest of the diocese to serve as "personal representative of the bishop" or "diocesan director of hospital affairs." That official should be considered as a special consultant to every institutional ethics committee in the diocese (or archdiocese). If the diocese has organized a diocesan ethics committee, that individual would be most valuable in keeping the members of all institutional ethics committees in touch with diocesan needs, plans and policies with regard to moral-medical issues.

Sample models for institutional ethics committees, as well as similar committees on the diocesan and multi-institutional level are provided in the published proceedings of the workshop on ethics committees in September, 1983 (cosponsored by the Pope John Center and the Catholic Hospital Association).[573] Many aspects of organizing an ethics committee must be decided on the local level: quorum requirements for regular meetings; number of members required for urgent, emergency meetings; the assigning of each member to one of the standing or subcommittees based on his or her interests and expertise; the keeping of all patient-records as confidential; means of letting the hospital community and patients know that the committee is "at their service," etc. Among the extra dividends of an ethics committee (not reflected in the functions above) is that a well-functioning ethics committee will provide insulation against possible legal suits, and will minimize the need of having medical matters decided by the civil courts.

Professional Medical and Spiritual Consultation

Every Catholic health facility has a right to seek assurance both of the promotion of the "total good of the patient" and the faithful observance of the *Ethical and Religious Directives* by insisting on adequate consultation. This right has a special urgency in two situations: one (in behalf of the Directives) arises when there is a doubt regarding the morality of a procedure; and another (in behalf of the patient) arises when the proposed procedure involves serious

---

[573]*Ibid.*, pp. 113–144.

consequences. A well-functioning ethics committee can be of definite value in both situations. There is also need, however, of ongoing doctor-to-doctor consultation. One such situation of more frequent occurrence is presented in doubtful pregnancy cases preliminary to any procedure which might be abortive in effect (cf. Directive 24). The many illustrations of the application of the Principle of the Double Effect in chapter seven also involve situations when a conscientious physician needs the consultative services of professional colleagues on a proposed medical procedure and/or the consultative services of a moralist or of an ethics committee on the morality of a procedure.

If the physician truly has the best interests of the patient at heart, there will be occasions when he will realize the need of seeking consultation on medical matters either at the request of the patient (or family members), or because he faces a difficult or doubtful dilemma, or because he is determined to be satisfied with only the highest quality of medical service possible. There is sometimes the possibility that the consulted or referral physician will take advantage of the situation by tempting the patient to transfer to his or her professional care. A highly-motivated physician must be willing to take that chance. The Code of Ethics of the American Medical Association requires him to do so:

> A physician should seek consultation upon request; in doubtful or difficult cases; or whenever it appears that the quality of medical service may be enhanced thereby.[574]

If the attending physician is asked to recommend a consultant, he would benefit by looking upon the request not as a sign of diminished confidence on the part of the patient, but as an opportunity to shed new light on the case— and possibly even as a learning experience for himself. The latter advantage would materialize especially if the consultant is a specialist in some field of medicine. If the consultant is to be selected by the attending physician, however, he might be tempted to favor a colleague merely on the basis of friendship rather than medical expertise, or to try to enhance his own reputation by instructing the consultant to corroborate his own diagnosis and treatment, or to persuade the consultant to split the consultation fee. Such behavior, in all three instances, would be immoral and unworthy of the medical profession.[575] A physician who cooperates fully in the matter of seeking consultation is worthy of high commendation. By doing so, he does risk the possibility of

---

[574]Reiser, Stanley J., MD, Ph.D., "Codes of Medical Ethics," in *Health Matrix,* Summer, 1984, p. 47.

[575]Rizzo, Dr. Carlo, in *Dictionary of Moral Theology* (cf. note 346), pp. 308, 309.

being accused of having erred in his diagnosis and/or treatment. If some error of medical judgment clearly amounts to illegal or unethical practice, the consultant would have to abide by the Code of Medical Ethics and "expose, without hesitation, illegal or unethical conduct" of this fellow-member of the medical profession.[576]

Another reference to consultation, but of the family-to-physician variety, is when there is doubt as to how seriously ill a loved one might be with regard to the need of summoning the chaplain to administer the sacrament of the anointing of the sick (Directive 41). Scrupulosity in this matter is not to be encouraged. The sacrament can be administered based on any probable or prudent judgment as to the seriousness of the illness. There is no need to wait until the patient is in danger of death (cf. Cann.1004,1005).

Hospital chaplains and pastoral care personnel also must be vigilant in anticipating the need of spiritual consultation and counseling. A young couple may be in a crisis of conscience because they are inclined to withdraw life-support from an infant who is the victim of some type of congenital malformation. Family members or a spouse may be in a state of confusion, doubt and anxiety regarding the options open to them for the treatment of an incompetent and seriously-ill husband or father. Spiritual counseling can help to free such individuals from emotional conflict, and often from unconscious guilt feelings which add to the anxiety over the treatment of incompetent loved ones. Finally, a word must be added about the obligation of chaplains, pastors, and priests generally, to consult their moral-theology sources or some qualified moralist when in doubt as to the moral implications of any impending or proposed medical procedure. When approached for spiritual or moral-medical guidance, it is far better to say: "I will look it up for you," than to give in to the temptation to hazard a guess.

Directive 7: Adequate consultation is recommended, not only when there is doubt concerning the morality of some procedure, but also with regard to all procedures involving serious consequences, even though such procedures are listed here as permissible. The health facility has the right to insist on such consultations.

---

[576]Reiser, Stanley J. (cf. note 574), p. 45.

Consultations Among Theologians, Physicians and Other Scholars

In his address to the participants at the workshop on ethics committees in September, 1983, Archbishop Daniel E. Pilarczyk of Cincinnati referred to scholarly consultations which took place previous to the approval of the present *Ethical and Religious Directives for Catholic Health Facilities* at the annual meeting of the National Conference of Catholic Bishops and the United States Catholic Conference in November, 1971,—and also referred briefly to consultations which took place after 1971 as follows:

> Some theologians reacted to certain parts of the code; some physicians counterreacted. Eventually several questions arising from the code on tubal ligation and material cooperation were presented to the Holy See, and the Roman response together with a commentary was published in 1977. Although some of the code was revised in 1975, the code today is basically the code that was approved by the bishops in 1971.[577]

The Roman response and commentary to which the archbishop refers will be found in the appendix of this book, along with the July 3, 1980 statement of the National Conference of Catholic Bishops on tubal ligation. This is a case where consultation resulted in reaffirmation of Directives 18 and 20 on sterilization and an explicit statement on material cooperation.

The other controversial directives (in addition to directives 18 and 20) which certain theologians and lay groups insist "must be changed" are Directive 19 on contraception, Directive 21 on artificial insemination and masturbation, and Directive 22 on hysterectomy (when the mother's uterus is in a serious pathological condition due to repeated cesarean sections). In view of the reaffirmation of Directives 18 and 20 (paragraph above), it is unreasonable to expect a change whereby tubal ligations and vasectomies would be allowed. In view of the repeated reaffirmation of the doctrine emphasized in Pope Paul VI's encyclical letter "Humanae Vitae" (1968), it is likewise unreasonable to expect a change in the matter of contraception (Directive 19). Directive 22 (hysterectomy after repeated cesarean sections) has ceased to be a prime issue of contention. As mentioned in chapter six, ongoing consultation and discussion among theologians has made that a closed question (not recommended, but permissible to the extent that it may be approved by the bishop of the diocese in particular cases). That leaves only Directive 21 on

---

[577] *Ethics Committees: A Challenge for Catholic Health Care* (cf. note 226), p. 19.

artificial insemination and masturbation as a logical objective of those who seek and advocate significant changes in the directives.

Returning to the address of Archbishop Pilarczyk referred to above, his explanation of the binding force of the directives merits serious reflection. After stating that these Catholic health facilities directives were approved by the American bishops "through a discernment process that included suggestions and reactions from the theological and medical communities," he added:

> The *Directives* reflect the ordinary teachings of the Church that Church members are obliged to accept and that local bishops are responsible for upholding and fostering. The local bishop is also charged with interpreting the code and directing its application in specific situations that arise in his diocese. Here again, the bishop is not free to accept or reject basic teaching, since the teaching reflects the teaching of the Church universal. His task as interpreter is to make a prudent judgment on how the *Directives* fit into the complexities of individual situations that arise in Catholic health care facilities in his jurisdiction. He exercises this responsibility not as hospital administrator or as a rulemaker, but as spokesman for the Church's teachings.[578]

There is no extensive evidence of a ground swell for change in the rest of the directives (excluding those mentioned above) except for minor changes, suppressions or additions which would not affect basic teachings or principles. Some authors may feel that innovative procedures should be included in the directives (for example, embryo transfer, surrogate motherhood, new tests for pregnancy, etc.). Others may feel that certain procedures which today are somewhat outmoded should be excluded. Discussion, dialogue and consultation on commendable changes is encouraged. The effectiveness of such modes of communication with the appropriate committees of the United States Catholic Conference was demonstrated abundantly in the prolonged process which led to the approval of the present hospital directives in 1971 (cf. Chap. I, and the opening pages of chap. X).

Unfortunately, not even the most open dialogue, communication and consultation can lead to the resolution of all concerns or to the unlimited approval of all concerned. Unless loyalty to the magisterium of the Church is cultivated and practiced, the lack of full satisfaction with the results of the communication process can leave a damaging residue of bitterness and resent-

---

[578]*Ibid.,* pp. 19, 20.

ment. Realistic members of the faithful will call to mind many times that even the Good Lord Himself can answer prayers in two ways; either "yes," or "no." Men and women of faith pray for the strength to accept either an affirmative or a negative response with the conviction that "He knows best." In a declaration of 1967, following the changes of Vatican II, the German Catholic Bishops encouraged a similar attitude of "So be it" with regard to the official teachings and positions of the Church:

> We do not need to fear that in adopting the positions of the Church . . . we are failing to respond to the claims of our own age. Often enough the serious questions raised for us by our own age, and which we are called upon to answer on the basis of our faith, make it necessary for us to think out the truths of our faith afresh. It is perfectly possible that in this process fresh points will come to be emphasized. But this is not to call the faith itself in question. Rather it contributes to a deeper grasp of the truths of divine revelation and of the Church's teaching. For we are firmly convinced, and we see that experience confirms us in this, that we need neither deny any truth for the Catholic faith, nor deny the Catholic faith for the sake of any truth, provided only that we understand this faith in the spirit of the Church and seek always to achieve a deeper grasp of it.[579]

Preamble, paragraph 7: In addition to consultations among theologians, physicians and other medical and scientific personnel in local areas, the Committee on Health Affairs of the United States Catholic Conference, with the widest consultation possible, should regularly receive suggestions and recommendations from the field, and should periodically discuss any possible need for an updated revision of these *Directives.*

8.3 PROMOTING THE COMMON GOOD

Within the scope of the mission of healing, individuals and groups have

---

[579]*Readings in Moral Theology, III,* ed. by Charles E. Curran and Richard A. McCormick, S.J. (New York, N.Y.: Paulist Press, 1982), p. 116.

responded to the call to personal responsibility and sacrifice in behalf of the common good—associations and movements such as Pro-Life, the American Cancer Society, the Muscular Dystrophy Association, etc., have illustrated the variety of ways in which men and women of good will can help afflicted members of the human community to "achieve their own fulfillment in a relatively thorough and ready way." Several avenues of such commendable collaboration for the common good through personal sacrifice are highlighted in the hospital Directives.

Contributing to the Common Good

Medical science depends to a considerable extent upon the results of post-mortem anatomical examinations (autopsies) which are performed in most cases with respect for the wishes of the deceased and with the cooperation of the next of kin. The survivor of the criminal attack of a rapist is challenged to make every effort to protect the new life which was conceived in flagrant violation of her personal dignity. Some generous individuals will even volunteer to submit their disease-ridden bodies to experimental procedures with minimal hope of improvement in their own physical condition. Other self-sacrificing individuals come to the aid of victims of disease by offering a healthy organ of their bodies for transplant purposes.

1) The Transplantation of Human Organs (Homografts)

A *homograft* differs from a *heterograft* in that the former involves the transfer of human tissue from one human body (whether living or deceased) to another, while the latter refers to the transfer of tissue between individuals of different species. The most outstanding heterograft on the contemporary scene took place on Oct. 26, 1984, when Dr. Leonard L. Bailey of Loma Linda, Cal., replaced the defective heart of Baby Stephanie Fae (then only 2 weeks old) with the matched-size heart of a seven-month-old female baboon. The celebrated infant died three weeks later. Dr. Bailey provided the parents of the infant with a full explanation of the risks and benefits of other reasonable options and alternatives; the parents were under no illusions as to the "quality of life" and longevity of the infant as a result of this procedure; the expertise of Dr. Bailey in the field of transplant surgery and his sensitivity to their right to deny permission for the procedure provided an adequate basis for their *informed* consent to the procedure. Hence the procedure could not be regarded as immoral.

Pope Pius XII spoke of the morality of such heterografts in an address to a group of eye specialists on May 14, 1956. He approved of the transplanting

316

of eye corneas from a non-human being to a human being, as well as the transplanting of living tissues from non-humans to humans in cellular therapy. He explained, however, that approval would depend upon the type of tissue: "The transplantation of the sexual glands of an animal to man is to be rejected as immoral."[580] This would prohibit any transplanting of non-human gonadal glands in human beings for purposes of generation. If non-human gonadal tissue could be effective, however, in restoring endocrine balance in a human being (a purely theoretical question), such a procedure would not seem to come under the ban mentioned by Pius XII.[581] There are various other types of transplants known as "static" (because the tissue is supportive, rather than incorporated into the human host) which are employed in contemporary medical practice: non-human bone, cartilage, blood vessels, muscle tissue. These non-human tissues serve rather as struts or mechanical supports on which the host tissue can grow.

Human Transplants From a Living Person

In discussing the Principle of Totality, it was mentioned that this principle would not justify the donation of an organ of the human body in behalf of a member of the community who is in serious need of an eye, a kidney, a lung, a heart, etc. Pope Pius XII made it clear that the Principle of Totality concerns the physical integrity of the human body, and that neither the state nor the individual himself or herself has unlimited direct dominion over the physical body. By virtue of *indirect* dominion, the state may limit or curtail the exercise of the human rights of citizens for appropriate reasons by requiring payment of taxes, military service, observance of just laws, etc.,—and an individual may allow a restriction or curtailment of physical integrity if the good of the whole body requires the excision of an organ or part of the body which threatens the life of the whole body. The Principle of Totality does not confer that unlimited *direct* dominion over the body whereby either the state or a human individual as a "whole" has any natural right to "dispose of the parts." A person cannot say even for the highest of motives (based on the Principle of Totality): "Here, you can have one of my kidneys . . ."[582] As noted below, however, such a magnanimous donation could be made on the

---

[580]*The Human Body* (cf. note 61), p. 374.

[581]O'Donnell, Thomas, S.J., *Medicine and Christian Morality* (cf. note 31), p. 107.

[582]Pope Pius XII rejects the concept of sacrificing a particular member (hand, foot, kidney, liver, etc.) to the organism "man" lest this might justify a conclusion that it would likewise be permitted to sacrifice a particular member to the organism "humanity" (such as one who is sick or suffering). Cf. *The Human Body* (cf. note 61), p. 375.

basis of the Principle of the Common Good.

Article 75 of *The Church Today* refers to the common good several times. The following statement is of special relevance: "Citizens should develop a generous and loyal devotion to their country, but without any narrowing of mind. In other words, they must always look simultaneously to the welfare of the whole human family . . ." The *Commentary On The Documents of The Second Vatican Council* has a fitting reflection on this passage: "Citizens in general are recommended to cultivate "pietas erga patriam," that is, the virtue by which we owe love, reverence and obedience to God, our parents and our native country; this *pietas erga patriam* is not a narrow-minded patriotism, but generously takes into account the well being of the whole human family."[583]

The same love of God and country and concern for the common good which obligates a citizen to submit to limitations in the exercise of personal rights (taxes, military service, etc.) can be compared to the virtue of love of God and neighbor and concern for the common good which inspires any member of the community (especially a Christian) to limit his or her personal physical integrity by offering a human organ in behalf of a seriously ill or incapacitated individual. Going one step higher—and recalling the relationship of the Principle of Totality to the Principle of Personal Integrity as a means to a common end (chapter 6,)—that same sacrifice of a human organ in behalf of another human individual may be intended for the spiritual advancement of the donor.[584] In effect, this is yet another application of: "Whatsoever you do for one of my least brothers . . ." (Matthew,25:40).

The need for organ transplants is on the rise. According to figures from the American Council on Transplantation (as of 1983), 7,000 people are waiting for kidney transplants (6,116 performed during that year), 175 are waiting for liver transplants (163 performed), 50,000 could benefit from heart transplants (172 performed) and 5,000 could benefit from pancreas transplants (218 performed).[585] Although 80,000 Americans are on renal dialysis today, only about 10% are listed as "clinically suitable" or candidates for a transplant due to the shortage of available kidneys.[586]

When the donor is a living person (this would apply mostly to kidney donors) the anticipated benefit to the recipient must be proportionate to the harm done to the donor. In view of the urgent need of kidney transplants so

---

[583]*Commentary on the Documents of Vatican II, Vol. V* (cf. note 42), p. 322.

[584]Cf. Kelly, Gerald, S.J., *Medico-Moral Problems, Part III*, pamphlet edition (St. Louis, Mo.: Catholic Hospital Association, 1951), pp. 22–28. Cf. also O'Donnell, Thomas, S.J., *Medicine and Christian Morality* (cf. note 31), pp. 109, 110; Healy, Edwin, S.J., *Medical Ethics* (cf. note 46), pp. 140, 141.

[585]*Time*, Dec. 10, 1984, p. 70.

[586]Annas, George, JD, M.P.H. in *Law, Medicine and Health Care*, Feb., 1985, p. 7.

that only the most serious cases are on the waiting list ("clinically suitable"), there is no doubt about the substantial benefit to the recipient. If the donor is in good health with no indications of any kidney or kidney-related problems, the donation of one kidney would not put the donor in substantial danger. Every potential donor should reflect, however, that he or she might forfeit life or at least substantial functional integrity if something happened to the one remaining kidney. Individuals who are in poor health, *especially* if their condition is kidney-related, would not be justified in volunteering the donation of one of their kidneys. An exception might be made if the seriously-ill patient has a close relative who insists on being the donor even though he or she is not in robust health, provided that such a generous individual enjoys normal kidney function. Otherwise, in the words of *Directive 30,* the donor would be in danger of being deprived "of life itself [or] of the functional integrity of his body."[587]

If all aspects of commercialism are avoided, there would be no objection to reimbursing the donor for expenses involved in hospitalization, surgery, absence from gainful employment, etc., plus a modest financial token of appreciation. Anything beyond that would make the organ donation an immoral transaction. The financial incentive could tempt a financially embarrassed or unemployed individual who is not in good health to put his or her life in substantial danger. In the words of several transplant experts of the medical profession: "It is immoral to offer someone an incentive to undergo permanent change."[588] A moderate financial offering is considered appropriate, however, to donors of renewable anatomical elements such as blood transfusions and skin grafts. It should be moderate enough to indicate that it is not "payment," but rather a token of appreciation for time and inconvenience involved in the procedure.

Human Transplants from Cadavers

Most organ transplants are obtained from human cadavers. Dr. C. Everett Koop, the U.S. Surgeon General, has emphasized the sad fact that more organs are available than are being harvested (actually excised for transplant).

---

[587]For a brief review of theological debate on this subject, cf. Healy, Edwin, S.J., *Medical Ethics* (cf. note 46), pp. 139–142. Cf. also O'Donnell, Thomas, S.J., *Medicine and Christian Morality* (cf. note 31), pp. 107–110. Pope Pius XII did not condemn the donation of human organs "inter vivos" but saw the importance of pointing out that it could not be justified on the basis of the principle of totality.

[588]This opinion of several transplant physicians which appeared in the correspondence section of the Feb. 9, 1984, edition of the *New England Journal of Medicine,* p. 395, is of special significance, because it was expressed as the opinion "of most physicians engaged in transplantation."

An increasing number of Americans have signed donor cards, indicating that specific organs or all organs and tissues of their bodies can be harvested after death. As a very general rule, however, hospitals will not attempt to excise and use the organs without the permission of the next of kin. The Uniform Anatomical Gift Act, drafted in 1968 by the National Conference of Commissioners on Uniform State Laws, and adopted in every state and the District of Columbia by 1971, made such "postmortem" donations possible. Permission of the next of kin is not required. There are three good reasons, however, to explain why hospitals will not use the organs without that permission: 1) the danger of legal disputes between the family and the physician and/or hospital; 2) the fact that medical personnel in 25 states believe it is morally wrong to ignore the objections raised by the family, and 3) the spectre of bad publicity which would make transplant coordinators "look like vultures."[589]

Because of this sensitive "next of kin" problem, some authors favor a "presumed consent" policy whereby "physicians, acting with state or federal authority, would simply take needed tissues and organs from cadavers unless an individual carried a card prohibiting such tissue transfer, or unless the deceased person's next-of-kin objected."[590] Such a policy could defeat rather than promote effective after-death utilization of human organs. Certain aspects of such a program would be immoral. It would be immoral to remove cadaveric organs if the deceased, while living, had expressed opposition to such a procedure. It would be immoral to disregard the objections of the next of kin unless the deceased had signed a donor card while living or had clearly indicated that he favored the donation of his bodily organs in behalf of others.

Presumed consent means "taking;" voluntarism means "voluntary donation and consent." Several authors appropriately conclude: ". . . considerable support for voluntarism continues to exist because the principles of giving rather than taking are maintained."[591] In order to make such a policy effective, however, it is highly recommended that police personnel and hospital personnel be authorized legally to institute a prudent and respectful search for donor cards at the scene of an accident or when the victim of an accident is brought to the hospital. The Church also could advance a policy of voluntarism by motivating the faithful to sign such cards as an expression of love of

[589]Overcast, Thomas D., JD, Ph.D., et al., "Problems in the Identification of Potential Organ Donors," in *Journal of the American Medical Association*, March 23/30, 1984, pp. 1561, 1562. The article (pp. 1559–1562) was based on a survey of organ procurement programs and district attorneys' offices in 50 states and in the District of Columbia.

[590]Caplan, Arthur L., *The Hastings Center Report*, Dec. 1983, p. 23. Article entitled "Organ Transplants: The Costs of Success," pp. 23–32.

[591]Sadler, Alfred M., MD, and Sadler, Blair L., JD, "Organ Donation: Is Voluntarism Still Valid?," in *The Hastings Center Report*, Oct., 1984, p. 9.

God and neighbor and out of concern for the common good.

The greatest obstacle to an effective transplant program is not the organ-procurement aspect, but the cost factor. When the U.S. Congress decided in 1972 to pay 80% of the cost of kidney transplants and dialysis for anyone with kidney failure, the expected yearly total was nearly $140 million. Within a decade, that cost has soared to $2 billion (10% of all Medicare payments for physicians).[592] The actual cost of surgery in organ procurement is a minor item. In heart and liver transplants, the cost of surgery in general amounts to only 5% of the total cost. The most costly item is the number of days spent in the Intensive Care Unit.[593] Hence even if the problem of organ procurement could be solved through voluntarism and intensive donor-card campaigns, the cost factor is bound to limit the expansion of the transplant program. On a more positive note, medical science may solve the transplant problem for some victims of renal failure. As of late 1985, nine medical institutions throughout the nation (including four in Boston) were involved in a new therapy featuring controlled low-protein diets with a special nutrition supplement. The report states that such a therapy "could delay or even replace the need for kidney dialysis among many of the more than 70,000 patients whose kidneys work with less than 10 percent efficiency."[594]

Directive 30: The transplantation of organs from living donors is morally permissible when the anticipated benefit to the recipient is proportionate to the harm done to the donor, provided that the loss of such organ(s) does not deprive the donor of life itself nor of the functional integrity of his body.

---

2) Experimentation With Patient's Consent

Human experimentation from a moral viewpoint refers to relatively untested and usually more innovative medical and surgical procedures which, although often unrelated to the interests of the patient (but related to the class of patients of which the individual is a member) are applied (always with the consent of the patient) primarily as a means of contributing to the common good in the interests of humanity through anticipated progress in medical science. The term "common good" is not here understood as an end in itself, as if the state or individuals possessed unlimited direct dominion over human

---

[592]*Time*, Dec. 10, 1984, p. 72.
[593]Annas, George J. in *Law, Medicine and Health Care*, Feb., 1985, p. 6.
[594]Cf. footnote 335.

bodies which might be sacrificed for the good of humanity. The term is understood rather as a means to an end, whereby individuals can submit to such experimental procedures for the love of God and neighbor.

Due to the tragic evidence of unlimited and inhuman research and experimentation particularly under the Nazi regime in Germany prior to and during World War II, the nations of the world have taken steps to submit all experiments on human subjects to strict ethical controls. One author mentions that the ethics of human experimentation have been formalized into at least 33 different codes since World War II, and lists five basic guidelines which appear to be generally accepted. These guidelines are listed below,[595] interspersed with related quotations from several addresses of Pope Pius XII to various medical groups:

Proposed guideline (1):
"A research subject must be a person who volunteered on the basis of having all the necessary information for his decision to be an informed one." *Pope Pius XII* would stretch the limits of consenting even to doubtful cases "when the known methods have failed, [and] a new and insufficiently tried method offers, along with elements of great danger, appreciable chances of success."[596] This applies only if the person freely consents to the procedure.

Proposed guideline (2), referring to the research subject:
"He should be allowed to withdraw from the research at whatever point he wishes." Obviously *Pope Pius XII* would not question the validity of this guideline.

Proposed guideline (3):
"All unnecessary risks should be eliminated in the design of the research and through prior animal experimentation." *Pope Pius XII* calls it an "obvious law" that the "application of new methods to the living person must be preceded by research on the dead body or the laboratory model, and by experimenting on animals."[597]

---

[595]These 5 guidelines are proposed in *Human Subjects in Medical Experimentation* by B.H. Gray (New York, N.Y.: John Wiley and Sons, Inc., 1975), p. 7. Similar guidelines are presented by Alexander Morgan Capron in the *Encyclopedia of Bioethics*, II, Warren T. Reich, ed. (New York, N.Y.: The Free Press, 1978), pp. 696, 697.

[596]Address to Histopathologists, Sept. 13, 1952, in *The Human Body* (cf. note 61), p. 207.

[597]*Ibid.*, p. 207.

Proposed guideline (4):

"The benefits of the experiment, either to the subject or to society should outweigh the risks to the subject." *Pope Pius XII* admitted that the practice of prior-experimentation might sometimes be impossible or simply inadequate. Except for a truly exceptional situation as in his quotation under guideline (1) above, however, he insists that there must be limits to what the moral law can allow:

> Doubtless, before authorizing new methods according to moral law, the total exclusion of all danger and of every risk cannot be demanded. This is beyond the possibilities of human nature, and would paralyze all scientific research, and would very often turn to the detriment of the patient. The appreciation of the element of danger must be left, in these cases, to the judgment of an experienced and competent doctor. There is, however, . . . a degree of danger which the moral law cannot permit.[598]

Proposed guideline (5):

"Finally, an experiment should be conducted only by individuals qualified to do so." Surely this guideline would be considered of basic importance by *Pope Pius XII.*

Moral Guidance in Human Experimentation

If available evidence indicates that the proposed experimentation will lead to serious injury, mutilation or death, no one (not even members of the medical profession) would be justified in volunteering to submit to the experiment regardless of his or her dedication to the common good. For other types of human experimentation, a distinction must be made between *healthy* and *incurable patients, and sick* patients. The healthy and incurable patients cannot benefit by the experimentation, although some benefit might accrue to the common good (testing a vaccine, confirming a medical hypothesis, etc.). Experiments on a *sick* person, however, may serve a double purpose; one on behalf of the subject (recovery or improvement in condition) and one as a possible dividend for the common good (advancing medical knowledge).[599]

A healthy or incurable patient (more logically a "subject" in the case of a healthy person who becomes a "patient" in the experiment) may submit to an

---

[598]*Ibid.*, p. 207.
[599]McFadden, Charles, O.S.A., *The Dignity of Life* (cf. note 65), pp. 206, 207.

experiment if there is reasonable hope that medical science will benefit in the process and evaluation of the experiment. This applies, however, only if *all* of the five guidelines mentioned above—including the quotations from Pope Pius XII—are strictly observed. With the same proviso, a sick person may submit to an experimental procedure if that procedure is not in violation of any of the conditions required by the Principle of the Double Effect. In this regard, special attention must be given to the condition that there is no reasonable and available alternative to bring about the desired and intended good effect—and the condition that there must be a due proportion between the good effect intended and the foreseen evil effect which is merely permitted. That due proportion here is between the good to humanity in advancing medical knowledge (the common good) and the evil of possible injury to an individual member of society.[600]

Of course, the intended good effect also includes the possibility of curing or improving the condition of the patient; but this will not suffice to justify the procedure if the danger to the patient is of serious proportions. This would tip the balance in favor of a direct dominion of the common good over the welfare of an individual. This is the core of the difficulty in delineating the moral limits of human experimentation. In the address referred to above, Pope Pius XII reminded his audience that man does not exist for society, but that society exists for man. A contemporary author expressed the same need of caution and reserve when he wrote: "The basic ethical problem in human experimentation . . . is that experimentation is the use of one person by another to gather knowledge or other benefits that may be only partly good, if at all, for the first person; that is to say, the experimental subject is not simply a means but is in danger of being treated as a mere token to be manipulated for research purposes."[601]

Within appropriate moral limits, the Church approves of legitimate research and human experimentation. Pope Paul XII stated in his audience on September 13, 1952, that he wished to become the "interpreter of the moral conscience of the research worker, of the expert, of the practitioner;"—and spoke in glowing terms of their work:

> The spirit of research, bold and determined, urges one to set out
> on newly discovered paths, to extend them further and further, to

---

[600]Cf. O'Donnell, Thomas, S.J., who makes the following important observation in *Medicine and Christian Morality* (cf. note 65), p. 96: ". . . a possible contribution to the common good, though not without its importance, weighs lightly against serious harm to a given individual. This is so because society in general, or the common good, exists for the individual, not *vice versa*." Cf. also remarks at the beginning of this chapter.

[601]Capron, Alexander Morgan, *Encyclopedia of Bioethics, II* (cf. note 595), p. 694.

create other itineraries, to overhaul methods . . . research and the acquisition of truth with a view to arriving at new knowledge and a new, more vast, more profound comprehension of this same truth, are in themselves in harmony with the moral order.[602]

There are higher moral values, however, which indicate "well-defined frontiers" for human experimentation. As examples of those higher values, Paul XII mentions "The relationship of confidence between doctor and patient, the right of the patient to life, physical and spiritual, in its psychic or moral integrity. . ."[603]

Clinical Research on the Unborn

The question of prenatal research with regard to genetic diseases has been discussed in the chapter on the Principle of the Right to Life (cf. 3.6). High-risk prenatal experimental procedures (properly called "therapeutic") may be undertaken only in those particular cases when such a procedure is a last available measure to try to save the life of the unborn infant. Other types of fetal research which are conducted as a means of advancing the frontiers of medical science (hence called "non-therapeutic") are illicit. The recent *Instruction on Respect for Human Life In Its Origin and On the Dignity of Procreation* as issued by the Congregation for the Doctrine of the Faith on February 22, 1987, addresses this important issue as follows:

> *If the embryos are living, whether viable or not, they must be respected just like any other human person; experimentation on embryos which is not directly therapeutic is illicit.*
> No objective, even though noble in itself, such as a foreseeable advantage to science, to other human beings or to society, can in any way justify experimentation on living human embryos or foetuses, whether viable or not, either inside or outside the mother's womb . . . To use human embryos or foetuses as the object or instrument of experimentation constitutes a crime against their dignity as human beings having a right to the same respect that is due to the child already born and to every human person.[604]

The Code of Federal Regulations (45 CFR 46) of the Department of Health and Human Services et al. on the *Protection of Human Subjects* were

---

[602] *The Human Body* (cf. note 61), pp. 195 and 197.
[603] *Ibid.*, p. 197.
[604] Cf. Appendix II, Chapter I,n.4.

revised as of March 8, 1983. Section 46.208 on "Activities directed toward fetuses in utero as subjects" reads as follows:

> (a) No fetus *in utero* may be involved as a subject in any activity covered by this subpart unless: (1) The purpose of the activity is to meet the health needs of the particular fetus and the fetus will be placed at risk only to the minimum extent necessary to meet such needs, or (2) the risk to the fetus imposed by the research is minimal and the purpose of the activity is the development of important biomedical knowledge which cannot be obtained by other means.
>
> (b) An activity permitted under paragraph (a) of this section may be conducted only if the mother and father are legally competent and have given their informed consent, except that the father's consent need not be secured if: (1) His identity or whereabouts cannot reasonably be ascertained, (2) he is not reasonably available, or (3) the pregnancy resulted from rape.[605]

These regulations are well in harmony with Catholic moral standards. It is also important to note that prenatal experimental procedures are primarily observational rather than procedural, due to the accompanying danger of bringing about an unintentional spontaneous abortion.

It would be beyond the purpose of this chapter to go into the theological discussions on the subject of fetal experimentation. The reader will find that subject adequately treated in two publications of the Pope John Center.[606] Various other aspects of prenatal manipulation ("in vitro" fertilization, embryo transfer, insemination by donor, etc.) have been discussed in the chapter on the Principle of Human Dignity (Chap. II). There is no need to repeat the moral aberrations involved in these attempts to circumvent the role of conjugal love in God's plan of "increase and multiply." The most recent condemnation of such vagaries of medical science was pronounced by Pope John Paul II in his address to a group of scientists in October, 1982. After words of approval of appropriate experimentation on animals, and on artificially culti-

---

[605]*OPRR Reports,* "Protection of Human Subjects," 45 Cfr. 46 (Washington, D.C.: U.S. Gov. Printing Office, 1983), p. 13.

[606]*An Ethical Evaluation of Fetal Experimentation: An Interdisciplinary Study,* ed. by Donald G. McCarthy and Albert S. Moraczewski, O.P. (St. Louis, Mo.: Pope John Center, 1976), 137 pages; and *Genetic Counseling, The Church and the Law,* ed. by Gary M. Atkinson and Albert S. Moraczewski, O.P. (cf. note 188), 259 pages.

vated human tissues which can lead to the cure of diseases related to chromosomal defects, the Holy Father said:

> I condemn, in the most explicit and formal way, experimental manipulations of the human embryo, since the human being, from conception to death, cannot be exploited for any purpose whatsoever.[607]

Directive 27: Experimentation on patients, without due consent is morally objectionable, and even the moral right of the patient to consent is limited by his duties of stewardship.

---

3) Postmortem Examinations (Autopies)

Autopsy (from the Greek "aut opsis," or "seen by oneself"—more logically, "seeing for yourself") poses no problem for the Church providing that the human cadaver is treated with due respect. It is not permissible if it is done merely out of curiosity or for a trivial reason, or if it is done contrary to the express wishes of the family or next of kin. The family members or next of kin should be motivated to give their consent in the interests of the common good. It would also be immoral if the hospital or the undertaker, or both in tandem, would badger the family members to give consent to the procedure by not releasing the body for embalming over a protracted period of time, or by accusing the family members of being unreasonable or selfish in their attitude, or by taking advantage of the illiteracy of the family member(s) by having them sign a form which is unintelligible to them. In addition, both hospital and undertaking personnel must be careful to avoid disfigurement of the face and head except when the family members have agreed to a "closed coffin" wake.

The advantages of an autopsy in many cases are as important to the family members as they are in the interests of medical science. They can thus be cautioned against any diseases or conditions that may "run in the family;" they are comforted by knowing that everything possible was done for their loved one. They should understand that a prime reason for autopsies is to help the hospital and its staff to become more proficient in the diagnosis and care of the sick.

---

[607]*St. Louis Review,* Oct. 29, 1982, p. 8.

If the hospital staff has an accurate autopsy report, they can check it against detailed hospital records and evaluate the accuracy of the diagnosis and the propriety and effectiveness of the treatment which was administered. There is also the possibility of discovering new evidence of the origin and metastasis of certain diseases, and of arriving at a deeper understanding of the management and control of adverse factors in the future. The hospital authorities are also expected to look for any evidence that professional standards may have been overlooked or neglected in the diagnosis or treatment of a particular individual (perhaps a hasty diagnosis—or insufficient consultation with patient or professional colleagues—or too much reliance merely on test results—or faulty laboratory service, etc.). Authorities of top-ranked hospitals value the autopsy program as a rich and necessary learning experience. The American Medical Association understandably gives high ratings to a hospital with a high percentage of autopsies throughout the year.

"Definition of Death" Criteria

An autopsy may not be performed until it is morally certain that the person is dead. To proceed with an autopsy on the basis of a "high probability" that the patient is dead means that there is "some probability" that the patient is still alive. This would be tantamount to taking a chance of causing directly the death of an innocent person. The determination of the time of death must be made "in accordance with responsible and commonly accepted scientific criteria" (*Directive* 31). A similar phrase concludes the proposed Uniform Determination of Death Act which was formulated in May, 1980, at a meeting of the Executive Director of the *President's Commission* with representatives of the American Bar Association, the American Medical Association and the National Conference of Commissioners on Uniform State laws:

> An individual who has sustained either (1) irreversible cessation of circulatory and respiratory functions, or (2) irreversible cessation of all functions of the entire brain, including the brain stem, is dead. A determination of death must be made in accordance with accepted medical standards.[608]

Although most of the individual states in the U.S.A. have adopted a definition-of-death statute which includes the brain-death stipulation, the exact calculation of the moment of death is left to the "accepted medical standards" and the law in each jurisdiction. The *President's Commission* favors the

---

[608]*Defining Death,* a report of the *President's Commission* (cf. note 332), p. 73.

view that "death should be viewed not as a process but as the event which separates the process of dying from the process of disintegration."[609] The proposal of the *President's Commission* above is saying that a person can be declared dead either by *cardiopulmonary* criteria (n. (1) above), or by *neurologic* or brain-based criteria (n. (2) above). Based on investigations of the *President's Commission* which focused on respirator-assisted comatose patients, the report of the commission stated: "Clearly, cardiopulmonary criteria remain the predominant basis for determining that death has occurred, even in patients on respirators."[610] In all calculations as to the moment of death (whether based on cardiopulmonary or neurologic criteria), the "accepted medical standards" are of prime importance.

Perhaps the earliest of such standards for the determination of brain death were those formulated by a special committee of the Harvard Medical School in 1968—known and respected as the *Harvard Criteria*. In accord with these criteria, the diagnosis of death cannot be given in brain-death cases until all of the specified tests (including a flat electroencephalogram) have been repeated at least 24 hours later with no change.[611] It is safe to suspect that the *Harvard criteria* are more respected than adopted for general use in practice. It is reassuring to know, however, that in diagnosing brain death, and depending upon problematic aspects of the case, the recommended waiting period after the first application of the various tests is within the range of 6 hours, to 12 hours, and even to 24 hours—followed by re-application of the tests and a confirmatory electroencephalogram. In other cases, using the cardiopulmonary criteria, the waiting or observation period to establish the irreversible cessation of circulatory and respiratory functions may be as little as a few minutes, for example, "in clinical situations where death is expected, where the course has been gradual, and where irregular agonal respiration or heartbeat finally ceases."[612]

It is also reassuring to know that medical science is well aware of complicating conditions which require additional tests and/or extended observation. These conditions are listed as a) drug and metabolic intoxication, b) hypothermia (which can "mimic brain death by ordinary clinical criteria and can

---

[609]*Ibid.*, p. 77. *The Handbook of 1985 Living Will Laws* (New York, N.Y.: Society for the Right to Die, 1986) reports that as of March 6, 1986 (when South Carolina enacted a "Death with Dignity" act), 37 states have enacted "living will" legislation (p. 5, plus an inserted addendum on the South Carolina act).

[610]*Ibid. (Defining Death)*, p. 100.

[611]The Harvard Committee conclusions are presented in *Death, Dying and Euthanasia*, ed. by Dennis J. Horan and David Mall (Washington D.C.: University Publications of America, Inc., 1977), pp. 42 and 43 (footnote 11).

[612]*Defining Death* (cf. note 332), pp. 162–165.

protect against neurologic damage due to hypoxia"), c) children younger than 5 years (who may have "increased resistance to damage and may recover substantial functions . . .") and d) patients who are in shock.[613] Finally, according to the report of the *President's Commission*, the rather common impression that the brain death criteria were formulated primarily to facilitate the early removal of donated human organs, does not correspond to fact:

> Indeed, considerations such as respect for the dead and a desire to make scarce resources available to those whom they might benefit are today more important incentives for the use of brain-based criteria when traditional criteria for determining death cannot be applied.[614]

Evaluation of "Definition of Death" Criteria

It is significant that Pope Pius XII provided clear papal teaching on the subject of the moment of death over 20 years before the prevailing formulation of the "Uniform Determination of Death Act" as proposed and reported by the *President's Commission*. The occasion was his address to the International Congress of Anesthesiologists on Nov. 24, 1957. He contemplated the situation "when the blood circulation and the life of a patient who is deeply unconscious because of a central paralysis are maintained only through artificial respiration and no improvement is noted after a few days," and then stated the question as follows:

> Has death already occurred after grave trauma of the brain, which has provoked deep unconsciousness and central breathing paralysis, the fatal consequences of which have nevertheless been retarded by artificial respiration? Or does it occur, according to the present opinion of doctors, only when there is complete arrest of circulation despite prolonged artificial respiration?

He then answered the question by saying:

> Where the verification of the fact in particular cases is concerned, the answer cannot be deduced from any religious and moral principle, and, under this aspect, does not fall within the competence

---

[613]*Ibid.*, pp. 165, 166.
[614]*Ibid.*, p. 101.

of the Church. Until an answer can be given, the question must remain open. But considerations of a general nature allow us to believe that human life continues for as long as its vital functions—distinguished from the simple life of organs—manifest themselves spontaneously or even with the help of artificial processes. A great number of these cases are the object of insoluble doubt, and must be dealt with according to the presumptions of law and of fact of which we have spoken.[615]

In making the distinction between vital body functions manifested spontaneously "or even with the help of artificial processes," and the "simple life of organs," he anticipated the day when, after the diagnosis of death, organ functions would be maintained through artificial processes only so that certain organs of the deceased might be excised and guarantee longer life to the living. There are no theological obstacles to the acceptance of the Uniform Determination of Death Act of 1980. There is basis for justifiable apprehension that the prescribed determination of death "in accordance with accepted medical standards" may be treated lightly in the haste to salvage human organs for transplant. Distinguished members of the medical profession insist that the cessation of total brain function, whether irreversible or not, is not necessarily linked to total *destruction* of the brain or to the death of a person. In order to obviate the possibility of excising organs for transplant while the subject is still alive, they would propose the following determination-of-death standard (emphasizing the *destruction* of the brain):

No one shall be declared dead unless respiratory and circulatory systems and the entire brain have been destroyed. Such destruction shall be determined in accord with universally accepted medical standards.[616]

Hopefully, the published professional opinions of the "loyal opposition" as above will influence the members of the medical and scientific community to arrive at *"universally* accepted medical standards" (cf. quotation above) in

---

[615] *The Pope Speaks,* spring, 1958, p. 398.

[616] Byrne, Paul A., MD, O'Reilly, Sean, MD, Quay, Paul M., S.J., Ph.D., and Salsich, Peter W., Jr., JD, "Brain Death—The Patient, The Physician, and Society," in *Gonzaga Law Review,* 1982/83, n. 3, pp. 429–516, Quotation, p. 515. Cf. also "Brain Death—An Opposing Viewpoint," by the first 3 authors mentioned above, in the *Journal of the American Medical Association,* Nov. 2, 1979, pp. 1985–1990. The report of the *President's Commission, Defining Death,* responds to the arguments of these distinguished scholars on pages 75, 76 and 81, 82 (cf. note 332).

determining the moment of death. The following facts cannot be denied: that the Uniform Determination of Death Act of 1980 was a timely response to an urgent need; that it is indeed a "fait accompli;" and that it has been incorporated into legislation in a majority of states of the nation. Furthermore, it agrees substantially with the "Definition of Death" as proposed in the final report of the Pontifical Academy of Sciences, which was prepared for Pope John Paul II, and released at the Vatican on October 30, 1985 (and awaits the formal approval of the Holy Father):

A person is dead when he has suffered irreversible loss of all capacity for integrating and coordinating physical and mental functions of the body.

Death has occurred when: A) Spontaneous cardiac and respiratory functions have irreversibly ceased; or B) There has been an irreversible cessation of all brain function.

From the discussion it appears that cerebral death is the true criterion of death, since the definite cessation of cardio-respiratory functions leads very rapidly to cerebral death.

The group thus analyzed the various clinical and instrumental methods to ascertain this irreversible cessation of cerebral functions. In order to be sure, by means of the electroencephalogram, that the brain has become flat, that is, that it no longer shows any electric activity, the observation must be made at least twice within a six-hour interval.[617]

In view of the fact that "getting used to" the prevailing concept of brain death presents emotional difficulties for family members of the deceased donor in organ transplant situations as well as for professional participants in the transplant procedure, there is an urgent need for information and education on the scientific and medical aspects of total brain death. This is emphasized in a recent article by Stuart J. Youngner, MD, and 7 collaborators entitled "Psychosocial and Ethical Implications of Organ Retrieval" which appeared in the Aug. 1, 1985 issue of *The New England Journal of Medicine*. Just one quotation from this article might be presented to illustrate the poignancy of the situation:

---

[617]"The Artificial Prolongation of Life and The Exact Determination of the Moment of Death," in the *St. Louis Review*, Nov. 8, 1985, p. 11.

Maintaining organs for transplantation actually necessitates treating dead patients in many respects as if they were alive. . . . Should the "patient" have a cardiac arrest, even resuscitation is considered essential. It is no wonder that intensive-care-unit personnel may feel confused about having to perform cardiopulmonary resuscitation on a patient who has been declared dead, whereas a "do not resuscitate" order has been written for a living patient in the next bed.[618]

In order to avoid a "conflict of interests" position, the physician or physicians of the donor-patient who just expired should not be members either of the organ-procurement team or of the organ-transplant team. Rare exceptions could be made at the express request of the family of the donor (for example, their interest in autopsy results) or at the request of the family of the intended recipient of the transplant organ (for example, the physician is a close relative of the recipient).

Directive 31: Post-mortem examinations must not be begun until death is morally certain. Vital organs, that is, organs necessary to sustain life, may not be removed until death has taken place. The determination of the time of death must be made in accordance with responsible and commonly accepted scientific criteria. In accordance with current medical practice, to prevent any conflict of interest, the dying patient's doctor or doctors should ordinarily be distinct from the transplant team.

---

4) Victims of Rape

A young girl or woman who is the victim of rape is justified in doing whatever she can to repel the attack and to prevent the ejaculation of semen into her vagina when she is attacked. It is a case of justifiable self-defense against shameful and unjust aggression. As a social crime, rape is on the

---

[618]The article (pp. 321–324) originated at the University Hospitals and Case Western Reserve University School of Medicine, Cleveland, Ohio. Quotation on p. 321.

increase. Statistically, the chances of pregnancy after rape are low. Some of the reasons for this low statistic are the following: the woman is in a state of shock when attacked; the aggressor often seeks not vaginal union but perverted sexual contact (oral or anal); the woman is pregnant at the time, or sterile due to venereal disease, surgery (tubal ligation), contraceptives, etc. In one survey of 170 convicted offenders, 34% experienced some type of sexual dysfunction in the actual assault (impotence, premature ejaculation, etc.).[619] There is also evidence that some rapists are motivated not by a desire for sexual pleasure, but to assert hostile feelings and to humiliate the victim. Whatever the motive or the outcome, the victim of rape is always entitled to kind and sympathetic treatment by hospital personnel, without any hint of harboring preconceived notions of blame, shame or guilt.

In order to shield the victim of rape from emotional trauma and embarrassment, the first emphatic need is to have the hospital chaplain or a member of the pastoral care department provide psychological and spiritual support and guidance. This will be needed before the other steps of the rape-victim program are initiated, and also as a follow-up treatment. Medical treatment should include attention to any physical injuries or abrasions, use of spermicidal douche or powders or other medications to control infections and prevent venereal disease, and treatment as required to avoid pregnancy. The argument of "doing this for the common good" can be effective in winning her cooperation in these procedures, and especially in submitting to a rather extensive examination of the vagina, pelvic area, and clothing in a search for evidence which will be needed in apprehending and prosecuting the rapist— and especially in motivating her to protect the new life within her body in the rare event that pregnancy results from the tragic encounter.

The Ethical Problem of Preventing Pregnancy

After the attack of the rapist has occurred, the semen within her genital tract can be considered a continuance of the unjust aggression. A spermicidal douche or powder may be administered immediately after the attack to expel the semen. If this is done more than 5 to 10 minutes after the attack, however, it would probably be ineffective in expelling the semen. Within that short span of time, the sperm may well have travelled as far as the fallopian tubes. An intrauterine douche is not recommended due to the danger that the fluid could flow through the fallopian tubes into the peritoneal cavity and cause

---

[619]Groth, A. Nicholas, Ph.D., and Burgess, Ann Wolbert, R.N., "Sexual Dysfunction During Rape," in the *New England Journal of Medicine*. Oct. 6, 1977, p. 765.

infection. The physician may suggest dilation of the uterus and curettage of the lining of the uterus. This would be immoral, for it would render the uterus inhospitable to the implantation of a conceptus which may result from the rape, or could dislodge an embryo implanted in the uterus from a prior act of intercourse and subsequent fertilization (even though the woman may not realize that she is pregnant).

Contraceptive pills which have been designed primarily to *prevent ovulation* (to be discussed presently) could be used in rape cases if circumstances warrant their effectiveness, even though there is some possibility that such pills may prevent implantation. In view of the known primary effect of diethylstilbestrol (DES) as an abortifacient, however, plus other damaging side-effects, it would be immoral to use it in rape cases.[620] Diethylstilbestrol is described as a "crystalline synthetic estrogenic substance capable of producing all the pharmacologic and therapeutic responses attributed to natural estrogens." In addition to substantial adverse effects of such estrogen treatment for the woman, there is evidence that the use of DES (in some cases with "only a few days of treatment") can result in congenital anomalies for the infant. The *Physicians' Desk Reference* (1986) emphasizes the following precaution:

> If diethylstilbestrol is administered during pregnancy, or if the patient becomes pregnant while taking this drug, she should be apprised of the potential risks to the fetus and of the advisability of pregnancy continuation.[621]

If DES is administered after fertilization (with the same danger of the adverse effects to the woman as mentioned above), it will prevent the implantation of the fertilized ovum (now a "morula"). An eminent obstetrician-gynecologist, William A. Lynch, M.D., emphasized this anti-implantation effect in an article published in the *Linacre Quarterly* in 1977. He quoted Dr. John McLean Morris (whom he called "perhaps the recognized authority on the use of DES in preventing pregnancy") as follows:

> More recently, it has been observed that estrogens administered to women in very much higher doses after ovulation will prevent implantation. The term interception has been suggested for the

---

[620]In an article entitled "Medication to Prevent Pregnancy After Rape," published in the Aug., 1977, issue of the *Linacre Quarterly* (pp. 210–221), Father Donald McCarthy, Ph.D., of the Pope John Center, investigated the possibility of using DES to prevent ovulation in application of the Principle of the Double Effect.

[621]*Physicians' Desk Reference* (cf. note 67), p. 1046.

process of preventing implantation after fertilization has occurred.[622]

Even if the dosage is light and presumably not effective in preventing implantation, there is the probability of congenital defects in the offspring as mentioned above.

Based on the information presented above, the administration of DES, like curettage of the uterus to prevent implantation, must be considered as "morally equivalent to abortion." The reference to high-dose administration of estrogen (DES) is a description of the popular "morning after" pill which is designed to be taken for a set number of days after fertilization has occurred, so that the endometrium of the uterus will be rendered inhospitable to implantation. Clearly, it is an abortifacient.

As a general rule, pills which are described in the *Physician's Desk Reference* as having a "primary mechanism" of altering the cervical mucus and exerting "a progestational effect on the endometrium, interfering with implantation . . ." (for example, the pill listed as "NOR-Q-D," as well as "Ovrette Tablets") may not be used to protect the victim of rape because they are abortifacients.[623] The same moral evaluation would apply to the so-called "mini-pill" (which is described as a low-dose progesterone-only pill) provided that such a type of pill is listed by qualified pharmacologists as designed primarily to prevent implantation. In his scholarly report entitled "Report on the Use of the IUD and Mini-pill" in 1983, Father Jack Gallagher, C.B.S., Director of the Cardinal Carter Centre for Bioethics, made the following statement (with regard to the low-dose, progesterone-only pill): "It is generally agreed that this type of pill usually operates by preventing implantation after fertilization."[624]

Of the 55 types of oral contraceptives listed in the 1986 edition of the *Physicians' Desk Reference,* however, it appears that most of them are classified as combination pills—that is, composed of a combination of estrogen and progesterone. In describing the "Demolen-Ovulen-Enovid" series (9 types of pills), for example, the manufacturer states that the "primary mechanism of action is inhibiting ovulation;" without denying, however, that a side effect

---

[622]"Comments on 'Medication to Prevent Pregnancy After Rape' in the *Linacre Quarterly,* August, 1977, p. 226.

[623]*Physicians' Desk Reference* (cf. note 67), pp. 1794 and 1966.

[624]Quotation on p. 4 of a 111-page mimeographed report which was based on the scholarly research of Suzanne R. Scorsone, Ph.D., Director of the Office of Catholic Family Life of the Archdiocese of Toronto, Canada. This report (to be referred to as *Canadian Report*) was prepared at the request of Cardinal Carter of Toronto, Canada.

could be one of "reducing the likelihood of implantation."[625] Since most medications have unfavorable side-effects (hypertensive drugs, for example), however, the medication should be judged by its primary purpose and effectiveness (which is intended) and not (in keeping with the Principle of the Double Effect) by a possible unfavorable side effect (which is not intended but merely permitted or tolerated).

It must be stressed again that the use of abortifacient contraceptive pills could not be justified morally if there are positive reasons to believe that fertilization may have already occurred, thus raising the possibility of the prevention of implantation of the conceptus.[626] Presuming that such is not the case, and that the primary effect of the pills is the prevention of ovulation, they may be used in the treatment of a victim of rape if relevant. Such medications probably would not inhibit ovulation if they are started after day 8 of the woman's menstrual cycle; some authors would stretch that time element to the 10th day of the cycle. The variables which apply in such situations are stated by Lloyd Hess, Ph.D., in an article entitled "Treatment for Rape Victims in Catholic Health Facilities," as follows:

> We need to keep in mind that there are three principle variables for any survivor: 1) the time of her cycle at which the rape occurs, 2) ovulation time, and 3) sperm viability. A second group of important variables that need to be observed or otherwise determined include the presence of sperm (absent in 50% of rapes), age, contraceptives or preventatives such as the IUD. Pregnancy preventions would not be indicated for most rapes in consideration of these variables alone.[627]

As inferred above, therefore, the situation is quite different if there are no reasons to judge that fertilization may have already occurred. Such would be the case if there is definite evidence that the woman had not ovulated and that (depending on the day of her cycle) ovulation could not coincide with the administration of postcoital contraceptives. In such a situation, there would be no basis for concern over the possible abortifacient effects of postcoital contraceptives. Hence even pills which have been designed primarily to inhibit implantation could be used if the physician judges that they may have a

---

[625]*Physicians' Desk Reference* (cf. note 67), p. 1680. Cf. also, *Canadian Report* as above (note 624), pp. 59, 60.

[626]Ashley-O'Rourke, *Health Care Ethics* (cf. note 80), pp. 293, 294. Cf. also McCarthy, Donald (cf. note 620), pp. 212 ff.

[627]Hess, Lloyd W., *Ethics and Medics* article, January, 1986, p. 4.

significant anovulant effect. With the same proviso, this could apply also to the prescription on the progesterone-only "mini pill." This could not apply, however, to the "morning after" pill which is described as containing diethylstilbestrol (DES) (cf.footnote 628). This prohibition is based not primarily on the abortifacient effect of DES, but on the serious risk involved for the woman and for her infant (just in case the rape victim happens to be pregnant at the time of the assault, or becomes pregnant while taking DES).

Another important point which bears repetition is that no contraceptive pills of any kind may be administered to the victim of alleged rape if there is any indication that the woman may be pregnant at the time of the assault. Furthermore, there would be no advantage in administering contraceptive pills to the victim of rape when warranted (that is, she has not ovulated, etc., as above) if she is already on a regimen of birth control at the time of the assault.

The task for the physician in arriving at a judgment as to which contraceptive pills are primarily anovulant and which ones are primarily abortifacient is not an easy one. The current edition of the *Physicians' Desk Reference* should provide basic guidance. The *Canadian Report,* however, states that even pills of the same kind may differ from each other in their mode of action because of the differences in the women using them; also that the mode of action of a particular pill often is difficult to discover. Several "valid generalizations" are stated as follows:

> It is generally agreed that combination pills with a high dosage of estrogen, in the large majority of cases, prevent pregnancy by preventing ovulation. It is generally agreed that, other things being equal, the lower the dosage the less likely it is that the pill will prevent ovulation. The critical level of Estrogen appears to be about fifty micrograms. At this or higher dosage, ovulation appears to be prevented effectively. Below this level (e.g., thirty or thirty-five micrograms) it appears that ovulation is not consistently prevented, so some other mechanism must be operative. There is a considerable body of evidence to suggest that the mech-

---

628*Canadian Report* (cf. note 624), pp. 4, 5. The reference to the "morning after pill" above requires some comment on the report of the British Catholic Bishops (cf. *Origins,* March 13, 1986, pp. 633–638) wherein they seem to approve of the "morning after pill" if ovulation did not take place previous to the rape assault or would not coincide with the administration of postcoital contraceptives. Based on the understanding that this particular pill as known in the U.S.A. contains diethylstilbestrol (DES), however, the use of the "morning after pill" in any American rape-treatment program would be unwarranted.

anism is the prevention of implantation. However, since dosage by weight is not the only factor influencing the mode of action of the combination pills the above generalizations may not hold in every instance.[628]

Other Aspects of the Rape Problem

Fathers Ashley and O'Rourke, O.P. refer to Pope John Paul II's observation of the sinfulness of the husband who approaches his wife for sexual union with what might be called a rape mentality—whereby the husband "considers his wife a mere sexual object without regard for her free personhood."[629] This question was explored recently by Father Edward Bayer, STD, of the Pope John Center staff in a book entitled "Rape Within Marriage." The author presents cogent arguments in proposing as a solidly probable opinion today "that there may indeed be cases where a wife may use even artificial means of avoiding pregnancy without having to fear that she is going against the teaching of the Church regarding contraception."[630] Of relevant significance is the fact that religious Sisters and other women caught in the Belgian Congo uprisings of the early 1960's were allowed to use anovulant drugs for temporary sterilization against the danger of rape.[631] A study of references of Pope Pius XII in particular with regard to conjugal union, reveals that the pontiff characterizes conjugal union as "voluntary," and "freely chosen" and based on a "desire to have relations,"[632]—expressions which are quite the contrary of sexual union imposed by a partner with the rape mentality.

In going from theory to practice, however, it is evident that efforts to put the theory into practice in individual cases could be subject to confusion, misunderstanding and rampant abuse. A situation might be imagined in which the wife is convinced that the three or four small children in the home need the supportive care and attention of a father-husband who has the rape-mentality in his "love" life, but who is otherwise very loving and attentive with regard to the children. Even in such a situation, however, it is difficult to see how the wife could have a proportionate reason for resorting to contraceptive pills on a regular basis, (not to mention the possible "break-up" of the marriage), when they present such a significant danger to her own health.

---

[629]*Health Care Ethics* (cf. note 80), p. 291.
[630]*Rape Within Marriage, Moral Analysis Delayed* (cf. note 140), pp. 126, 127.
[631]*Ibid.*, pp. 63 and 88 ff.
[632]*Ibid.*, pp. 63–67.

The 1986 edition of the *Physicians' Desk Reference* emphasizes the following "boxed in" warning:

> The use of oral contraceptives is associated with increased risk of several serious conditions including venous and arterial thromoembolism, thrombotic and hemorrhagic stroke, myocardial infarction, visual disorders, hepatic tumors, gallbladder disease, hypertension, and fetal abnormalities.[633]

No woman should be expected to pay such a price in order to assert her "freedom" with regard to conjugal union. If all efforts to make the husband see the error of his ways end in failure, the better solution might be to seek an ecclesiastical and civil separation "from bed and board,"—or, as one noted canonist put it, "a mensa et a tauro." There is even the possibility of an annulment of the marriage on the basis of the husband's radical incapacity to assume the essential obligations of marriage "due to causes of a psychic nature" (Can.1095,3).

A recent "letter to the editor" published in the *New England Journal of Medicine* again drew attention to the possibility that a Catholic hospital might face civil action for not administering the "morning after pill" after rape. The physician-correspondent allowed that "Church-affiliated hospitals have a right to their moral convictions," but insisted that "insofar as they act as public emergency facilities, they must provide rape victims who do not subscribe to the same moral code the right to choose immediate anti-pregnancy prophylaxis, as is indicated for optimal medical care."[634] The correspondent may be excused for not knowing that, in Catholic teaching, the "morning after" pill is not anti-ovulation but rather anti-life or abortive prophylaxis.

Fortunately, as of the present, all civil cases brought against a Catholic health facility for prohibiting certain procedures on the basis of Catholic values and standards have been decided in favor of the Catholic health facility. Typical of such decisions is a 1973 case, *Taylor vs. St. Vincent's Hospital* (Chicago) in which the defense relied on the "Church amendment" to the Health Program Extension Act of 1973. This Act states that even if a health facility had received any grant, contract, loan or loan guarantee by virtue of civil legislation, this does not empower any public authority or public official to require the hospital to "make its facilities available for the performance of any sterilization procedure or abortion if the performance of such procedure or abortion is prohibited by the entity on the basis of religious beliefs or moral

---

[633]Cf. note 67; p. 1681.

[634]Issue of Dec. 20, 1984, p. 1637. the correspondent was John J. Goldenring, MD, M.P.H. of Hermosa Beach, Cal.

convictions . . . ."[635]

Every Catholic health facility must exercise supreme caution, prudence and circumspection in emphasizing dedication to the *Ethical and Religious Directives For Catholic Health Facilities* in the base document of any incorporation procedures, and in inserting provisions in corporate articles and bylaws whereby all professionals are required to adhere to the *Directives*.[636] Detailed discussions of these essential aspects of civil incorporation are found in a 1983 publication by Bishop Adam Maida, JCL, JD, and Nicholas P. Cafardi, JD, entitled *Church Property, Church Finances, and Church-Related Corporations*.[637]

Directive 24: In all cases in which the presence of pregnancy would render some procedure illicit (e.g. curettage), the physician must make use of such pregnancy tests and consultation as may be needed in order to be reasonably certain that the patient is not pregnant. It is to be noted that curettage of the endometrium after rape to prevent implantation of a possible embryo is morally equivalent to abortion.

8.4 PRACTICES AND PROCEDURES CONTRARY TO THE COMMON GOOD

Ghost Surgery

The practice of ghost surgery obviously is contrary to the common good. It means that the physician who actually does the surgery is an "unknown" to the patient. For example, the patient is prepared for surgery with the definite impression that the surgery will be performed by Dr. Z, his family physician. In reality, Dr. X performs the surgery as an agent of Dr. Z without the knowledge of the patient. Sometimes the patient is not only not informed of the identity of the surgeon, but is deceived as to the identity of the surgeon. In such instances, Dr. Z may be a general practitioner who lacks skill and experience in that particular type of surgery, and persuades Dr. X, a skilled surgeon, to substitute for him with an agreement to split the fee. Thus Dr. Z shares in the more substantial revenue of the skilled surgeon. The patient,

---

[635]*In Defense of Values,* by the Division of Legal Services of the Catholic Health Association (St. Louis, Mo.: Catholic Health Assoc., 1984), p. 7.

[636]*Ibid.,* pp. 19–22.

[637]Published in St. Louis, Mo. by the Catholic Health Association, 1984. Cf. especially pp. 155–170.

ignorant of the substitution, never sees Dr. X. The latter sees the patient only when he or she is under anesthesia.

Such a practice is immoral primarily because it involves deliberate deceit—a flagrant violation of the rights of the patient. Other aspects of immorality on the basis of injustice are the following: The substitute surgeon has no opportunity to check the diagnosis of the patient's doctor; the patient is deprived of the post-operative examination and care-supervision of the skilled surgeon; the patient's physician (Dr. Z) has no right to a portion of the surgical fee. Futhermore, the common good is violated inasmuch as such arrangements bring the medical profession into disrepute. The medical code of ethics of the American Medical Association (section 7) appropriately disapproves of ghost surgery:

> In the practice of medicine a physician should limit the source of his professional income to medical services actually rendered by him, or under his supervision, to his patients. His fee should be commensurate with the service rendered and the patient's ability to pay. He should neither pay nor receive commission for referral of patients.[638]

It is in the interests of the common good, however, that hospitals have adequate residency training programs. Such programs are designed to provide essential training in professional experience and techniques and in personal responsibility to the trainees. Every patient, however, whether a paying patient or an indigent person, has a right to be protected from any unnecessary risk. Such a risk would be present if the operating surgeon in a residency training program were to allow a trainee to do all of the surgery without supervision, and this without the knowledge and consent of the patient. This would be ghost surgery.

With regard to a paying patient who enters into a formal contract with a specified surgeon, the surgery must be performed by that specified surgeon, with whatever professional assistance as required in the situation. In a residency training program, however, some additional participation by a trainee under the direct supervision of the surgeon would be allowed only if such an arrangement is expressed or clearly implied in the physician-patient relationship. With regard to an indigent patient (providing that no unnecessary risk is involved), the patient should be informed that adequate care by competent professionals will be provided, but that it may be necessary to employ the

---

[638]Reiser, Stanley, "Codes of Medical Ethics" (cf. note 116), p. 46.

assistance of one or more trainees of the residency training program under appropriate professional supervision. If the indigent patient agrees to such a condition, either explicitly or implicitly (after having received an explanation of the purposes of the residency training program), there is no violation of Catholic moral standards.[639]

Contemporary Health Maintenance Organizations (HMO's) usually specify that expert surgical services will be provided but without an option on the part of an enrolled member to choose the physician or surgeon. The reason for this understanding is reflected in lower financial rates for membership in an HMO. It can be presumed that the enrollee agrees to this limitation as to choice of physician, with the understanding that all medical and surgical service will be provided in accord with high standards of adequacy and competency. In such cases, the HMO sponsors reserve the right to assign the physician or surgeon, as the case may be. Again, no violation of moral standards is involved.

> *Directive 32:* Ghost surgery, which implies the calculated deception of the patient as to the identity of the operating surgeon, is morally objectionable.

Euthanasia

The advocates of euthanasia (also called "mercy killing" and "death with dignity") are organized worldwide. One publication of late 1984 lists euthanasia societies in twenty nations—three in the U.S.A. (Concern for Dying, Hemlock Society, Society for the Right to Die).[640] When a group of five French physicians announced in September, 1984, that they had helped some of their patients to die, one of their group made it very clear that he had not only withdrawn support from patients at their request, but had also taken active measures aimed at ending their lives, including the administration of drugs.[641] In other words, he practiced both *passive or negative* euthanasia (voluntary omission of an ethically obligatory life-preserving action) and *active or positive* euthanasia (voluntary commission of a life-terminating action).

---

[639]For an interesting review of discussions within the medical community on the subject of ghost surgery, cf. O'Donnell, Thomas, S.J., *Medicine and Christian Morality* (cf. note 31), pp. 78–82.

[640]Supplement to *Human Life Issues,* Nov./Dec., 1984, pp. 12, 13. Publication of the Human Life Center, University of Steubenville, Steubenville, Ohio.

[641]*Ibid.,* p. 4.

The *Declaration on Euthanasia* from the Holy See on June 27, 1980, amounted to a comprehensive condemnation of euthanasia:

> Euthanasia here means an action or omission that by its nature or by intention causes death with the purpose of putting an end to all suffering. Euthanasia is, therefore, a matter of intention and method. We must firmly state once again that no one and nothing can in any way, authorize the killing of an innocent human being, whether the latter be a fetus or embryo, or a child or an adult or an elderly person, or someone incurably ill or someone who is dying.
>
> In addition, no one may ask for such a death-dealing action for oneself or for another for whom one is responsible, nor may one explicitly or implicitly consent to such an action. Nor may any authority legitimately command or permit it. For such an action is a violation of divine law, an offense against the dignity of the human person, a crime against life and an attack on the human race.[642]

The crime of contributing to the death of infants by active and passive means both in the prenatal and postnatal periods was discussed in the chapter on the Principle of the Right to Life (cf. 3.6). As to the pleas of the seriously ill who may beg at times to be "put to death," the document quoted above states that such pleas "are hardly to be understood as conveying a real desire for euthanasia," but rather as "anguished pleas for help and love" (cf. p.118).

One factor that should temper the zeal and enthusiasm of all advocates of euthanasia is the record of the tragic and diabolic disregard for human life in official programs designed to eliminate the opposition and to "purify the race" in Adolph Hitler's Third Reich from 1933 to 1945. Lucy Dawidowicz, a noted historian of the Holocaust, described the overall program as one of positive eugenics (to increase the population of racially pure "Aryans") and negative eugenics, with a view to Nazi-German domination of the world:

> Positive eugenics was a program designed to increase the population of persons who were regarded as racially pure "Ayrans" (and good Nazis as well). Negative eugenics was a program designed first to halt the procreation of persons or categories of persons

---

[642]Issued by the Sacred Congregation for the Doctrine of the Faith, June 27, 1980. Cf. *The Pope Speaks*, 1980, p. 292.

[compulsory sterilization enacted, July 14, 1933] who did not meet the standards of racial purity through sterilization and then eventually to kill them and to kill those who were regarded as the racial enemy—the Jews and the Gypsies.[643]

One can at least hope that the haunting Nazi disregard for human life was a tempering influence in the discussions and deliberations of the members of the *President's Commission* on the subject of life-sustaining treatment. At any rate, the commission refrained from providing a "guidebook of morally correct choices for patients and health care providers who are facing such a [life-sustaining] decision." The report (which, incidentally, "generated the greatest public response of any the Commission produced") emphasized generalities such as the following:

-The importance of respecting the choices of individuals competent to decide to forego even life-sustaining treatment;
-The importance of providing mechanisms and guidelines for decision-making on behalf of patients unable to do so on their own;
-The importance of maintaining a presumption in favor of sustaining life;
-The importance of improving the medical options available to dying people;
-The importance of providing respectful, responsive, and supportive care to patients for whom no further medical therapies are available or elected;
-The importance of encouraging health care institutions to take responsibility for ensuring that adequate procedures for decisionmaking are available to all patients.[644]

The advocates of euthanasia cloud the reality of their aspirations by using euphemisms such as "death with dignity," and "Right to Die" and "Mercy killing;" they would argue that what they recommend [release from suffering] is for the common good. Without meaning to be offensive, some of them may use the argument that the same humane consideration should be manifested for a hopelessly-ill and incurable human being as would be manifested for an incurably ill and acutely-suffering animal: "Put it out of it's misery." The

---

[643]"Biomedical Ethics and the Shadow of Naziism," a 20-page supplement to *The Hastings Center Report*, Aug., 1976, p. 3. Cf. also *Experimentation With Human Beings*, by Joe Katz, 2nd, ed (New York, N.Y.: Russell Sage Foundation, 1973), pp. 283 ff.

[644]*Summing Up*, Final report of the *President's Commission* (Washington D.C.: U.S. Gov. Printing Office, 1983), pp. 32-34.

argument that God alone has direct ownership over human life is unintelligible to them. In their mode of thinking, pain and suffering are absolute human evils—without any redeeming purpose or utility. Since those characterized as "hopelessly ill" are going to die anyhow, many advocates of "death with dignity" are inclined to look upon hastening death as the lesser of two evils. If they lack convictions with regard to supernatural life and the prospect of eternal life beyond this fleeting terrestrial life (with emphasis on "trial"), it would be useless to approach them with arguments based on "taking up the cross" in following the Divine Savior (Luke,9:23), or on St. Paul's reminder that "whom the Lord loves, he disciplines" (Hebrews,12:6).

The obligation of each individual to guard and protect his or her physical life is not absolute. Although those who are seriously ill are *not* to be taken seriously when they beg to be "put to death", yet these same patients may renounce treatments which "can only yield a precarious and painful prolongation of life" when death is imminent and inevitable (cf. pp.164 ff.). Although no human individual may be expected to endanger his or her life in the interests of medical experimentation without some hope of improvement in physical health (cf. pp.321,322), yet there are words of high praise for those who *voluntarily* endanger their lives by submitting to a medical or surgical procedure which redounds uniquely to the common good and the cause of progress in medical science, with little or no hope of an improvement in their personal physical condition. The Holy See's *Declaration on Euthanasia* extolls such generosity as follows:

> Suicide must be carefully distinguished from the sacrifice of life in which men and women give their lives or endanger them for some noble cause such as the honor of God, the salvation of souls or in the service of the brethren: 'There is no greater love than this: to lay down one's life for one's friends' (John,15:13).[645]

This would apply not only to those who endanger or give their lives in testimony of their faith in God, and to those who are willing to make the supreme sacrifice for love of God and country through military service, but also to contemporary examples of voluntary submission to professionally-managed innovative procedures (for example, recipients of mechanical hearts) which give reasonable promise of progress in mankind's enduring struggle against human misery, illness and disease.

---

[645] *The Pope Speaks*, 1980, p. 291.

Directive 28: Euthanasia ("mercy killing") in all its forms is forbidden. The failure to supply the ordinary means of preserving life is equivalent to euthanasia. However, neither the physician nor the patient is obliged to the use of extraordinary means."

CHAPTER IX

Principle of Confidentiality

If you once forfeit the confidence of your fellow citizens, you can never regain their respect and esteem . . .[646] (Abraham Lincoln)

PRINCIPLE: EVERY PERSON HAS A RIGHT TO KNOW THOSE THINGS WHICH, IN JUSTICE AND IN CHARITY, SHOULD BE TOLD—AND EVERY PERSON HAS A RIGHT TO HIS SECRET. THIS LATTER RIGHT IS FOUNDED EITHER ON THE OWNER-SHIP THAT EACH ONE HAS OVER THE FRUITS OF HIS OWN THOUGHTS, INDUSTRY AND TALENTS, OR ON THE RIGHT THAT EACH ONE HAS TO HIS GOOD NAME. A SECRET, THEN, BELONGS TO ITS OWNER, AND NO ONE MAY STEAL THAT SE-CRET (Adapted from *Medical Ethics,* by Edwin F. Healy, S.J., p. 46).

---

[646]Cf. *Familiar Quotations,* John Bartlett, ed. (cf. note 132), p. 542.b. The rest of this quotation is familiar to millions of Americans: "It is true that you may fool all of the people some of the time; you can even fool some of the people all of the time; but you can't fool all of the people all of the time."

Webster's Collegiate Dictionary defines *deceit* as "an attempt or disposition to deceive: a trick; fraud." The same source defines *confidence* as the "state of one who confides; trust; reliance" (from the Latin "confidere;"—to have faith in, to trust). A person in whom others confide loses or forfeits that confidence basically in two ways: by deceiving or fooling others through lies, hypocrisy or trickery, and by betraying a secret. The words of St. Paul to the Corinthians come to mind: "Rather, we repudiate shameful, underhanded practices. We do not resort to trickery or falsify the Word of God" (II Corinthians, 4:2). Deceit and betrayal of secrets are violations of the virtues of justice and of charity: of justice, because every person has a right to the truth and to reciprocal trust and to the preservation of his or her secrets; of charity, because both deceit and betrayal of secrets amount to using a neighbor instead of loving a neighbor.

9.1 USING OTHERS THROUGH DECEPTION

Veracity or truthfulness is a virtue which inclines a person to speak the truth appropriately. The word "appropriately" means that an individual is not obliged to tell everything he knows, nor is he free to tell the truth on just any occasion. Veracity is violated by hypocrisy, double-dealing, trickery or any other diversions which are used to deceive another person or other persons. All of these are variations of lying—of expressing falsehoods. A lie is a deliberate word or sign expressing something which is contrary to what is on the mind of the communicator. *Deliberate* means that the communicator knows what he is saying or doing; *word or sign* means that falsehood can be expressed by a nod of the head, a wave of the hand or some other non-verbal mode of communication; *contrary to what is on the mind* means that there is a sense of definite opposition between what the communicator is thinking and what he expresses by word or deed (contrary, that is, to one's knowledge and judgment in the matter). Since lying is an abuse of the very purpose of human communication and hence contrary to the natural law, it is always immoral. In the words of the Book of Proverbs (12:22): "Lying lips are an abomination to the Lord, but those who are truthful are his delight."

Although lying is considered to be *intrinsically* evil (that is, sinful by its very nature), and cannot be justified by even a noble end or purpose, it is not, in itself, a serious sin. The gravity of the sin of lying in particular cases depends upon the extent to which another virtue besides veracity is violated, for example, against the virtue of justice, religion, love of neighbor, etc. There are *malicious* lies which involve the intention or at least the foresight of deceiving another; there are *officious* lies, which are told for one's own advantage or that of another; and there are *jocose* lies which are told for the sake of amusement or diversion. St. Thomas states that the intention of deceiving does not pertain to the essence of lying (II-II,Q.110,art.1). Examples of seriously-sinful malicious lies would be telling a deliberate falsehood which results in serious harm to another (loss of good name, loss of opportunity to achieve a substantial goal or ambition, serious financial loss), or which results in serious harm to the common good (perjury, dereliction of duty with serious consequences) provided that the lying individual intended to deceive or cause harm or at least could be held responsible for foreseeing the evil consequences.[647]

The Validity of Mental Reservations

Lying can be particularly cruel and harmful in the mission of healing. There are situations, however, when the communication of knowledge must be limited or tempered by a consideration of the best interests of the patient, or by the questioner's right to know, or by the respondent's obligation to preserve a secret, etc. In such situations—and always, providing that there is a proportionate reason for concealing the truth—a person could be justified in resorting to what is known as a mental reservation. A mental reservation is an act of the *mind* whereby an individual conceals the truth by restricting the meaning of words or signs to something different than the obvious meaning of the words or signs used. An ambiguous statement (amphibology) is similar to a mental reservation (the word "beat," for example, can refer to physical harm or to winning a card game). A *strict* mental reservation, in which no clue is given to a secondary meaning, is equivalent to a lie. If a young man comes home with $10 which he had taken by stealth from the local gas station, and answers his mother's question, "did you steal that money?" with a simple "No," but with an unexpressed mental reservation, "not with my left hand," he is guilty of lying. A *broad* mental reservation, whereby a prudent person can gather the intended meaning from the surrounding circumstances or from customary usage (as in the example below) can be allowed. Broad mental reservations should be used sparingly—and always with a proportionate reason.

Some authors claim that Jesus' words in John 7:8 could be interpreted as a broad mental reservation. In that passage from the Gospel of St. John, Jesus told some of His followers: "Go up yourselves [to Jerusalem] to the

---

[647]Cf. any standard manual of moral theology such as Merkelbach, Benedict Henry, O.P., *Summa Theologiae Moralis, II* (Paris: Declée de Brouwer, 1935), nn. 857 ff.; Genicot-Salsmans, S.J., *Institutiones Theologiae Moralis, 14th. ed., I* (cf. note 186), nn. 413 ff.; Arregui, Antonio, S.J., *Summarium Theologiae Moralis, 13th. ed.* (Westminster Md.: Newman Bookshop, 1944), n. 426.

festival. I am not going up to the festival because the time is not yet ripe for me." Yet later, He went up to Jerusalem "but as if in secret" (John,7:10). He gave the clue to the reserved meaning of His words when He said: "the time is not ripe for me." Jesus knew that "some of the Jews were looking for a chance to kill Him" (John,7:1), and He was saying that His "going up" would not be for the purpose of fulfilling His Father's will through His suffering, death and resurrection—"His time," His great sacrifice on the cross, would come later. A physician or nurse might use a similar broad mental reservation in the following case: a mother and her teen-age son are both in critical condition in the hospital as the result of a tragic auto accident; the son dies during the night; next morning, the critically-ill mother asks "How is my son?;" fearing that the full truth would retard the mother's recovery, the nurse or physician answers: "Don't worry about him; he is in good hands." The import of the response is that the son is in God's hands. No falsehood is involved. There is a proportionate reason for concealing the full truth.

The proportionate reason for using a mental reservation could be some legitimate utility or advantage for oneself or for others. In a court of law, for example, the accused, even though under oath, is required to reveal the truth only insofar as the law obliges him to do so. He can resort to evasive statements in order to avoid incriminating himself. Likewise, in order to observe confidentiality, the physician may use a mental reservation to answer a questioner who has no right to know. People should know that physicians are bound to professional secrecy, and that a physician's answers to questions about his patient are to be interpreted in the light of that obligation to secrecy. The hospital visitor (who has no right to know) might ask: "And how is Mrs X coming along?" Even though Mrs X has not shown any improvement in several days, the physician would be justified in saying "She's doing all right." Even if the visitor is a close friend of Mrs X and asks "does she have cancer?," the physician may answer: "we are doing our best for her" (in unspoken words: "I cannot tell you").

Informing Patients of Their Condition

The physician's quandary of "how much to tell," "when to tell it," etc. with regard to questions from his patients was discussed at length in the chapter on the Principle of Informed Consent (cf. especially pp. 198–200). The recommendation of one panel of 20 physicians was that practically all patients, even disturbed ones, are better off knowing the truth.[648] Putting that

---

[648]Wanzer, Sidney H., MD, et al., "The Physician's Responsibility Toward Hopelessly Ill Patients," in *The New England Journal of Medicine*, April 12, 1984, p. 957.

guideline into practice, however, calls for finesse, feeling, warmth, empathy, etc. with regard to how much?—when?—how? as noted in chapter V (Informed Consent). If the patient asks "Is it cancer, doc?", and the physician judges that it is too early for a definitive diagnosis (results of confirming test not received as yet, plans to consult with a colleague, patient in a highly emotional state at the time), the physician may answer: "Let's worry more about how to get you back into circulation again." If the patient knows that cancer is the definitive diagnosis, and asks "How long do I have, Doc?", the physician might say "you will still be around many months from now, and a lot longer than that if my diagnosis proves to be wrong." With the rapid progress in medical science today, the physician often could be justified in saying: "Just "hang in there," and "we might come up with a few surprises for you."

The obligation of the physician to inform the patient who is near death regarding the inevitability of death, either personally or through another, bears repeating. As mentioned in Chapter V on the Principle of Informed Consent (pp. 199,200), fulfilling that obligation could be unnecessary (patient well aware of impending death and well prepared), or it might be considered either useless (patient would ignore the information completely) or harmful (would drive the patient to despair, thoughts of suicide, etc.). In the last two situations ("useless" and "harmful"), the physician still is obligated to fulfill the obligation either personally or through the chaplain or close relatives.

In addition to the right to know about the approach of death, every patient who is reasonably in danger of cardiac arrest has a right to adequate information about the life-or-death implications of the cardiac-pulmonary resuscitation procedure (CPR). The survey mentioned in chapter V (p.157) regarding the reluctance of physicians to discuss this subject in time with their patients illustrates the urgent need of open lines of communication between physician and patient. Physicians who are inclined to think that "it is the doctor's responsibility to make decisions about resuscitation for patients," or who excuse themselves for not initiating the subject with their patients because it would be "too threatening a subject for most acutely ill patients," or who might feel exonerated from discussing CPR because "the (cardiac) arrest is totally unexpected," should reflect on their overall obligation to advance the best interests of their patients.[649]

There are cases when the physician may be justified in giving more information to the members of the family than to the patient. Such exceptions may

---

[649]The propriety of such excuses is discussed by Susanna E. Bedell, MD, and Thomas L. Delbanco, MD in an article entitled "Choices About Cardiopulmonary Resuscitation in the Hospital," *The New England Journal of Medicine*, April 26, 1984, pp. 1091, 1092.

well be covered by the rule of "primum, non nocere" (above all, do not cause harm). The general rule, however, is that the competent patient sits in the driver's seat, and makes the decisions; the incompetent patient's previously-expressed wishes must be respected. Patients who are left in the dark, or left isolated from what they have a right to know as a basis for decision making, are victims of injustice. They are being denied the means to advance their autonomy and self-determination. One member of the medical profession explains the inadequacy of saying: "But I talked it over with close family members:"

> How can we square this practice with the rights of patients to self-determination? In talking first, and sometimes solely, with the family of a competent adult, physicians infantilize the patient and so undermine his autonomy. Without information he cannot participate in decisions. Perhaps more important is the isolation of the patient that occurs in the special case of a protracted fatal illness during which the family is systematically kept better informed than the patient. In this situation, the family may try, often with relentless good cheer, to maintain that the patient is getting better, while the patient pretends to be oblivious to any evidence to the contrary. This dissembling takes place at precisely the time when the patient most needs the companionship of being able to talk honestly about his concerns with those he loves. He is thus isolated from both his physician and his family.[650]

9.2 The Right to Guard Secrets

Poetess Charlotte Bronté speaks of secrets of the human heart as "treasures, in secret kept, in silence sealed; . . . whose charms are broken if revealed."[651] The Book of Sirach (27:16 and 21) has stronger words of reproach for violators of secrecy;

> He who betrays a secret cannot be trusted, he will never find an intimate friend. . . A wound can be bound up, and an insult forgiven, but he who betrays secrets does hopeless damage.

A secret is hidden knowledge which may not be revealed. If Vatican II's

---

[650]Angell, Marcia, MD, "Respecting the Autonomy of competent Patients," in *The New England Journal of Medicine,* April 26, 1984, p. 1116.

[651]*Familiar Quotations,* John Bartlett, ed. (cf. note 132), p. 586,b.

pastoral constitution on *The Church Today* (n.71) can refer to ownership or dominion over material goods as "an extension of human freedom," what must be said of each individual's ownership and dominion over the fruit of personal thoughts, ideas, industry, creativeness, talents, etc.? In his address to the Congress of the International Association of Applied Psychology on April 10, 1958, Pope Pius XII referred to "an area of the intimate psychism"—in particular, tendencies and dispositions—when he said:

> And just as it is illicit to appropriate another's goods or to make an attempt on his bodily integrity without his consent, so it is not permissible to enter into his inner domain against his will, whatever is the technique or method used.[652]

St. Paul infers that every individual must some day render an account for "the reflections and thoughts of the heart" (Hebrews,4:12 and 13), but until that judgment day dawns, every individual's thoughts, reflections, hopes, memories, etc., must be respected by others as extremely personal possessions and treasures.

In addition to the right of each individual to possess and protect these innermost private possessions, there is also the right of each individual to a good name. Since every human individual has not only comforting and enriching personal thoughts, reflections, etc., but also similar outpourings of the human mind and heart which are unpleasant, embarrassing and even revolting, the connection between revealing the secrets of others and the loss of their good name should be abundantly clear. Once incriminations and aspersions have been made by the revelation of the secrets of another, it is practically impossible to restore that good name to its pristine goodness.

There are *natural* secrets, so called because the natural law binds the possessor to keep the secret (for example, knowledge that a certain person is illegitimate); there are *promised* secrets which a person binds himself to keep *after* the knowledge is revealed to him (for example, "promise me that you will not tell anyone what I have just confided to you"); there are *entrusted* secrets which are revealed *only on condition* that the one to whom the knowledge is about to be revealed agrees explicitly or at least tacitly to keep the secret. Since the discussion here involves primarily entrusted secrets, the other two categories can be relegated into the background of the present discussion by saying that revealing a promised secret (which binds under the virtue of fidelity) ordinarily is a venial sin—unless it leads to serious consequences for

---

[652] *The Pope Speaks*, Summer, 1958, p. 15.

others. The revelation of a natural secret (which binds under the virtue of justice) ordinarily is a serious sin. The revelation of any type of secret is also a violation of the virtue of charity. There is no sin involved, however, in the revelation of any type of secret if the person who reveals the secret has a proportionate reason for doing so.[653]

Confidential knowledge which is made known to professionals such as physicians, lawyers, pastors, civil officials, etc., is known as an *entrusted* secret (secrets). The unjustifiable revelation of an entrusted secret is a violation of the virtue of justice. The most binding of all entrusted secrets is the sacramental secret of the seal of confession. The Code of Canon Law states that the seal of confession is "absolutely inviolable," and that it is a crime for a confessor "in any way to betray a penitent by word or in any other manner or for any reason whatsoever" (can.983,1). In fact, even when all danger of disclosing or revealing the information in any way is excluded, the confessor is "absolutely forbidden to use knowledge acquired in confession when it might harm the penitent" (can.984,1). The penalty for directly violating the seal of confession is an automatic excommunication which is reserved to the Holy See (can.1388,1).

With regard to all secrets (except the sacramental seal of confession), the general rule is that the obligation of keeping the secret ceases when the guarded knowledge becomes common knowledge, or when the one to whom the secret was confided can justly presume that the individual concerned would give permission to reveal the information. Thus a physician who knows from professional knowledge that his patient has a venereal disease may presume permission to discuss the situation with the young man's uncle who learned about his nephew's plight from another source. A special situation arises at times with regard to entrusted secrets,—due to a conflict between the rights of the patient and the rights of others. The physician is justified in revealing secret information when such a revelation is necessary to avert serious harm to the common good, to an innocent third party, or to either the one who revealed the secret or to the one "to whom revealed."

Valid Exceptions to Keeping Professional Secrets

By virtue of the principal that the common good takes precedence over

---

[653]Public officials and others who are obligated professionally not to reveal secret knowledge (physicians, priests, etc.) are not only justified in saying "I don't know" to those who have no right to know, but may also make such an affirmation under oath if necessary. For a review of other sensitive situations (testimony in court, commercial and political issues, etc.) cf. Merkelbach, Benedict, O.P., *Summa Theologiae Moralis, II* (cf. note 647). nn. 871–874.

the good of the individual, the physician is required to report instances of certain *communicable diseases*. This applies only between the physician and the civil agencies which have a "right to know" (federal, state or local). The importance of this regulation is illustrated in the struggle of medical science against the spread of Acquired Immunity Deficiency Syndrome (AIDS) which has assumed epidemic proportions. A less dramatic example could be that of an elderly patient with active pulmonary tuberculosis who has signed up for a protracted group excursion. If this gentleman refuses to inform the tour or excursion conductor of his condition, the physician would have an obligation to do so. Is the professional genetic counselor required to inform the members of the family or others of his patient's communicable genetic disease? If the answer is in the affirmative, the patient may be refused employment or suffer embarrassment within his family and relationship. If the answer is in the negative, the risk of transmitting the disease (for example, cystic fibrosis, Huntington's disease, etc.) through procreation constitutes a threat to the common good.

The members of the *President's Commission* did not take a clear stand on this sensitive subject. They concluded that "under certain, limited circumstances a genetic counselor may be justified in overriding a patient's desire for confidentiality in order to protect identifiable relatives from severe and otherwise unavoidable harm."[654] This dilemma was addressed by Pope Pius XII in his presentation to the Italian Medical-biological Union of St. Luke on November 12, 1944:

> Another of the duties which derive from the eighth commandment is the observance of the professional secret, which must serve and serves the good of the individual and even more of society. In this sector too, there can arise conflicts between the public and private interests, or between different elements and aspects pertaining to the common good. In these conflicts it will often be very difficult to measure and weigh justly the pros and cons for speaking out or keeping silent. In such a dilemma, the conscientious doctor seeks his norm in the basic tenets of Christian ethics, which will help him to pick the right course. These norms, in fact, while they clearly affirm the obligation on the physician to preserve the professional secret, above all in the interest of the common good, do

---

[654]*Summing Up* (cf. note 644), p. 37.

not concede to this an absolute value. For that very common good would suffer were the professional secret placed at the service of crime or injustice.[655]

With regard to "speaking out or keeping silent" when the patient or client has been diagnosed definitely as having a genetic disease, there is seldom question of an obligation to report the fact to a government agency unless the disease is dangerous to the general public. The only ones with a right to know (in addition to the client or patient) are the spouse or fiancee of that person and (to some extent) members of the immediate family of both parties. The patient or client cannot be denied the right to a basic knowledge of his condition as well as of possible consequences through procreation for those who have a right to know—unless circumstances are such (suicidal tendencies, deep depression, etc.) that it is necessary to reveal the condition gradually over a period of time, or to enlist the help of others (family member, pastor, etc.) to reveal and/or explain the patient's condition. The physician or genetic counselor should impress upon the patient the importance of informing his spouse or fiancee (and others, as required), but the degree of persuasion required would depend on the type of disease, the family background, the age of the parties, the patient's financial and employment stability, etc. In some cases the physician might make his point and leave it up to the patient to communicate the information to others. In other cases with more drastic consequences for the families involved, he might have to resort to saying: "I am willing to communicate this information to your loved ones with your permission. If you deny me that permission, I may have to do it on my own."

The quotation of Pope Pius XII above furnishes a general guideline: "the conscientious doctor [or counselor] seeks his norm in the basic tenets of Christian ethics, which will help him pick the right course." He would also be justified in consulting with a professional colleague, or with the pastor of the patient, in an effort to fulfill his obligation. Solving this conflict between obligations of confidentiality to the patient and obligation to societal considerations is not an easy matter. Possible legal complications can develop in some cases.[656] A reminder from Pope Pius XII is of prime importance: "The interests of science, of the individual, and of the community are not, after all,

---

[655] *The Human Body* (cf. note 61), p. 63 (n. 62).

[656] For an extended discussion of this issue, cf. *Genetic Counseling, the Church, and the Law*, by Gary M. Atkinson, Ph.D., and Albert S. Moraczewski, O.P., Ph.D. (cf. note 188), pp. 29–51.

absolute values and do not necessarily guarantee respect for all rights."[657] The situation calls for a careful balancing of the pros and the cons as well as prudential foresight and discretion.

Should the patient or client be advised to avoid the procreation of children? All factors mentioned above (type of disease, family background, etc.) would have to be taken into consideration. On the one hand, the marriage contract does not confer the right to have children (cf. chapter II,p.60). On the other hand, advice not to have children (if appropriate) should be given with a sense of assurance that the use of legitimate means of avoiding conception such as Natural Family Planning will not alienate the couple from God's love and God's grace. There may even be a possibility of adopting children. If the physician or counselor senses that the patient and his spouse or fiancee are absolutely determined to have a family, he should content himself with having done his duty of informing them of the likely prognosis and leave them decide for themselves. Any effort to fulfill his duty as a professional counselor by furnishing information on sinful alternatives (even without approving of them) such as abortion or sterilization would amount to sinful cooperation in the evil of others. Unfortunately, other agencies would be only too willing to furnish such information to the patient and/or the couple.

Marriage with an AIDS-infected Partner

A very sensitive situation arises if one of the parties to a proposed marriage has been diagnosed as having the Acquired Immunity Deficiency Syndrome (AIDS). Other sexually transmitted diseases such as syphilis and gonorrhea can respond to medical treatment and be cured. As of the present, there is no cure for the highly-infectious AIDS disease nor for the AIDS infection which is a prelude to the "full-blown" AIDS disease. There is no doubt that it would be morally wrong for the individual who is contemplating marriage and who suspects that he or she may carry the AIDS virus HTLV-III (*H*uman *T*-cell *L*ymphotropic *V*irus, type III) to fail deliberately to submit to the AIDS testing procedure, or to withhold the secret of his or her infected or diseased condition from the proposed marriage partner after the AIDS diagnosis has been made. In the event of a positive diagnosis, the more urgent and delicate problem arises as to how the medical and pastoral counselor should proceed in discussing the prospect of marriage with the AIDS victim and with his or her proposed marriage partner.

---

[657]Address to the International College of Neuro-psychopharmacology, Sept. 9, 1958; *The Pope Speaks,* autumn, 1959, p. 436.

According to the Code of Canon Law, all persons who are not prohibited by law can contract marriage. This means that all persons who are not prohibited by divine law or by ecclesiastical law are free to enter a marriage covenant. Pope Pius XII commented on this right to marriage in his address to the members of the Roman Rota on October 3, 1941:

> In the first place, considering the right to marriage, Our glorious Predecessors Leo XIII and Pius XI taught that "no human law can deprive men of the basic natural right to marriage." Because this right, in fact, was given to man by the Author of nature Himself, the supreme Lawgiver, it cannot be denied to anyone unless it is proved either that he has of his own free will renounced this right, or that he is incapable of contracting matrimony because of some mental or bodily defect.[658]

Pope Pius XII returned to the subject in his address to the First Symposium on Genetic Medicine on September 7, 1953. After his discussion of individuals who might be incapable of contracting marriage because of a mental or physical defect, he added:

> Outside of these cases, the banning of marriage or of marital intercourse for biological, genetical or eugenical motives, is an injustice, no matter who it is who issues that prohibition, whether a private individual or a public authority.

> Certainly it is right, and in the greater number of cases it is a duty, to point out to those whose heredity is beyond doubt very defective, the burden they are about to impose upon themselves, upon their marriage partner, and upon their offspring. The burden might perhaps became unbearable. To advise against, however, is not to forbid. There might be other motives, especially of a moral or a personal nature, which are of such importance as to authorize the contracting of marriage and its use, even in the circumstances just mentioned.[659]

Five years later, in his address to the Seventh International Hematological Congress on September 12, 1958, the same Pius XII furnished another guideline with regard to progeny for individuals who can transmit a serious

---

[658] *The Human Body* (cf. note 61), pp. 49, 50.
[659] *Ibid.*, p. 259.

disease through marriage when he said: "From the moral point of view it can be said in general that a person has no right to disregard real risks of which one is aware."[660]

The Reality of the Risks in an AIDS-related Marriage

A clear distinction must be kept in mind between the *AIDS infection* and the *AIDS disease* (approximately 21,000 cases reported in the U.S.A. as of May, 1986). The latter is also referred to as "full-blown AIDS," as manifested (in accord with the Centers of Disease Control criteria) by the *presence* of a "reliably diagnosed disease at least moderately predictive of cellular immune deficiency," and the *absense* of an "underlying cause for the immune deficiency or of any defined cause for reduced resistance to the disease."[661] The total cases of *AIDS infection* can only be estimated. This is due to the fact that only a small percentage of American adults have submitted to the AIDS virus blood test. A further distinction should be made between *AIDS exposure* and *AIDS infection*. "Exposure" means that an opportunity for AIDS virus infection took place; for example, through sexual contact with an AIDS-infected individual, or the sharing of a needle with an AIDS-infected person. Such "exposed" individuals should submit to the AIDS virus blood test sequence. "Infected" means that the individual has been confirmed as positive in the AIDS blood test sequence ("sequence" referring to the fact that individuals are considered as "infected" only after repeated positive results of the so-called ELISA test as confirmed by the more specific Western blot test).[662]

The AIDS virus belongs to the "retrovirus" family. Members of this killer-germ family (which includes HTLV-I which has been identified as the primary cause of human cancer) are remarkable for their virulence (deadly nature) and for their endurance. In the words of Dr. William Haseltine of Harvard University: "Once infected, a person is infected for the rest of his life. Once infected, a person is *infectious*. It's not safe to assume otherwise."[663]

---

[660]*The Pope Speaks,* VI, (1959–1960), p. 397.

[661]Slaff, James I., MD, and Brubaker, John K., *The Aids Epidemic* (New York, N.Y.: Warner Books, Inc., 1985), pp. 268–270. Two of the primary diseases which are considered "at least moderately predictive of cellular immune deficiency" are *Kaposi's sarcoma* (a previously rare form of skin cancer which causes cancerous lesions on the skin which often spread to the lining of the mouth, the lymph glands, and many internal organs), and *Pneumocystis carinii* (a parasite that "attacks the lungs of most AIDS patients causing pneumonia . . . and is often part of the cause of death."). *Ibid.,* pp. 18, 19.

[662]*Ibid.,* pp. 46, 47 and 51, 52.

[663]*Ibid.,* p. 28.

The problem is complicated by the fact that there can be an apparent period of "latency" between infection with the AIDS and the production of measurable antibodies which provides evidence of the presence of the virus. This latent period, which was generally believed to be from two to eight weeks, has been measured to be longer than six months.[664] This emphasizes the importance of periodic testing for all individuals who may have reasons to suspect that they may have been exposed to the virus.

Although the AIDS epidemic is worldwide, the prognosis of infection in the U.S.A. alone is of horrendous proportions. Since 1981, when AIDS was officially defined, the *estimated* number of individuals infected *per month* has risen from 3,600 (1981) to 22,500 (1984). In June of 1985, Dr. James Curran of the Centers for Disease Control in Atlanta, Ga., estimated the number of infected Americans to be between 500,000 and 1 million. Others would raise that estimate to well over 1 million. In congressional testimony on July 22, 1985, Dr. Dani Bolognesi of the Duke University Medical Center said:

> Current estimates indicate that as many as 2 million people in the United States alone have already been infected . . . and are therefore at risk for developing the disease. Until preventive measures, such as vaccines, are available, this number is expected to double each year.[665]

If the more conservative figure of 1 million infected individuals as of 1985 is accepted, along with the prospect of doubling each year, the cumulative total of infected AIDS cases could exceed 30 million by the year 1990. This would mean ("quod Deus avertat," or "God forbid") that approximately 1 out of 10 Americans could be infected by the year 1990!

Since the scientific community can base predictions only from 1981 onwards (when the AIDS infection was officially defined), it is difficult to predict just how long the AIDS infection may lie dormant, or to predict how many who are diagnosed as *infected* may later develop the AIDS disease ("full-blown" AIDS). Indications are that at least 5% and perhaps 20% or more will develop the AIDS disease within 5 years of infection. An additional 25% will develop some form of what is known as the *AIDS-related complex* (ARC)

---

[664]*Ibid.,* pp. 179, 180. One of the issues which obtained the consensus of the International Conference on Aids at Atlanta, Ga., in April, 1985, was the following: "Third, most individuals remain symptomless for at least a year following infection." *Ibid.,* pp. 139, 140.

[665]*Ibid.,* p. 160. Statistics on the estimated number of people infected are found on pp. 156–159.

with symptoms such as swollen glands, persistent fever, weight loss, and diarrhea. Some of these (with ARC symptoms) will later develop the AIDS disease.[666] In other words, attention must be focused on a 3-stage possibility: the symptomless carrier of the AIDS infection, the individual with symptoms of ARC (Aids-related Complex) who has been diagnosed as infected, and the individual who has been diagnosed as having "full-blown AIDS" (AIDS disease).

Although the majority of AIDS *infection* and AIDS *disease* cases in the U.S.A. are found among homosexual and bisexual men, there is basis for the haunting fear that the epidemic may spread significantly through *heterosexual* transmission. In Africa, for example, the ratio in transmission of AIDS is approximately 50% man to woman, and 50% woman to man. Experts are divided as to whether or not a significant transmission through heterosexual contacts could happen in the U.S.A. The noted Dr. Robert Gallo of the National Cancer Institute has taken the cautious and sobering view: "Clearly the virus can go man-man, woman-woman, woman-man, and I don't think there is a single bit of interest in the mode of sex."[667]

A heart-rending risk in AIDS-related marriage is that an infection-free wife can be infected by her husband (even if symptomless and hence not diagnosed as infected), and the wife can communicate the AIDS infection to her unborn infant through the placenta or through infected mother's milk. As of October, 1985, 191 cases of AIDS among children 12 years of age or under had been reported to the Centers for Disease Control. Of this number, 143 had been infected either prenatally or perinatally through their mothers. The other cases were linked to causes such as blood transfusions, hemophilia, etc.[668] If this happens within the family, it can mean either that the parent (or parents) may not be around for long to rear the child (children), or that the infected child (children) may face death at a tender age. The risk of "full-blown" AIDS for parent and/or child cannot be denied. If that risk materializes, the statistics as established since 1981 will apply: "Statistics show that 80% of the people diagnosed as having "full-blown" AIDS will die within

---

[666]*Ibid.*, pp. 73, 74. Cf. also *The Aids Epidemic*, Kevin M. Cahill, MD, ed. (New York, N.Y.: St. Martin's Press, 1983), pp. 86, 87; chapter on "Parasitic Infections" by Kevin M. Cahill, MD.

[667]Slaff-Brubaker, *The AIDS Epidemic* (cf. note 661), p. 5. On the reality of the heterosexual spread of the AIDS virus, cf. also *The AIDS Cover-Up*, by Gene Antonio (San Francisco: Ignatius Press, 1986), pp. 81–89; *Understanding and Preventing AIDS*, by Chris Jennings (Cambridge, Ma.: Health Alert Press, 1985), pp. 17–18.

[668]Marwick, Charles, "AIDS-associated Virus Yields Data to Intensifying Scientific Study," in the *Journal of the American Medical Association*, November 22/29, 1985, pp. 2865–2870. Cf. p. 2867. Cf. also *The AIDS Epidemic*, by Slaff-Brubaker (cf. note 661), pp. 72, 73.

three years of the diagnosis, and the rest will die within five years."[669] AIDS is not compatible with marriage and family life.

In the words of Pope Pius XII as quoted above, "to advise against is not to forbid." If a law were enacted that all prospective brides and grooms must submit to the AIDS blood test sequence, and that those diagnosed as positive (hence AIDS infected) would be barred from entering a marriage contract, such a law would be, in effect, a prohibition of marriage pending the discovery of a cure for AIDS. Such a law would be a violation of human rights. Such legislation would also be of limited value in preventing the spread of AIDS since it would not detect the presence of the infection in those who are symptomless carriers of the AIDS virus ("latent" or "dormant" cases of the infection). The control of the AIDS epidemic can be promoted effectively only through adequate information, education and motivation (above all, spiritual motivation) with regard to the virulence ("deadly nature") and the risk of the transmission of AIDS, and by prudent but persistent persuasion with regard to the risks of AIDS-related marriage and procreation.

All individuals who are contemplating marriage, and who have any positive reasons for suspecting that they may have been exposed to the AIDS virus (for example, through sexual intimacy with an infected person or through needle-sharing with an infected person) should feel obligated, in justice and in charity, to submit to the AIDS blood test sequence, and to share the results of that testing procedure (if diagnosed as AIDS infected) with the prospective spouse in all honesty. If the prospective bride or groom agrees to the marriage despite the diagnosis of AIDS, the couple must be urged to seek both medical and pastoral counseling so as to receive realistic and adequate knowledge of the risks involved. The pastoral counselor will have the important and delicate task of motivating the couple (if they insist on marriage) to have recourse to Natural Family Planning so as to avoid the risk of transmitting the AIDS infection to the next generation. It should be added that if the AIDS-infected party to the marriage is unaware of the infection at the time of marriage (ignorance) or withholds knowledge of a diagnosed AIDS infection from the prospective spouse of set purpose (deceit), the marriage nevertheless would stand as valid and binding.[670]

---

[669]*Ibid.* (*The AIDS Epidemic* by Slaff-Brubaker), pp. 64, 65 and p. 73.

[670]In his address to the Seventh International Hematological Congress in Rome, Sept. 12, 1958, Pope Pius XII anticipated this question as to the validity of marriage by saying: "Aside from cases in which a party has laid down as a condition [new Code of Canon Law, Can. 1102] the absence of all hereditary disease, neither simple ignorance, nor fraudulent hiding of a hereditary defect, nor even positive error which would have halted the marriage if it had been known, is sufficient to render a marriage invalid." *The Pope Speaks,* VI (1959–1960), p. 398.

Other Exceptional Reasons for Revealing an Entrusted Secret

In some circumstances, the revelation of an entrusted secret could be required so as to avoid serious harm for an innocent third party. A young man who is intent on marriage, for example, may find out in the course of his premarital physical examination that he has primary syphilis. The scheduled wedding is only 5 days away. Unless the young man promises to inform his girlfriend and fiancée personally or to find some legitimate excuse for postponing the wedding until the disease can be cured, the physician is obligated in charity (as a last resort) to inform the young bride-to-be. Another solution might be to meet with the couple and—if a postponement of the wedding is impossible—to persuade them not to engage in marital intercourse until the disease has been brought under control.

Another reason for revealing an entrusted secret could be based on the danger of causing serious harm either to the person revealing, or to the recipient of the secret, by remaining silent. The "person revealing" could be, for example, a young man under treatment for genital herpes who had revealed to his physician the source of this infection: that he had been out of town on a specific night with a prostitute. Later on, this same young man is accused of a robbery and sent to jail. The physician realized that the night of the robbery was the very night of the young man's out-of-town episode with the prostitute. By volunteering that information to the authorities (and revealing the secret) he would save the young man from prosecution. An example of avoiding serious harm to the "recipient" could be the situation of a lawyer who is accused of misappropriating large sums of a corporation's money. One of his clients, however, had told him confidentially that he (the client) was guilty of the crime. By revealing this information to the authorities (and revealing the secret), the lawyer would protect himself from prosecution.

Privacy and Confidentiality

The phrase "right of privacy" as such is not found in the U.S. Constitution, but is gleaned from several amendments to the constitution. Within the scope of health care, the right of privacy can be described as the "interest in independence in making certain kinds of important decisions."[671] In the noted *Quinlan* decision, the New Jersey Supreme Court gave a broad interpretation to the right of privacy so as to encompass the patient's decision to decline

---

[671]*Deciding to Forego Life-Sustaining Treatment* (cf. note 215), p. 31.

medical treatment under certain circumstances—a right exercised in this particular case through the father of Karen Quinlan. With the growth of the movement for womens' rights, other court decisions expanded the scope of the right to privacy. In the *Griswold v. Connecticut* decision (1966) the U.S. Supreme Court held that a married couple has a constitutional right to use contraceptives, and indicated that the source of the right to privacy is found in the 1st, 4th, 5th, 9th and 14th amendments to the constitution.[672] Just for the record, it may be well to present "recall lines" with regard to these amendments:

(1st) Congress shall make no law respecting an establishment of religion or prohibiting the free exercise thereof . . .

(4th) The right of the people to be secure in their persons, houses, papers and effects against unreasonable searches and seizures shall not be violated . . .

(5th) No person shall be held to answer for a capital, or otherwise infamous crime, unless on a presentment or indictment of a Grand Jury . . .

(9th) The enumeration in the Constitution of certain rights, shall not be construed to deny or disparage others retained by the people . . .

(14th) . . . no state shall make or enforce any law which shall abridge the privileges or immunities of citizens of the United States . . .

The unfortunate landmark decision *Roe v. Wade* (Jan. 22, 1973) was based, in part, on the *Griswold v. Connecticut* decision, which it listed as having established the right to privacy "in the penumbras of the Bill of Rights." The court then proceeded to vindicate a woman's right to have an abortion as follows:

This right to privacy, whether it be founded in the Fourteenth Amendment's concept of personal liberty and restrictions upon state action, as we feel it is, or . . . in the Ninth Amendment's

---

[672]*Ethics in Medicine*, Stanley Joel Reiser et al., ed. (cf. note 334), p. 160.

> reservation of rights to the people, is broad enough to encompass
> a woman's decision whether or not to terminate her pregnancy.[673]

This brief background provides evidence of the need of caution in approaching issues which are said to be based on that nebulous "right of privacy." The concept can be twisted and expanded out of all due proportion in order to serve the interests of unscrupulous advocates of secular humanism.

Confidentiality serves the right of privacy as an important means of controlling, facilitating and protecting communications about intimate and sensitive information. This role includes not only concern for the privileged nature of communications between patient and physician, but also the accurate recording of such information and the effective control of access to patient records. The consultants to the *President's Commission* explained the relationship between the right of privacy and confidentiality as follows:

> Privacy is a concept that applies to *individuals* with respect to others; confidentiality is a concept that applies only to *relationships* between or among persons and institutions. Privacy concerns control over access and disclosure in the first instance; confidentiality concerns only redisclosure of information previously disclosed. Privacy is normally controlled by the individual; confidentiality by the person for/to whom the individual's privacy is relinquished.[674]

Once the patient has laid aside the prerogative of privacy to reveal innermost thoughts and feelings, the obligation to "keep it confidential" extends both to custody of the tongue and to custody of records.

It is generally agreed today that the confidential custody of medical records is more difficult in this age of computerized files and data banks. Furthermore, the proper functioning of important agencies such as ethics committees means that more individuals must be authorized to review the record files. Add to this the spectre of having the records consulted by attorneys in malpractice cases, and an argument can be made for keeping records down to a minimum—"the less said, the better." This, however, is a very dangerous and fallacious attitude. It is not only grossly unfair to the patients,

---

[673]*Ibid.*, p. 408. Cf. also *Aborting America* (cf. note 115) where Dr. Bernard Nathanson, once a leading advocate of abortion, states: "We cited in particular the *Griswold v. Connecticut* ruling striking down the anti-birth control laws on privacy grounds." P. 196.

[674]*Summing Up* (cf. note 644), p. 36.

but could be damaging to the financial status and to the reputation of the hospital. The best protection that hospitals, physicians, and health professionals have in civil malpractice cases comes from accurate, complete, and trustworthy records.[675]

Faulty and inadequate record-keeping is unfair to the patient. The physical pieces of paper, cards, books or computer "soft-wear" which constitute the hospital records clearly are the property of the hospital. The patient has a right to say, however, "that is MY record,"—and even "that record is my lifeline for future treatment." That record is the most (and perhaps the only reliable) probatory record of care rendered to the patient. Future diagnosis and treatment may depend on reliability of information, particularly when the record is used by physicians or other health personnel who do not know the patient, or were not involved in the patient's previous care. The welfare of the patient must be first and primary in the maintenance, care and custody of hospital records. If such records are complete, legible, unaltered and properly authenticated, they will also serve the material and financial interests of the hospital adequately when subjected to the scrutiny of government reimbursement programs, regulatory and accrediting agencies, malpractice attorneys, etc. Concern for the patient as a primary concern will guarantee these important dividends. Competent hospital administrators cannot afford to neglect the records department. Prudent record policies and regulations must be established and monitored accordingly.[676]

As important as the principle of denying access to hospital records to those who are not authorized to see them, is the principle that the patient has a right of access to his or her medical record. In the absence of legislation to the contrary, the patient may exercise that right to access directly without the intervention of an attorney. The hospital may limit the right with respect to matters which may be harmful to the patient or to others, but must bear the burden of providing adequate justification for whatever limitations it imposes. The hospital should take reasonable precautions in complying with a patient's request for access to his or her records. This would include seeking reliable information and identification of the patient (or his or her agent), a requirement that the request be made in writing and duly signed, and a prohibition against allowing the record to leave the hospital.[677]

---

[675]"The Medical Record as a Legal Document," in *Hospital Law*, John F. Horty, ed. (Pittsburgh, Pa.: Action Kit for Hospital Law, 1981), Jan., 1985, p. 1.

[676]*Ibid.*, PP. 1 and 10 (includes a recommended hospital policy for records).

[677]*Hospital Law* (cf. note 675), "Patient's Right of Access to His Medical Records," March, 1978, pp. 8, 9.

9.3   The "Theft" of Personal Secrets

The moral law forbids not only the unjustified disclosure of a secret, but also any voluntary effort to steal the secret of another. Dishonest means which could be used to accomplish such a purpose might be eavesdropping, opening personal letters, planting of electronic recording devices, use of drugs, bribery, torture, etc. The focus here is on the use of drugs to probe the innermost feelings, dispositions and recollections of the patient in the treatment of the mentally ill. The word "theft" is used in parentheses to indicate that there is no inference that the psychologist or psychiatrist is operating like a "Grand Inquisitor," exacting secret knowledge by force or fear. Within the patient-physician relationship, there is the assumption that inner knowledge and revelations are sought in the hope that such knowledge will shed light on the proper avenue to be pursued in restoring the patient to health. Yet, in line with the common definition of stealing as "taking without right or permission," there is an element of "theft" to the extent that there are things that no one has a right to know, and secret knowledge which the patient has no right to reveal.

Primitive peoples used narcotic potions to uncover secrets or to obtain confessions from suspected criminals. With the discovery of barbiturates, civilized nations resorted to narcoanalysis (from the Greek "narkoun," meaning to benumb) in probing for the truth and in the treatment of the mentally ill. As the drug (usually Sodium Aymtal) is slowly administered, the patient is asked to recite numbers aloud; this induces sleep and indicates when the patient is in sleep. One neuropsychologist describes the procedure as follows:

> Doctors make use of the pre-narcotic phase to [begin] questioning; this is also resumed and filled out by suitable suggestions and psychotherapeutic advice for the post-narcotic passage from sleep to awakening. During these twilight pre- and post-narcotic periods, spontaneous statements reveal complexes and feelings usually locked up in the subconscious; whatever is said, along with the gestures or mimicking expressions that sometimes accompany the recall of a painful event, is carefully noted down, since this represents material for further questioning, interpretation, suggestions, on which the psychotherapeutic action of the doctor will be based.[678]

---

[678]Rizzo, Dr. Carlo, *Dictionary of Moral Theology* (cf. note 346), p. 1109.

The effects of narcoanalysis were closely related to hypnosis. It had an advantage over hypnosis, however, because it could be administered to persons who could not be hypnotized. According to one expert, the results of narcoanalysis were of no value in about half of the cases "in the sense that the questioning during pre- or post-narcotic phases reveals nothing helpful to the diagnosis, neither changes of the emotions, nor appreciable results in the treatment."[679]

The 1955 version of the *Ethical and Religious Directives for Catholic Hospitals* included a directive (n.45) on "the use of narcosis or hypnosis for the cure of mental illness" [not included in the present Directives] which allowed such procedures with the consent "at least reasonably presumed of the patient" and "provided due precautions are taken to protect the patient and hospital from harmful effects, and provided the patient's right to secrecy is duly safeguarded."[680] The same 1955 version also had a directive (n.46) on "psychoanalysis or any other form of psychotherapy." That directive included "cautions as to sound morality" as follows (Cf. Deddens, *op cit.*, p.190):

> The psychiatrists and psychotherapists, however, must observe the cautions dictated by sound morality, such as: avoiding the error of pan-sexualism; never counseling even material sin; respecting secrets that the patient is not permitted to reveal; avoiding the disproportionate risk of moral dangers.

Pope Pius XII and Psychotherapeutic Practices

The "cautions as to sound morality" listed above undoubtedly were based in part on several addresses of Pope Pius XII to scientific groups in the 1950's. In his address to the First International Congress of Histopathology on Sept. 13, 1952, he branded as "untrue" several postulates of "the pan-sexual method of a certain school of psychoanalysis."[681] In his address to the Congress of Psychotherapy and Clinical Psychology on April 15, 1953, he spoke of the danger of "bringing to the level of consciousness of all the imaginations, emotions, and sexual experiences which lie dormant in the memory and the unconscious, and which are psychically experienced."[682] In the same

---

[679]*Ibid.*, p. 1109. Cf. also *Psychiatry and Catholicism*, by James H. Vander Veldt, O.F.M., Ph.D., and Robert P. Odenwald, MD, F.A.P.A. (New York, N.Y.: McGraw-Hill Book Co., Inc., 1952), pp. 69, 70.

[680]Kelly, Gerald, S.J., *Medico-Moral Problems* (cf. note 22), p. 282.

[681]The Human Body (cf. note 61), p. 200.

[682]*Ibid.*, p. 233.

address, with regard to the safeguarding of secrets in psychoanalytic treatments, he stressed the principle of discretion as applying to both the patient and the therapist:

> From the moral standpoint, and first and foremost for the common good, the principle of discretion in the use of psychoanalysis cannot be sufficiently stressed. Obviously it is not primarily a question of the discretion of the psychoanalyst, but of that of the patient, who frequently has no right whatever to give away his secrets.[683]

There may be personal secrets about an individual which *that specific individual* should "keep to himself" or "keep to herself" forever. The thought of Pope Pius XII on the prime responsibility of the patient NOT to reveal such secrets, is clarified in his address to the Congress of the International Association of Applied Psychology on April 10, 1958. Referring to the "right of the person to protect his inner world," he speaks of moral obligations to maintain a sense of a religious spirit, self-esteem, modesty, decency. The psychologist or therapist is not acting morally if he probes into these areas of moral obligations without first examining each individual case to determine "whether one of these motives of the moral order does not stand in the way of his intervention and, if so, precisely, to what extent."[684]

Pius XII admits that professionals such as physicians and psychologists have either an explicit or implicit right to subject a person to certain tests even though such tests may "run the risk in certain cases of arousing immoral thoughts," but he adds: "the use of such tests becomes moral when proportionate motives justify the danger risked."[685] The general rule is that it is immoral to penetrate into the conscience of anyone unless the therapist has a right to do so (consent), and has a proportionate motive or reason for doing so. Father Gerald Kelly, S.J. explores this problem, and emphasizes the importance of being treated by a conscientious psychologist or psychiatrist—a professional who will not in any way try to influence the conscience of the patient.[686]

---

[683] *Ibid.*, p. 234.

[684] *The Pope Speaks*, summer, 1958, p. 16.

[685] *Ibid.*, p. 18.

[686] *Medico-Moral Problems* (cf. note 22), pp. 286, 287.

Contemporary Psychiatric Treatment

One reason why procedures such as narcoanalysis, lobotomy, etc. are not mentioned in the present hospital Directives presumably is because they have been superceded by more effective treatments and techniques. The difference between neurosis and psychosis is no longer confusing to the average American. People understand quite generally that the neurotic person (whose name is "legion") is affected by relatively minor disorders of the psychic constitution which does not affect his or her general behavior pattern—and that the psychotic person suffers from a more pervasive and prolonged behavior disorder (including schizophrenia, and manic-depressive states). Those of the neurotic variety might even look upon having their own psychiatrist or psychologist as something of a status symbol. The need of psychotherapeutic guidance and treatment has simply expanded with the hectic pace of contemporary living.

Even for the management of the chronically ill schizophrenic patient, the trend has been away from prolonged and continuous inpatient treatment and hospitalization to a regimen of repeated brief hospitalizations for recurrent episodes of illness. The locale for treatment is shifting away from large state-owned and state-operated hospitals to treatment settings in local communities.[687] Many of the former treatments such as lobotomies are now regarded as old-fashioned.[688]

For the treatment of schizophrenia in a hospital setting, the emphasis today is on a three-pronged "psychotherapeutic management" including individual, group and family involvement with emphasis on chemotherapy.[689] For non-schizophrenic patients with an affective disorder, medication may include lithium, phenothiazines or tricyclic compounds. For patients with neuroses and personality disorders, the tri-level approach of efforts and interaction between the individual, the family, and group involvement (group psychotherapy) is pursued, with reliance on drug therapy as required.[690] These trends are more protective of personal secrets than the former narcoanalytic approach to mental illness. To the extent that the contemporary use of drugs may involve probing into the "inner world" and conscience of the patient,

---

[687]Glick, Ira D., and Hargreaves, William, *Psychiatric Hospital Treatment For the 1980's* (Lexington, Ma.: D.C. Heath and Co., 1979), p. 1.

[688]"Physical Manipulation of the Brain," in the *Hastings Center Report,* special supplement, May, 1972, pp. 13, 14.

[689]Glick/Hargreaves (cf. note 687), pp. 3, 4.

[690]*Ibid.,* p. 26.

however, the guidelines outlined by Pope Pius XII should be found valid and helpful.

It is safe to suspect that secrets may be revealed more readily and frequently by the individual who is "under the influence" of drugs. A recent edition of the *Journal of Health and Human Resources Administration* reports that well over 30 million Americans consider drugs to be a needed part of their existence. This category includes business men and professionals, housewives and career women, teenagers and old folks, sports heroes and the disabled. The report adds that "alcohol is now the constant accompaniment to virtually every other drug."[691] The drugs used include not only cocaine, marijuana, heroin and inhalants (spray paint, airplane glue, hairspray, gasoline) but also prescription drugs. The culprits include the over-prescribing physician and the pharmacist who knowingly fills questionable prescriptions.[692] Two encouraging efforts to stem the tide of drug abuse are the self-help movement known as Narcotics Anonymous, and the Parents Movement (supported by First Lady Nancy Reagan). The following statement expresses both a reproach and a promise: "A recognition of what voluntarism and self-help have to offer has been late in coming."[693]

Directive 9: The obligation of professional secrecy must be carefully fulfilled not only as regards the information on the patients' charts and records but also as regards confidential matters learned in the exercise of professional duties. Moreover, the charts and records must be duly safeguarded against inspection by those who have no right to see them.

---

[691]Winter issue, 1985, p. 398.

[692]*Ibid.*, p. 400.

[693]*Journal of Health and Human Resources Administration*, Winter, 1985, p. 407.

CHAPTER X

The Principle of Material Cooperation

The Congregation, while it confirms this traditional doctrine of the Church (on direct sterilization), is not unaware of the dissent against this teaching from many theologians. The Congregation, however, denies that doctrinal significance can be attributed to this fact as such, so as to constitute a "theological source" which the faithful might follow and thereby abandon the authentic magisterium, and follow the opinions of private theologians which dissent from it (Reply of the Sacred Congregation for the Doctrine of the Faith, March 13, 1975.)

PRINCIPLE: THE TRADITIONAL DOCTRINE REGARDING MATERIAL COOPERATION, WITH THE PROPER DISTINCTION BETWEEN NECESSARY AND FREE, PROXIMATE AND REMOTE, REMAINS VALID, TO BE APPLIED WITH THE UTMOST PRUDENCE, IF THE CASE WARRANTS. IN THE APPLICATION OF THE PRINCIPLE OF MATERIAL COOPERATION. . . GREAT CARE MUST BE TAKEN AGAINST SCANDAL AND THE DANGER OF ANY MISUNDERSTANDING BY AN APPROPRIATE EXPLANATION OF WHAT IS REALLY BEING DONE (*Ibid*).

The problem of material cooperation has been a primary concern of the American Catholic hierarchy, of hospital authorities and of moralists throughout the past twenty years. Well in advance of the formal approval of the present *Catholic Hospital Directives* by the National Council of Catholic Bishops (NCCB) and the United States Catholic Conference (USCC) in November, 1971, representatives of the hierarchy, hospital authorities and the theological community joined forces to address questions which involved basically a trend towards an expanded application of the Principle of Material Cooperation. The sequence of events was outlined by Msgr. Harrold Murray, then Director of the Department of Health Affairs of the USCC, in his report to the annual convention of the Catholic Hospital Association (CHA) in Atlantic City, N.J. on June 11, 1971. He described the background of growing concern as follows:

> At Board of Trustees meetings of the Catholic Hospital Association in 1965–1966, I began to detect a few rumblings of concerns—questions, informal comments about the need to restudy some directives in light of theological and medical advances. It was about this time that many other changes were taking place in society and in the Church—Vatican II, race, poverty, Vietnam, captured the headlines and front pages . . . This also marked the beginning of serious inquiries from the field regarding sterilization, family planning centers, formal and material cooperation, abortion and the role of the Catholic health facility in the one-hospital community.[694]

10.1 HISTORICAL BACKGROUND, OCTOBER, 1967, to NOVEMBER, 1971

The events which led up to the approval of the present Catholic hospital directives were sketched only in broad outline in chapter I. The original intention was to present a more-or-less complete scenario of those events in this chapter. Limitations of space will allow nothing more, however, than a summary listing of dates, deliberations and/or decisions. Also in the interests

---

[694]"Historical Reflections" (cf. note 8), p. 5.

of brevity, abbreviations will be used as follows when referring to certain agencies:

NCCB = The National Conference of Catholic Bishops
USCC = The United States Catholic Conference
CHA = The Catholic Health Association
CCHA = The Commission on Church Health Affairs
Directives = *The Ethical and Religious Directives for Catholic Health Facilities.*

1) October, 1967, the CHA Board of Trustees agreed to seek the guidance of the American hierarchy with regard to the "application of Catholic doctrine to the complex questions arising from the changing legal and social character of our private, Church-related hospitals." Later that year, the USCC established the CCHA, which was to operate under the sponsorship of the USCC Bureau of Health and Hospitals.[695] One of the first objectives of this new commission was to explore the status of Catholic hospitals by organizing first a meeting of scholars and experts to discuss the *legal* aspects of the issues involved, and then a second meeting of other scholars and experts to discuss the *theological* aspects.

2) March, 1968, the 5-member CCHA arranged a 2-day meeting in Washington, D.C., with a *panel of 6 attorneys,* plus resource persons from the fields of theology, medicine and canon law. The meeting resulted in a cautious but affirmative answer to the question: Does the Board of Trustees of a voluntary non-profit hospital, as a corporate entity, have the right to prohibit or restrict medical services and procedures which are legally and medically acceptable?[696]

3) February, 1969, the pre-planned meeting on the *theological* aspects of the question above was arranged by the CCHA. It took the form of a 2-day meeting in Washington, D.C., of a *panel of 5 theologians* plus resource persons from the field of medicine. In his *Historical Reflections,* Msgr. Harrold Murray stated that the theologians "lacked a consensus in their discussion of solutions of critical questions confronting Catholic-sponsored hospitals, such as sterilization procedures and family planning services." Motion #3 which resulted from this meeting (duly seconded and approved) drew attention to the Principle of Material Cooperation:

Inasmuch as strict adherence to the *Ethical and Religious Directives for Catholic Hospitals* brings serious moral dilemmas in contempo-

---

[695]*Ibid.,* p. 5.
[696]*Ibid.,* pp. 5, 6.

rary Catholic hospital administration and practice, immediate consideration should be given to provisions of the application of the Directives in a pluralistic situation, and more specifically to the role of the individual conscience and the question of cooperation, as a matter of priority.[697]

Representatives of both groups (nn.2) and 3) above on the "legal" and "theological" aspects) met the following July to draw up a report to the American hierarchy.

4) At the September, 1969 meeting of the USCC administrative board, the Department of Health Affairs (sponsoring group of the CCHA, formerly known as the Bureau of Health and Hospitals) was directed to proceed with the work of preparing recommendations for episcopal review and approval. The three theologians who were selected to prepare a draft revision of the *Directives*, Jesuit Fathers Richard McCormick and John R. Connery and Father Paul E. McKeever (then editor of the *Long Island Catholic*), were more intent on expanding the application of the Principle of Material Cooperation than on revising the 1955-version of the *Directives*. This was reflected in their proposed preamble to the *Directives* which was submitted to the episcopal chairman of the Committee on Health Affairs in October, 1970. The concluding paragraph of the preamble follows:

> The Catholic hospital should try, as in the past, to secure the implementation of the guidelines insofar as the situation permits, but it is important for hospital administrators to know the limitations which traditional principles place on their responsibility in this regard. Far from imposing an obligation to enforce the guidelines in all situations, these principles allow for material cooperation with procedures that might do more harm than good. So there is no thought of abandoning or compromising principles in any way. There is, however, a recognition of the changed situation of today which, at least in some hospitals, will warrant material cooperation more often than in the past. An attempt to apply the guidelines as strictly as in the past will not be realistic and might well undo much of the good that a particular Catholic hospital has

---

[697] *Ibid.*, p. 6. According to the files of the Pope John Center, the five theologians were: Msgr. Austin Vaughan (presently an auxiliary bishop of the Archdiocese of New York); Fr. Richard McCormick, S.J.; Fr. Warren Reich, M.SS.T.; Fr. Kieran Nolan, O.S.B; Fr. John Lynch, S.J.

achieved in a community for many years, and would hope to continue.[698]

5) The "behind the scenes" discussions and changes which must have taken place between 1970 and the approval of the present *Directives* in November, 1971, were merely inferred in Monsignor Murray's *Historical Reflections:*

> February 9, 1971 Bishop Guilfoyle sent a copy of the Ethical and Religious Directives approved by the Committee on Doctrine to the bishops for use in their dioceses if they so desired. Since publication, many bishops have adopted these Directives. These and others have made constructive comments on the document.
>
> On the occasion of the April, 1971 meeting of the National Conference of Catholic Bishops in Detroit, the episcopal members of the Committee on Health Affairs discussed the comments received thus far. Our meeting was attended by members of the Committee on Doctrine. As a result of that meeting, and in view of the limited agenda of the NCCB meeting, it was decided to study further the comments and suggestions received. The Committee on Health Affairs would then present any revisions agreed upon to the Committee on Doctrine for advice in sufficient time to send recommendations to all the bishops before the November meeting of the National Conference of Catholic Bishops. It is hoped that in November there can be a discussion of the Directives and a vote on adoption as the national code for use in each diocese remaining subject to the approval of the local bishop. This in no way affects those dioceses where the Directives have been officially adopted.[699]

Reactions to the Three-Theologian Revision

After the bishops throughout the nation had received copies of the revised *Directives,* comments and suggestions were forwarded to the Committee on Health Affairs. It became apparent that the proposed preamble as above

---

[698]Deddens, Clarence, *A Theological Analysis of the Ethical and Religious Directives for Catholic Health Facilities in the United States* (cf. note 17), p. 26. The quotation above was taken from a letter of Father Paul McKeever to Bishop Guilfoyle, dated October 9, 1970.

[699]"Historical Reflections" (cf. note 8), pp. 7, 8. Msgr. Harrold Murray was Director of the Department of Health Affairs of the USCC as well as a member of the Commission on Church Health Affairs.

would have to be changed. The new Chairman of the Committee on Doctrine, Archbishop John F. Whealon of Hartford, Conn. wrote a substitute version of the preamble.[700] In February, 1971, each bishop received a copy of the *Directives* as approved by the Committee on Doctrine for immediate use in each diocese as the Ordinary might decide.[701]

Expressions of disappointment came from several quarters. The Catholic Health Association people (then known as the Catholic Hospital Association) were unhappy because they wanted the *Directives* to be approved well in advance of the annual bishops' meeting in November. The attitude of the three theologians was, in effect: "without the preamble we proposed, why bother with a new code of regulations." Some of the Catholic physicians were apprehensive about one or the other of the *Directives*.[702] It was especially around this period when Father Thomas O'Donnell, S.J. became very helpful to the members of the Committee on Health Affairs in clarifying certain concepts which could have been subject to misinterpretation. He emerged as the guiding spirit of the revised code of hospital *Directives*. He was present, along with Msgr. Harrold Murray, at the meeting of the American bishops on November 16, 1971 to respond to any questions regarding the *Directives*. It was at this meeting that a motion was made "that the 'Ethical and Religious Directives for Catholic Health Facilities' be adopted as a national code and that it be up to the bishops to apply them in their dioceses." The motion passed by a written vote of: yes, 232; no, 7; abstain, 2."[703]

Reactions to the Revised Directives

It is worthy of special note that only 7 of the American bishops (out of a total of 241) had voted against the adoption of the revised hospital *Directives*. The guidance in moral-medical problems which administrators of Catholic

---

[700]Cf. Deddens, Clarence (cf. note 17), p. 34.

[701]*Ibid.*, p. 36. See also Msgr. Murray's comments on the previous page.

[702]*Ibid.* (Deddens), pp. 37–50. Father Deddens (*Ibid.*, pp. 61–71) presents a lengthy account of what he calls an "Attempt at a Third Version." Suffice it to say (as in the words of Msgr. Murray on the previous page) that the members of the Committee on Doctrine and of the Committee on Health Affairs reacted appropriately by taking the time to "study further the comments and suggestions received." By October 30, 1971, the final revision (including a third version of the preamble) was ready to be submitted to the Bishops at their November, 1971 meeting (Cf. Deddens, *ibid.*, pp. 70–72).

[703]*Ibid.*, p. 74.

hospitals had requested of the hierarchy 4 years previously was timely and appreciated. Members of the Catholic medical community also voiced their approval. At the November, 1971 meeting of the National Federation of Catholic Physicians' Guilds in New Orleans, John Brennan, MD defended the promulgation of the revised code, and echoed the words of an American Cardinal (John Cardinal Cody): "As teachers of the people and protectors of life, it is high time we make these norms obligatory."[704] Similar sentiments of commendation were expressed by the editor of the *Linacre Quarterly*, John Mullooly, MD: "Delegates to the annual meeting unanimously approved a resolution commending the U.S. Conference of Bishops for exercising their teaching authority."[705]

Unfortunately, the promulgation of the revised *Directives* did not serve to temper the pronouncements of those who had opposed the approval of the code. One influential theologian wrote that the bishops had failed "to deal adequately" with the "phenomenon of cooperation" and the "phenomenon of dissent."[706] The report of the Study Commission on Ethical and Religious Directives which had been established by the Catholic Theological Society of America in June, 1971 was very specific in pointing out just how the right of dissent would influence moral-medical decisions:

> It should also be noted that a substantial number of Catholic theologians believe that there can be legitimate dissent from several of the specific paragraphs in the recently promulgated code, including the following: the condemnations of contraception, direct sterilization, masturbation for seminal analysis, and artificial insemination with the husband's seed; the processes forbidden in the handling of extrauterine pregnancies; and the distinction between direct and indirect which is stated in terms of physical structure of the act itself.[707]

An underlying reason for such liberal views can be found in the divergent concept of the magisterium of the Church as a "multidimensional process"

---

[704]"Quicksands of Compromise," in *Linacre Quarterly*, Feb., 1972, p. 13.

[705]"From the Editor's Desk," in *Linacre Quarterly*, Feb., 1972, p. 5.

[706]"Not What Catholic Hospitals Ordered" by Richard A. McCormick, S.J. in *Linacre Quarterly*, Feb., 1972, p. 19.

[707]"Catholic Hospital Ethics" in *Linacre Quarterly*, Nov., 1972, pp. 246–268. Quotation found on pp. 266, 267. The chairman of the commission was Warren Reich, then with the Kennedy Center for Bioethics, Georgetown University, Washington, D.C.

involving various functions and lay participation on various levels:

> When these functions are related to individual persons in the
> Church, it might be possible to say that the magisterium is com-
> posed of three distinguishable components: the prophetic charism
> (very broadly understood as previously noted, so as to include
> many competences); the doctrinal-pastoral charism of the hierar-
> chy; and the scientific charism of the theologian. It is the interplay
> of these charisms that constitutes the full teaching function of the
> Church, and I would suggest that it is the proper and harmonious
> interplay of these functions that yields a healthy, vigorous, and
> effective magisterium.[708]

Such an interpretation of "He who hears you, hears Me" (Luke,10:16) represents a radical departure from the description of the magisterium of the
Church as found in Vatican II's *Dogmatic Constitution on Divine Revelation*
(n.10), and in the *Dogmatic Constitution on the Church* (n.25).

Commentary on the Historical Background

There is evidence that many of the theologians, Catholic attorneys and
health-care personnel and others who were involved in the hospital *Directives*
revision process actually labored under one or both of two hovering clouds of
doubt and apprehension: one was the influence of the route in moral-medical
problems as taken by the Canadian bishops; the other was a lack of faith in
the protective stance of the American legal system with regard to religious
health facilities.

1) Influence of the Route Chosen by the Canadian Hierarchy

For many years, the Catholic bishops of Canada shared the same standards on moral-medical problems as their counterparts to the south in the
U.S.A. A radical change in the Canadian view of the role of the Church in
the conduct of hospitals was announced by Archbishop J. Hayes of Halifax in
an address to the Atlantic Conference of Catholic hospitals, in October, 1968:

In its broad outlines the present situation would appear as follows.

---

[708]McCormick, Richard, S.J., *Health and Medicine in the Catholic Tradition* (cf. note 206), p. 68.
Cf. also Reich, Warren, "Policy vs. Ethics" in *Linacre Quarterly*, Feb., 1972, pp. 22-25; McBrien,
Richard P., *Catholicism*, 2 vols., I (Minneapolis, MN.: Winston Press, 1980), pp. 71, 72.

The practical necessity for the existence of specifically Catholic hospitals in society has been transformed into a practical impossibility of maintaining them. As the public conscience and the public authority assume responsibility, they assume corresponding rights of administration and direction which were formally [perhaps this should be "formerly"] exercised autonomously by the Church . . . In short, the Catholic hospital is being forced by its factual situation to accept the pluralism which characterizes the community it serves . . . The bearing of Christian witness and the promotion of Christian ethical standards will be the responsibility of the practitioner. Moral judgment and responsibility will be taken out of the hands of a specifically Catholic administration and will reside in the individual Christian conscience.[709]

This unfolding of what one Canadian theologian called the "New Approach to Morality" is well documented in a comparison of the preambles of the U.S. hospital *Directives,* and the Canadian "Medical-Moral Guide" (approved, April 9, 1970): definitely an illustration of the *objective* stance of the U.S. hospital code and the *subjective* stance of the Canadian "Medical-Moral Guide:"

U.S. Code	*Reflecting the Moral Teachings of the Church*	*Canadian Guide*
Any facility identified as Catholic assumes with this identification the responsibility to reflect in its policies and practices the moral teachings of the Church under the guidance of the local bishop.		But Christian moral life may not be viewed solely from the point of formal enactment of law and not even primarily from the standpoint of the imperative of the divine will. With such an approach, one cannot grasp the meaning of Christian moral life.

Binding Power of the Directives (Guidelines)

The Catholic sponsored health facility and its board of trustees . . . carry an overriding responsibility in conscience to prohibit those proce-		The Guidelines present a concise statement of these exigencies in the field of hospital work. They should be read and understood not as com-

---

[709]Address entitled "The Validity of a "Catholic" Hospital" (4 pages), in *Catholic Hospital Association of Canada Bulletin*, June, 1968, pp. 1, 2.

dures which are morally and spiritually harmful.

These directives prohibit those procedures which, according to present knowledge, are recognized as clearly wrong. The basic moral absolutes which underlie these directives are not subject to change.

mands imposed from without, but as demands of the inner dynamism of human and Christian life.

In certain complex situations, and owing as much to the difficulty as to the importance of the decision, personal conscience will benefit from the opinions of specialists.

Final Word in Difficult Situations

The moral evaluation of new scientific developments and legitimately debated questions must be finally submitted to the teaching authority of the Church in the person of the local bishop, who has the ultimate responsibility for teaching Catholic doctrine.

The Guidelines therefore propose the appointment of medico-moral committees whose work should be particularly important for the solution of concrete cases and for the continuing revision of the present Guidelines.[710]

There is no question here of sitting in judgment against the Catholic hierarchy of Canada. The point is that the bishops of Canada, in the words of Archbishop Hayes (quoted above), were convinced of the "practical impossibility of maintaining Catholic hospitals," presumably because of the peculiar situation of the Church and the "altered social condition" in Canada. The Catholic bishops of the U.S.A. see no insurmountable obstacle to preserving the apostolic quality of the Catholic mission of healing "by fidelity to the Church's teachings while ministering to the good of the whole person" (preamble). This was indicated as a resounding conviction in the November, 1971 vote to approve of the present *Directives* by a written vote of 232 "yes" to 7 "no" votes (and two abstentions). It would have been highly illogical for them to consider seriously the route taken by our Catholic neighbors to the north.

---

[710]Quotations from the Canadian *Medico-Moral Guide* (1970 edition). There is a similarity between the concepts conveyed in this *Medico-Moral Guide* and the arguments advanced in the final report of the commission established by the Catholic Theological Society of America as referred to in note 707 above. The Canadian *Medico-Moral Guide* was approved by the Canadian Catholic Conference (Canadian Hierarchy) at their plenary session in Ottawa, April 9, 1970.

2) Apprehension Over Legislative or Judicial Interventions

The cloud of apprehension lest legislative or judicial agencies might force Catholic hospitals to allow their facilities to be used for prohibited procedures can be magnified beyond reason. That danger could be very real in countries where the legal status and security of the Church depends upon the whim of a dictator or the decrees of a military junta or of a socialistic policy-bureau,— but the government of the U.S.A. is a government by law. Legal actions against a physician or against a Catholic hospital for not honoring a patient's demand for an abortion or for a sterilization procedure have been raised in the past, and undoubtedly will be raised in the future. If Catholic hospital policies with regard to such prohibited procedures are properly grounded in the civil incorporation process, however, they do not constitute grounds for governmental intervention (known as "state action"). A recent publication of the Division of Legal Services for the Catholic Health Association (1984) fortifies this confidence in government by law:

> Catholic hospitals have not been immune from these pressures, but to date attempts to force them to allow abortions or sterilizations on the basis of "state action" have been uniformly unsuccessful.[711]

In a leading case regarding refusal of a Catholic hospital to allow a woman to undergo a tubal ligation at the time of her cesarean delivery, the hospital relied on a pertinent portion of the "Church Amendment" to the Health Programs Extension Act of 1973, which reads as follows:

> Sec.401(b). The receipt of any grant, loan, or loan guarantee under the Public Health Service Act, the Community Mental Health Centers Act, or the Developmental Disabilities Service and Facilities Construction Act by any individual or entity does not authorize any court or any public official or other public authority to require . . . such entity to . . . make its facilities available for the performance of any sterilization procedure or abortion if the performance of such procedure or abortion in such facilities is prohibited by the entity on the basis of religious beliefs or moral convictions . . . .

---

[711] *In Defense of Values* (cf. note 635), p. 1.

The decision of the trial court, affirmed by the court of appeals, was in favor of the hospital. As to the rights of the patient who was denied the tubal ligation, the court found that any infringement of the patient's right to privacy "is outweighed by the need to protect the freedom of religion of denominational hospitals having 'religious or moral scruples against sterilizations and abortions.'" This important case is known as *Taylor v. St. Vincent's Hospital*. Of special significance is the fact that St. Vincent's Hospital was the ONLY health facility in that area which was able to provide the requested services.[712]

10.2 TRADITIONAL DOCTRINE ON MATERIAL COOPERATION

Before proceeding to explain the traditional doctrine of the Church with regard to material cooperation and its application to sterilization cases, it must be stressed that the Holy See and the members of the American hierarchy had gone to great lengths to clarify that traditional doctrine. Without doubt, the Holy See considered seriously the arguments of the opposition before issuing the definitive reply of March 13, 1975 "on Sterilization in Catholic Hospitals." That reply begins with an assurance that the Holy See had considered "diligently" not only the problem of contraceptive sterilization for therapeutic purposes "but also the opinions indicated by different people toward a solution, and the conflicts relative to requests for cooperation in such sterilizations in Catholic hospitals" (Appendix, lines 1–6). Undoubtedly, all of these "opinions" and "conflicts" were duly emphasized when Archbishop Quinn and several other members of the American Catholic hierarchy met with Pope Paul VI and also with the Sacred Congregation for the Doctrine of the Faith in early 1975 (p.15).

The Holy See took the time and the trouble to mention and reject three principal arguments which were used extensively to prevent the emergence of the revised directives as obligatory moral-medical hospital standards. These were the argument from the common good, the argument based on the Principle of Totality, and the argument based on the legitimate right to dissent.

The Rejection of Three Arguments for Direct Sterilization

The argument for the common good was multifaceted. It was based on deep sentiments that Catholic morality should not be imposed upon non-

---

[712]*Ibid.*, pp. 6, 7. Cf. also the Appendix, lines 134–138, *NCCB Commentary, 1977.*

Catholic patients; that a realistic recognition of pluralism requires a willing-ness to serve the medical needs of others in accord with their own moral values; that medical reasons such as a bad heart should entitle a woman to a directly-sterilizing operation if she has a subjectively-right intention; that civil authority might protect the citizens and the state from defective progeny by legislating sterilization for certain couples. Only the last two arguments above (*medical* reasons; *civil* legislation) were rejected verbatim in the Reply of March 13, 1975 (Appendix, lines 11–22). The first two arguments (imposing morals; pluralism) were answered effectively by Father Kevin O'Rourke, O.P. as follows:

> From a theological point of view, it is clear that principles and values of Catholic morality should not be imposed upon others. But by the same token, a person or an institution should not be forced to surrender important principles and values in the course of serving the public. Patients and physicians are not forced to use Catholic hospitals; if they chose to use these facilities, such hospi-tals have a right to provide services in accordance with their reli-gious beliefs. . . . The United States, according to its Constitution, is a pluralistic society, but it is not a secular society . . . In a secular society, religious organizations are not allowed a place in public life if their values conflict with those of the society.[713]

As to the argument for allowing direct sterilization based on the Principle of Totality, the responses of the Holy See (Reply of March 13, 1975) and of Pope Pius XII are presented in chapter III on the Principle of the Right to Life (pp.85,86). In its traditional sense, the Principle of Totality is restricted to the promotion and preservation of the *functional wholeness of the human body*. Several contemporary writers would extend the application of the Principle of Totality well beyond the functional wholeness of the human body to "an all-embracing concept of totality, the dignity and well-being of man as a person in all his essential relationships to God, to his fellow man, and to the world around him."[714] With such a view of totality, one might conclude that it would be for the overall good (physical, psychological, emotional, etc.) of a woman with a serious heart or kidney condition, if she could submit to a sterilizing procedure so as not to have another pregnancy. The Reply of March 13, 1975

---

[713]"An Analysis of the Church's Teaching on Sterilization," in *Hospital Progress,* May, 1976, pp. 70, 71.

[714]Häring, Bernard, C.SS.R., *Medical Ethics* (cf. note 60), p. 62.

is saying, in effect (Appendix, lines 11–29): "Do not call evil good. A tubal ligation or vasectomy in such a case would be evil because it would amount to deliberately depriving freely-chosen conjugal love of openness to new life." Disposing deliberately of that gift of the reproductive faculty for the "good" of the whole person would be sinful."[715]

As to the third argument rejected in the reply of the Holy See, that is, the one based on the legitimate right to dissent, it is clear from Vatican II's *Dogmatic Constitution on the Church* that submission of mind and will must be manifested in a special way to the "authentic teaching authority of the Roman Pontiff, even when he is not speaking ex cathedra." The quotation continues:

> That is, it must be shown in such a way that his supreme magisterium is acknowledged with reverence, the judgments made by him are sincerely adhered to, according to his manifest mind and will. His mind and will in the matter may be known chiefly either from the character of the documents, from his frequent repetition of the same doctrine, or from his manner of speaking (n.25).

Applying these standards to the Reply on sterilization of March 13, 1975, it should be apparent that Pope Paul VI went to extreme lengths to emphasize "his manifest mind and will." Such "manifestation" is clear from

(1) *"The character of the documents:"* the document resulted from a personal meeting of representatives of the American hierarchy with the Holy Father and with members of the Sacred Congregation for the Doctrine of the Faith; the document begins with a statement that diligent consideration had been given to opinions and conflicts regarding the problem of contraceptive sterilization; the document's doctrinal and theological significance is acknowledged and emphasized by the American hierarchy's *Commentary on the Reply of March 13, 1975* under date of Sept. 15, 1977 and their *Statement on Tubal Ligation* (July 3, 1980).

(2) *"His frequent repetition of the same doctrine:"* Footnote 1 of the Reply of March 13, 1975, which follows the definition of direct sterilization, refers to Pope Paul VI's encyclical letter "Humanae Vitae" (n.14) and to two of Pope Pius XII's addresses which stress the Church's traditional doctrine on direct sterilization (to the obstetricians or midwives, 1951, and to the hematologists in 1958). On the subject of "dissent against this teaching,"

---

[715]Cf. Ford-Kelly, *Contemporary Moral Theology*, II (cf. note 65), pp. 318 ff.

there is a footnote reference to Vatican II's *Dogmatic Constitution on the Church, article 25* (cf. quotation above).

(3) *"His manner of speaking:"* There is every indication that the reply was intended to settle a doctrine, hitherto controverted and disputed in some quarters, "in order that, with the uncertainties of the faithful cleared up, the bishops might more easily respond to their pastoral duties" (Appendix II, lines 64–67). The reply left no doubt that the "authentic magisterium" was speaking, and that the faithful could not look to the theologians who "dissent against this teaching" as a source of guidance and as an excuse for not following the "authentic magisterium" in the matter of direct sterilization (cf. quotation at the head of this chapter, and Appendix, lines 32–38).

Another proposed argument for disregarding the Reply on Sterilization of 1975 is that it is of questionable binding force because it did not come directly from Pope Paul VI but from one of the Roman congregations. In response to such an argument, it should suffice to recall that the doctrinal decrees of the Congregation for the Doctrine of the Faith as well as those of the Biblical Commission belong to the same category as papal encyclicals as expressions of the living magisterium of the Church.[716]

The Traditional Doctrine Regarding Cooperation in Evil

In its metaphorical sense, the word "formal" refers to the essential nature or constitution of a thing, concept, action, etc. When applied to cooperation, "formal" means a type of participation which pertains to the very nature or constitution of an evil action—that is, a sharing in the *intent* of the principal agent who performs the action. It is not merely something external to the evil action as in *material* cooperation, but an approval of the evil action. This might be called, in the words of Jesus, something that "emerges from within . . . from the deep recesses of the heart" (Mark,VII:20,21). The Reply on Sterilization of 1975 applies this concept of cooperation to the Catholic hospital situation:

> For the official approbation of direct sterilization and, *a fortiori,* its management and execution in accord with hospital regulations, is a matter which, in the objective order, is by its very nature (or intrinsically) evil. The Catholic hospital cannot cooperate with this for any reason (Appendix, lines 45–50).

---

[716]Ford-Kelly, *Readings in Moral Theology, No. 3* (cf. note 579), p. 4.

In *material* cooperation there is indeed some type of assistance which facilitates the performance of an immoral procedure, but there is no sharing in the intent of the principal agent. This type of cooperation can be allowed in certain circumstances if there is a proportionately serious reason for lending such assistance. If that type of assistance is so closely associated with the performance of the evil deed itself, however, so as to amount to actually joining the physician in performing the immoral procedure, it is more than mere material cooperation. Such a type of *immediate* cooperation in performing an immoral procedure amounts to *formal* cooperation. In the words of Father Thomas O'Donnell, S.J.: ". . . it is vacuous to say that a person in his right senses performs a criminal action without intending, in his will, to do so."[717] This explains why *immediate* cooperation (apart from exceptional cases such as forced participation in theft), is equivalent to *formal* cooperation in the strict sense.[718]

Even *mediate* material cooperation can become formal cooperation if the *reason for cooperating* is not something over and above the *medical reasons* as advanced in favor of the immoral procedure. In other words, the reason for cooperating must be the separate, proportionately serious reason which justifies the act of cooperation. The American bishops clarified this issue in their *Commentary on the Roman Reply of 1975* by saying that if a hospital cooperates because of the *medical reasons* advanced in support of allowing the procedure (that is, the "reasons for the sterilization"), "the hospital can hardly maintain under these circumstances that it does not approve sterilizations done for medical reasons, and this would make cooperation formal" (Appendix, lines 146–156). Other examples of sharing in the intent of the principal agent (hence, *formal* cooperation) would be the following: any service or accommodation on the part of the Catholic hospital whereby requests for immoral procedures are referred to other health facilities, agencies or individuals where such procedures are provided; any deliberate efforts on the part of individuals to induce another person to submit to an immoral procedure by means of threats, persuasion, etc.; any express approval of the plans of an individual who is determined to submit to an immoral procedure.

1) An Analysis of Mediate Material Cooperation

Cooperation in evil can be allowed in certain circumstances if it is *material* (no sharing of evil intent) and *mediate* (sufficiently removed from actually joining the principal agent in performing the procedure). In addition, the

---

[717]O'Donnell, Thomas, S.J., *Medicine and Christian Morality* (cf. note 31), p. 32.
[718]*Ibid.*, footnote 16, p. 295.

assisting or facilitating action or deed must be something which, in itself, is either good or at least indifferent, and there must be a proportionately serious reason for cooperating as well as serious consideration of the scandal element (to be discussed later). Since the cooperator does not share in the evil intent, he or she is not sharing in the sin of another. It is more accurate to say that the principal agent is using the good or indifferent act of the cooperator as an occasion of or assistance in the performance of the immoral deed. One author calls it the abuse of that good or indifferent act in order to accomplish an evil deed.[719]

St. Alphonse of Liguori (1696–1787) usually is credited with having refined the Principle of Legitimate Material Cooperation. He also explained why such cooperation is not contrary to the law of charity, despite the fact that it presents the occasion (but not the cause) of a sinful deed:

> The reason is because when you place an indifferent act without an evil intention, if the other person chooses to abuse it so as to accomplish his sin, you are not bound to prevent that sin except by the law of charity. And since charity does not obligate with a grave inconvenience, you do not sin by providing your cooperation with a just reason; then the sin of the other person does not proceed from your cooperation, but by the malice of that person who abused your act.[720]

The principle behind the exonerating effect of a "grave inconvenience" is that a person is not obliged to prevent harm from coming to another if in doing so, he or she would suffer equivalent harm himself or herself.

The basic elements in determining the morality of material cooperation in particular cases might be summarized in four questions: How *serious* is the evil procedure objectively considered? How *closely-related* and how *indispensable* is the action of the cooperator for the performance of that evil? How serious is *the reason* for cooperating in view of the answers to the first two questions. The fourth question (the scandal element) will be discussed at length later on in this chapter. As to the seriousness of the evil, objectively considered, the "sterilization of the faculty itself" is a greater moral evil than the "sterilization of individual acts" (Appendix, lines 15–18). Within the birth control category, the use of contraceptive means which are also abortifacient is more

---

[719]Prümmer, Dominic, O.P., *Handbook of Moral Theology* (cf. note 151), pp. 103, 104. Cf. also the quotation from St. Alphonse of Liquori below (note 720.

[720]*Theologia Moralis*, I, D. Leonardi Gaudé, C.SS.R., ed. (Rome: Ex Typographia Vaticana, 1905), p. 357.

seriously evil than the use of means which are designed to prevent conception.

The "How closely-related" question refers to the distinction between *proximate* and *remote* material cooperation. A more serious justifying reason would be required for functioning as the anesthetist in a sterilization procedure (*proximate* cooperation) than for functioning as the floor nurse who provided nothing more than routine nursing care for the patient (*remote* cooperation). The "How indispensable" question refers to the distinction between *necessary* and *free* cooperation. A more serious justifying reason would be required for the surgical nurse to prepare the patient for the immoral procedure if she were the only qualified nurse available to perform that service (*necessary* cooperation) than if there were one or more qualified nurses available who could prepare the patient if the assigned nurse simply refused to have anything to do with the procedure (*free* or "dispensable" cooperation).

2) The Application of the Principle of the Double Effect

In every case of *material mediate* cooperation, there is the good or morally indifferent action of the cooperator with a double effect. The good effect is intended; the evil side effect is foreseen but not intended. There is no need to explain the five conditions which must be verified in every double-effect situation. That subject was treated in chapter VII. One of the conditions bears repetition especially in material-cooperation situations, however, and that is the condition that *the good effect as intended is not otherwise attainable.* The good sometimes can be attained by "speaking up,"—for example, by going to the supervisor or administrator of the health facility and saying respectfully: "For reasons of conscience, I prefer *not* to be involved in immoral procedures in anyway." Such an individual would have a reasonable alternative to participating in the forbidden procedure, and hence would not have a seriously proportionate reason for cooperating. If the supervisor or administrator of the clinic or hospital refused to honor that nurse's conscientious objections, however, she could be justified in cooperating in the procedure in order to hold her job, or be eligible for promotion, etc.

It should be noted that the good effect intended through material cooperation could be either a *greater harm to be avoided* (e.g., to enable a nurse to hold her job), or a *greater good to be promoted.* Lay men and lay women who are employed in public and non-denominational hospitals may feel that they can be a power for good in persuading the administration to cut down the number of abortions, to enhance spiritual service to the patients, etc. They may see the need of cooperating more frequently even to a *proximate* degree when necessary, in order to maintain and build their power of influencing the administration and/or serving the patients in so many material and spiritual aspects of health care and medical practice. Such a nurse could exercise a type of apostolate through her employment in a non-Catholic hospital by summoning the priest for Catholic patients, by baptizing dying infants, by helping dying patients, both Catholic and non-Catholic, to make their peace with God.[721]

The same principles which apply to *positive* mediate material cooperation as discussed thus far, apply also to *negative* material cooperation. Negative cooperation is understood as cooperation in the sin of another by neglecting to exert a *deterring influence* on the potential primary agent (son, daughter, parish member, etc.) which is obligatory because of personal authority or official position. Such negative cooperation could even be formal by constituting approval of evil. It would apply, in varying degrees, to binding-in-conscience responsibilities of hospital authorities with regard to all patients (cf.*preamble* to the Directives, paragraph 2) as well as to similar in-conscience responsibilities of parents towards their children and to bishops and priests with regard to the faithful under their pastoral care.[722]

10.3 PRUDENCE IN APPLYING THE PRINCIPLE OF MATERIAL COOPERATION

The caution of "prudence in application" refers primarily to Catholic hospitals as health-care institutions. Hence the institutional aspect will be discussed first. Catholics who are employed in Catholic hospitals would face the material cooperation quandary on rare occasions only: for example, a physician or nurse might question the validity of the application of the Principle of Material Cooperation in a particular case and refuse to cooperate in any way. Catholics employed in non-Catholic hospitals and clinics, however, need guidelines in applying the Principle of Material Cooperation. Their situation merits extended discussion. Finally, Catholic hospitals today are challenged to promote efficiency and even at times to assure survival by considering various types of group ventures with Catholic or non-Catholic hospitals or agencies. That will constitute the third subject for discussion under the imperative of "prudence in application."

---

[721]Kelly, Gerald, S.J., *Medico-Moral Problems* (cf. note 22), pp. 134, 135.

[722]St. Thomas Aquinas, in his *Summa Theologiae* (cf. note 168), in Q.26 of part II-II, refers to Matthew 22:39 as evidence that we are to love ourselves more than others (art. 4), but that we are to love our neighbor with regard to his salvation more than we love our own bodies (art. 5). The order in loving others is to be based on their closeness to us (arts. 6 and 7), and those joined to us by blood ties have a greater claim on our love than others (art. 8).

1) The Institutional Aspects of "Prudence in Application"

Administrators of Catholic hospitals must keep in mind the following basic aspects of applying the Principle of Material Cooperation to immoral procedures:
- The principle can never be applied to abortion services (cf. *Directive 12*).
- The application of the principle to sterilization cases and other immoral procedures will be exceptional, and must be handled on a case-by-case basis.
- Such exceptions can never be allowed if the exception is made on the basis of the *medical reasons for sterilization* ("reason for the cooperation" must prevail, cf. p. 388).
- Consultation with the diocesan bishop or his delegate is required in each case.

The difficulty of arriving at a prudential judgment regarding the application of the Principle of Material Cooperation as above, should not be underestimated. One American archbishop describes the nature of such a challenge as follows:

> It is essential to note that what is at issue here is not necessarily a doctrinal rejection of one or more of the *Directives*. The *Directives* reflect standard Catholic teaching, which bishops are pledged to support and promulgate. What is at issue is the application of moral principles to the complexities of a local situation. This is what is called a prudential judgment. One weighs the principles against the situation and makes the best decision possible while respecting the demands of both. This is not always easy. Two prudent persons can conceivably come up with different responses to the same set of problems if the problems are sufficiently complex. Likewise, situations that appear similar may actually differ from one place to another and the same prudent man might come up with different responses to each. What we must remember is that we are dealing with highly specific situations that affect a small number of persons under Catholic health care . . .[723]

Despite the difficulty of arriving at a prudential judgment, however, it must be admitted that the doctrinal directives are loud and clear. On the other hand, the "pressure factor" on many hospital administrators is nothing less than formidable.

---

[723]"The Church as Teacher," by Archbishop Daniel E. Pilarczyk, in *Ethics Committees: A Challenge for Catholic Health Care* (cf. note 226), p. 20.

Pressure on Catholic Hospitals to Allow Sterilizations

There is no need to comment at length on the extremely-clear doctrinal positions enunciated in the Holy See's *Reply on Sterilization* (1975). Direct sterilization is clearly defined and cooperation in such a procedure is portrayed as approval of same and, as such, intrinsically evil. "Any cooperation so supplied is totally unbecoming the mission entrusted to this type of institution and would be contrary to the necessary proclamation and defense of the moral order" (Appendix II, lines 39–53). The Church is not denying that it would be comforting to a woman with a very serious heart condition to know that she would not become pregnant again. The Church is saying: "We are talking about something which 'in the objective order, is by its very nature (or intrinsically) evil.' We simply cannot approve of evil in order to realize even a good of the highest order."

The situation must not be confused with the application of the Principle of the Double Effect to cases of *indirect* sterilization, where contraception is not the purpose of the procedure. Thus, for example, a pregnant woman with cervical cancer who could not survive until her infant is viable, can submit to a hysterectomy in order to save her life. All who do cooperate in such a surgical procedure can be assured that the *reason for their cooperation* can be the same as the *medical reason* advanced by the physician in urging the woman to submit to the procedure. It is true that there is an evil side-effect; the premature delivery of a nonviable infant is always a bitter sorrow. The purpose of the hysterectomy, however—without which the procedure would never have been contemplated—was to save the mother from the scourge of cancer. There was simply no reasonable alternative for the physician in his determination to save the life of the mother. That good objective was realized through *directly-willed* good means (the removal of the source of the cancer) and not through the *indirectly willed and tolerated* (but foreseen) side-effect of terminating the life of an inviable infant.

In the case of a *direct* sterilization, where the procedure would never have been contemplated except for the desire to render conception impossible, the *reason for cooperation* cannot be the same as the *medical reason* as advanced by the physician, because it is evil at the outset (in the words of *Directive 19,* "to render conception impossible"). It is clearly a case of realizing a desired good through evil means. The necessarily-willed and intended effect, which is freedom from conception, is realized *through* the surgical elimination of the woman's (or man's) ability to generate new life. Furthermore, there are reasonable alternatives to sterilization besides the obvious route of sexual abstinence, such as recourse to the Natural Family Planning method (pp.74,75). These critical concepts are emphasized in the *Commentary on the*

Roman Reply as issued by the American bishops in 1977. The document stresses the prudence of a case-by-case mentality:

> In making judgments about the morality of cooperation, each case must be decided on its own merits. Since hospital situations, and even individual cases, differ so much, it would not be prudent to apply automatically a decision made in one hospital, or even in one case, to another (Appendix, lines 159–163, and the entire section on "Guidelines for Hospital Policy," lines 121 ff).

This same *Commentary on the Roman Reply* calls direct sterilization a "grave evil," and states that allowing material cooperation in extraordinary cases would have to be based "on the danger of an even more serious evil, e.g., the closing of the hospital could be under certain circumstances a more serious evil" (Appendix, lines 171–174). Very few situations of public pressure for expanded sterilization services would admit of a clear-cut, one-factor decision. First of all, any pressure to allow direct sterilizations on a general-category basis must be resisted. To capitulate to such pressure would be interpreted as allowing direct sterilizations for the *medical reasons* as advanced by the physician, and hence as formal approval. The "case-by-case" attitude is essential if the hospital is to be successful in projecting the proportionately serious reasons (the "reasons for cooperation") as the sole determinant in the decision to allow material cooperation in rare, particular cases. The civil right of the Catholic hospital to operate on the basis of Catholic values and standards must be vindicated at all costs.

As an illustration of the many factors, pro and con, which may have to be considered before arriving at a decision, one might imagine that a city of 20,000 staunch citizens (only 20% Catholic) organizes a movement to get more sterilization service from the Catholic hospital which they had funded as a community project 40 years previously. They informed the religious Sisters who own and sponsor the hospital, respectfully but firmly, that if they did not cooperate in allowing more sterilization procedures in the hospital, the citizens would explore seriously the possibilities of establishing a competing non-denominational hospital in the city. This likely turn of events would challenge the very survival of the Catholic hospital. Factors such as the following would demand serious consideration:

(a) *Con*–There are reliable indications that the pressure will disappear gradually with demographic changes: industry-wise, the trend is that the area will become primarily a retirement community. In other words, "ride out the pressure."

(b) *Pro*-There is convincing evidence that the area has the financial base and sustained economy to enable the general public to respond to the challenge to build and maintain a competing hospital. The pressure shows no signs of abating.

(c) *Con*-There is a confirmed probability that the state authorities would not grant approval for the construction of another hospital in the area (too many hospital beds in the general area, neighboring cities, etc.).

(d) *Pro*-There is definite information that the state authorities would allow the construction of another hospital, and that the prohibited procedures to be allowed would include abortions.

(e) *Con*-It is financially feasible that the Catholic hospital could survive by dropping all obstetric programs and services and substituting popular and community-centered services such as improved health-care services for the elderly, a fertility clinic, improved outpatient services, etc.; even with the foreseen probability that continued public pressure would continue for the construction of a professional clinic which would offer prohibited procedures including abortion services.

(f) *Pro*-The pressure for a competing hospital has proceeded to the point of a fund drive for that purpose. Funds are also being collected in a nearby city for a large non-denominational hospital which will specialize in obstetric and gynecological services. There are definite indications, however, that *temporary* compliance with the pressure for expanded sterilization services would dispose the local fund-raisers to promote the "nearby city" obstetrical health facility instead of a local competing hospital.

(g) *Con*-There is a solid probability that the principal promoters of the pressure group (possibly representing a dominant local industry) might be leaving the community relatively soon due to a significant change in management, or due to diminished prospects for industrial growth.

(h) *Con*-There is a very promising prospect of obtaining the support of community leaders as to turn the influence of the pressure group into a manageable minority movement. This countermovement could build on the many advantages enjoyed by the community in the past through the "Catholic presence" in the community (high moral values, concern for spiritual needs of patients, etc.).

A Catholic hospital which prides itself in a good public-relations image in the community might well be more successful in "riding out" any pressure for expanded sterilization services. The very element of community respect and appreciation for the Catholic hospital's presence and performance would dampen any pressure movement.

The *"pro"* factors considered in the aggregate may indicate that material cooperation in a particular case is warranted now and then. The *"con"* factors, again considered in the aggregate (both "pro" and "con") could indicate a decision to "hold the line" (against material cooperation) as the prudential position. The consideration of the "pro" and "con" factors can establish a basis for judging whether or not there is a serious reason for material cooperation—one which is proportionate to allowing an immoral procedure to take place in the Catholic hospital *including* the element of scandal (to be discussed at the end of this section). The former (reason for cooperation) must be more serious than the latter (allowing an immoral procedure, scandal possibilities included). To quote the American hierarchy's *Commentary on the Roman Reply,* material cooperation will be justified "only in situations where the hospital because of some kind of duress or pressure cannot reasonably exercise the autonomy it has (i.e., when it will do more harm than good)" (Appendix, lines 138–141 and 171–174).

Once the decision has been made, it is only fair to harbor the presumption that the decision was a legitimate application of the "traditional doctrine regarding material cooperation," and "was applied with the utmost prudence" (Appendix, lines 113–116). Those who contemplate such a decision only from the outside—who were not subject to the duress and pressure which precipitated the prudential decision—are not qualified to sit in judgment as required by regional reality.

It is especially because of the scandal element that "the bishop of the diocese or his representative must be involved in the decision" (Appendix, lines 142–145). This representative—often known as the Diocesan Director of Hospitals—should be chosen with great circumspection. He should be offered adequate training advantages and updating opportunities (workshops, conventions, etc.) so as to merit the full confidence both of the bishop and of the Catholic health facilities. If the diocese or archdiocese has more than 5 or 6 major Catholic health facilities, the bishop's representative can hardly measure up to his responsibilities if he is also assigned to full-time pastoral work or to a full-time teaching position. He must keep the bishop duly informed with regard to ethical and moral problems and solution-possibilities through his close contact with hospital sponsors and administrators, through his association with hospital ethics committees, and especially through his active participation as a member of the Diocesan Ethics Committee.

One of the frequent complaints heard from Catholic hospital sponsors and administrators is that they find it difficult (and sometimes all but impossible) to reach the bishop or his representative when faced with "on the spot" dilemmas. If this is true, every effort must be made to enlist the support of some influential intermediary who can bring this sad and "demoralizing" situation to the attention of the bishop.

Taking Positive Steps to Improve the Catholic Image

The general public is inclined to foster an impression of Catholic health care as somewhat insensitive to the needs of those who do not share the Catholic moral code. The media emphasize the Church's *negative* response to contraception, direct sterilization, artificial insemination, etc. Catholic hospitals can soften that negative image by promoting and publicizing *positive* programs for overcoming human infertility (pp.36 ff.); for facing the challenge of spacing births through the *Natural Family Planning* method, etc. The Church can hardly expect the news media or the professional medical agencies to publicize the fact that the Natural Family Planning method not only brings peace of mind and peace of conscience to millions of couples who regard contraceptive techniques as revolting and immoral, but that it carries a success-rating of 98% (p.89).

Catholic hospitals often neglect the advantages of "accentuating the positive." One survey indicated that 30% of Catholic hospitals that do offer Natural Family Planning programs list lack of funding as the primary obstacle in promoting the program.[724] Catholic hospitals often fail to take advantage of organizations such as the Couple to Couple League which could supply some of the funding and much of the publicity program by literally inundating physicians, nurses, social agencies and the general public with small eye-catching pamphlets which emphasize the success rate and the advantages (medical, social, psychological, spiritual) of Natural Family Planning. The dividends will become apparent when referrals to the NFP program begin to keep the hospital switchboard busy.

Since the desire to have a family has far more profound roots than the desire not to become pregnant, the wisdom of adding experts in human fertility to the Catholic hospital staff should not be overlooked or underestimated. This pro-life and pro-family emphasis unfolds an expertise where the Catholic faith, theologically, philosophically and apostolically is unequaled by any other human agency. In addition, the Catholic image can be refurbished by

---

[724]Martin, Mary Catherine, and Walker, William R., "Survey Discloses NFP Practices, Preferences in U.S. Catholic Hospitals," in *Hospital Progress,* Feb., 1983, p. 57. Cf. also "NFP Services in Catholic Hospitals," by Msgr. James T. McHugh, in *Linacre Quarterly,* August, 1983, pp. 246–250.

stressing other areas of unequalled Catholic achievement and dedication such as the promotion of improved programs for the elderly, increased concern for the basic health needs of the poor, research into the causes of defects among the pre-born and the newborn, specialized physical and spiritual care of victims of social diseases (such as the AIDS affliction), etc. When all of these achievements come to be associated with the name "Catholic," few fair-minded men and women will have any basis for perpetuating the view that Catholic health facilities are insensitive to the needs of humanity.

2) Proportionate Reasons Applying to Catholics As Individuals

The word "proportionate" means that, all things and aspects considered, there is a balance between the good effects as contemplated reasonably by the act of material cooperation and the evil effects as occasioned by the act of cooperation. As mentioned earlier in this chapter, the contemplated good effects must be at least somewhat more weighty than the evil effects.

Authors agree that when Catholic nurses and other Catholic health-care personnel apply for a position in a non-Catholic institution, they should state clearly and respectfully that they would have to be excused from assisting in prohibited procedures as a matter of conscience. If possible, this should be stated in writing as a matter of record if the Catholic individual is given employment. Such a precaution is even more urgent in seeking employment in a small clinic or physician's office where nurses often are expected to lend proximate assistance in office-type surgical sterilization procedures such as tubal ligations and vasectomies, and other directly contraceptive procedures (fitting diaphragms, IUD's etc.).[725] In many if not most cases, non-Catholic health facilities will respect and honor such conscientious objections.

Catholic moralists are not of one terminology in speaking of sufficient proportionate reasons for cooperation in moral-medical matters—and respected standard authors of the period before the 1940's rarely apply the Principle of Material Cooperation to hospital and medical situations. Reasons listed by some authors who do discuss moral-medical situations refer mostly to *proximate* mediate cooperation. Others prefer to speak of *proximate* and *very proximate* actions with only slight reference to *remote* actions. With due allowance for some variance in terminology, however, the following principles are

---

[725]Nurses may not lend *immediate* material cooperation in such cases. Cf. McFadden, Charles J., O.S.A., *Medical Ethics* (cf. note 17), pp. 306, 307; Connell, Francis J., C.SS.R., *Morals in Politics and Professions* (Westminster, Maryland: The Newman Bookshop, 1946), pp. 138, 139; same author, *Outlines of Moral Theology* (cf. note 462), p. 95.

representative of the accepted doctrine on proportionate reasons for cooperation as advanced by Catholic moral theologians.

(1) Actions which are *remote* with regard to facilitating the prohibited procedure but *not at all necessary* or indispensable to that end, are justified for
any *reasonable* cause. In such situations, a special reason is not required.
Such remote actions have no particular connection with the prohibited
procedure in question, but are performed rather as assigned duty for the
welfare of all patients as patients. Examples of such remote actions would
be the following: the routine nursing care of the patient, scrubbing down
and disinfecting the operating room for those who regularly are assigned
to cleaning duties, preparing the patient in the hospital room for the
scheduled procedure (pills, medications, etc.).

From one viewpoint, such dedication to duty with regard to all patients, regardless of the specific purpose for which they entered the hospital, is not only a normal part of the mission of healing, but also is
commendable from the admonition of the Lord Jesus especially with regard to those who may not share Catholic moral standards: "Be compassionate as your father is compassionate. Do not judge, and you will not be
judged" (Luke,6:36 and 37). If the Catholic hospital employee assigns
greater weight to the character of such ministrations as cooperation in
evil, however, her (his) right to decline to cooperate should be respected.
For such individuals, the reason for *not* refusing to perform such *remote*
actions of cooperation could be the risk of being ridiculed by fellow employees in the hospital, or the danger of being assigned to more menial
tasks by the hospital administration, etc.

(2) Actions which are *proximate* with regard to facilitating the prohibited procedure but *not at all necessary* or indispensable to that end, require a *serious
reason* for performing the act of cooperation. Examples of such *proximate*
actions would be the following: sterilizing the surgical instruments for
that particular prohibited procedure, laying out the surgical instruments
and/or preparing the operating table for that procedure; administering
the anesthetic in the operating room. The *serious reason* for performing the
act of cooperation could be one of the following well-founded dangers:
permanent termination of employment in that hospital (especially in an
area where job opportunities of similar employment and remuneration
are in very short supply); even temporary but relatively long-term loss of
employment (3 months or more) for an employee who is the sole support
of a family; definite indications from the hospital administration that such
a "refusing" nurse would either be demoted, or would lose all rights to

promotions (and hence substantial salary increases) in the future. Such Catholic employees are obligated to protest their involvement in such prohibited procedures even though there is slight hope that their protests would be respected and heeded.[726]

Catholic employees in non-Catholic health facilities who find themselves in such compromising positions with regard to *proximate* material cooperation not merely now and then but on a regular basis (sterilizations a "speciality" of the establishment) should make every effort to secure employment of similar status in some other health facility even though it may mean a change in occupation or a moderate decrease in salary and/or other benefits (retirement, insurance, bonuses, etc.).

(3) Actions which are *necessary or indispensable,*-and to the extent that the prohibited procedure would not take place at all without that act of cooperation—require a *very serious reason,* even if the act of itself is only remotely connected with the procedure. If the patient said, for example, "I will submit to the sterilization procedure only if my friend, Nurse "A" is assigned to take care of me in my hospital room before and after the surgery" (an example of *remote* cooperation), she would be indispensable for the procedure and could not accept the assignment unless she had a *very serious* reason for doing so.

In most cases, however, *necessary* or indispensable cooperation would be associated with proximate actions, for example, administering the anesthetic. The *refusal* of the nurse to cooperate to that extent might result in the cancellation of the procedure for one of several reasons: that the conscientious moral stand of the nurse inspires either the patient or the physician to "call off" the procedure, or that the physician will not proceed without a qualified anesthetist and there simply is no qualified anesthetist available to substitute for the Catholic nurse. Such fortunate turns in events, however, would be extremely rare. The nurse could not be allowed to cooperate in such a *proximate and necessary* manner unless she had an *extremely serious* reason. As an example of an extremely serious or "most grave" reason, Father Francis Connell, C.SS.R. mentioned "the well-founded fear that she might be dismissed from the hospital and be barred

---

[726]In addition to the authors mentioned in note 725, the following theologians may be consulted on the subject of material cooperation in evil: Davis, Henry, S.J., *Moral and Pastoral Theology,* I (New York, N.Y.: Sheed and Ward, 1943), pp. 341 ff.; Healy, Edwin, S.J., *Medical Ethics* (cf. note 46), pp. 101 ff; O'Donnell, Thomas, S.J., *Medicine and Christian Morality* (cf. note 31), pp. 31 ff.

from continuing her profession.'"[727] Other extremely serious reasons could be actual threats of serious physical harm to that nurse or to her loved ones (husband, children, parents), or serious threats to ruin her reputation in the community.

(4) Some cooperative actions must be classed as *very* proximate and also *necessary*. These are actions which come perilously close to being actual participation in the prohibited procedure itself. In reality, however, they are not ways of *participating* in the forbidden procedure, but of *facilitating* the performance of the procedure—for example, by standing by during the procedure and handing the surgical instruments to the physician, or by standing by to keep the patient quiet by administering anesthetics or narcotics as may be required during the procedure. Such cooperation would be necessary if such ministrations are considered indispensable, and if no other substitute is available or acceptable. For many surgical procedures in small clinics and in doctors' offices, the attitude of the physician might well be: "She is my nurse—we are accustomed to working together—I will not proceed without her."

Presuming that a Catholic nurse in such a situation clearly has expressed her disapproval of such demands on her services for conscience reasons, and considering not only the proximity and indispensability of her cooperation but also the *scandal* element, it is difficult to suggest a reason which might justify such cooperation in an intrinsically evil procedure. A distinction might be made between regular and irregular exposure to demands for such cooperation in sterilization procedures. If such procedures occur irregularly in the sense of now and then, and the nurse has protested in no uncertain terms *and* the physician respects her conscientious objections and promises to search for an additional staff nurse who would not object to such demands, it would seem that the Catholic nurse would be justified in continuing her cooperation in such infrequent and irregularly-scheduled procedures for an *extremely serious* reason (cf.n.(3)above) until the new nurse is available. If such a solution is not possible, however, and the physician continues to make such demands of

---

[727] *Outlines of Moral Theology* (cf. note 462), p. 95. If the cooperation is both proximate and necessary, involving serious harm to a third party, the extremely-serious reason for cooperating would have to be commensurate to the harm to that third party. Cf. O'Donnell, Thomas, S.J., *Medicine and Catholic Morality* (cf. note 31), pp. 34, 35. This would apply in all abortion procedures (the innocent 3rd party, the infant) and especially in cases of the permanent sterilization of husband or wife whereby the other spouse (third party) is deprived permanently of the prospect of progeny.

the nurse and no substitute is available or acceptable, only a definitely-established danger of serious physical harm to the nurse or to her immediate family members (major disfigurement, rape, kidnapping, etc.) could provide a sufficient and proportionate reason to justify her continued cooperation—and this *only* until she can find suitable employment elsewhere.

If such demands for *very proximate and necessary* cooperation are made of a Catholic nurse on a *regular basis,* however, it should be apparent that she is cooperating with a clinic or physician of unsavory reputation. The magnitude of the *scandal* element would be such that no "greater evil to be avoided" reason could justify such continued cooperation. There is the slight possibility that a "greater good to be fostered" reason could apply, however, in the unlikely situation that the Catholic nurse has been such a favorable influence on a particular clinic proprietor or physician ("doctor's office" procedure) that she can cherish a well-founded hope of dissuading that individual from offering such prohibited-procedure services within a reasonable period of time. Without doubt, the *scandal* element would present a serious obstacle, and the noble experiment would have to be terminated at the expiration of that "reasonable" period of time. This suggested solution illustrates the impossibility of making hard and fast rules of universal application in the matter of legitimate recourse to the Principle of Material Cooperation.

It can happen that a nurse or medical assistant truly is in doubt as to the morality of a particular procedure *after* the procedure has been initiated. Unless there is definite evidence to the contrary, the presumption should be that the physician is acting licitly. Doubts *before* the procedure is initiated should be settled in conference with the physician. Doubts *during* the procedure, however, should not prevent the nurse from exercising her professional responsibility. The matter should be settled definitely, however, after the procedure has been completed.[728]

3) Application to Joint Ventures

Efforts to increase efficiency in administration and even to guarantee survival may require collaboration with area hospitals, contracting for professional management services, etc. Catholic physicians also encounter challenges to their moral standards in their professional relationships. The

---

[728]Davis, Henry, S.J., *Moral and Pastoral Theology,* I (cf. note 726), p. 348; Healy, Edwin, S.J., *Medical Ethics* (cf. note 46), pp. 107, 108.

following situations illustrate the absolute need of dedication and caution in "holding the line" with regard to moral principles and values in the mission of healing.

The Catholic Hospital and its Own Office Building

If the Catholic sponsoring group owns and operates its own medical office building, the same high moral standards which apply in the hospital should prevail in the office building as well. If suites in the office building are made available also to physicians who are not on the staff of the hospital, they should be required to agree in writing that they will observe the Catholic moral standards as contained in the Catholic hospital directives . . . with express mention of abortion and contraceptive sterilizations. As an added assurance against violations of Catholic moral standards, the signed agreement might include a "termination clause,"—to the effect that "all rights and privileges of tenancy in this building are forfeited in the event of violation of Catholic medical-moral standards."

With regard to hospital staff members, all of whom are already pledged to compliance with Catholic moral standards in the hospital and in the office building, that same "termination clause" (which actually is designed to discourage a "material breach" of contract) could be added to the signed agreement whereby they become staff members. Without a protective clause of that type, it could be difficult to dislodge a pledge-breaking physician from his position in the hospital and/or in the office building. The reason is because the courts take the stand that once staff privileges have been granted, that physician has a property interest which cannot be terminated without full process of law.[729] It would be even more difficult to succeed in any legal action against a Catholic hospital staff member who performs direct sterilization procedures not in the Catholic hospital or its office building but elsewhere (clinic, private office, etc.). The reason is that the "conscience clause" is something of a two-edged sword—the physician could use it in defense of his actions outside of the hospital facilities.[730] If such a physician's outside activities became so scandalous, however, that the adverse effects on the Catholic hospital's reputation assumed damaging proportions, it might be possible to base legal action against him or her on the basis of the "disruptive physician"

---

[729]*Questions and Answers* prepared by the Division of Legal Services, the Catholic Health Association (St. Louis, Mo.: Catholic Health Assoc., 1985), pp. 17, 18.
[730]*Ibid.*, p. 18.

line of argument. As of the present, however, there is no applicable legal precedent for such an approach.[731]

The Catholic Hospital and an Office Building Based on a Land-lease

If the Catholic hospital does not own and manage the office building, special attention must be focused on two factors in particular: the proximity of material cooperation, and the gravity of the resultant scandal. It would be unrealistic—and restrictive of mankind's potential for doing good—to insist that all material cooperation must be avoided. Many positive advantages of moral value are derived, for example, from a Catholic physician's membership in the American Medical Association despite the fact that his membership in the AMA adds a certain amount of prestige to an association with a significant number of members who perform a wide variety of immoral procedures. The following land-lease agreements do *not* involve Catholic ownership of a professional medical office building, but there is foreknowledge that some of the tenants will perform immoral procedures—*with the exception of abortion*. It must be emphasized that a Catholic hospital may not allow its facilities (even on the basis of a land-lease agreement) to be used for abortion in any circumstances.

Two possible land-lease situations might be considered together: (a) Land owned by and adjacent to a Catholic hospital is leased to a professional management company which assumes full charge in the financing, construction and management of a medical office building; (b) Catholic hospital land is leased as above, but with a loan guarantee from the fixed capital of the hospital, thus providing a more favorable credit rating and a decrease in interest payments. In case (a), the cooperation relationship (remember, there is foreknowledge of some violations of Catholic standards) would be more remote than in case (b), due to the absence of a financial commitment (loan guarantee). In both cases the lessee-manager is required, both in the lease agreement and in the management agreement, to operate the facility in accord with Catholic moral standards. Protection against a material breach in both agreements is assured by a clause which states, in effect, that the hospital is entitled to assume operation and management of the facility if the management company fails to adhere to the moral standards as enunciated in Catholic hospital directives.[732] In both cases, the permission of the Holy See would

---

[731]*In Defense of Values* (cf. note 635), p. 17.

[732]*Church Property, Church Finances, and Church-Related Corporations* by Adam J. Maida, JD, JCL (now Bishop of the Diocese of Green Bay, Wis.) and Nicholas P. Cafardi, JD (cf. note 637), pp. 261–267.

be required on the basis of alienation of Church property if the amount is in excess of $1,000,000.[733] In case (b), the loan guarantee could constitute an additional reason for alienation procedures.

In case (a), the justifying reason for entering such a lease and management agreement could be the fact that the hospital lacks the personnel to manage the facility, in addition to their confidence that the reputable management company would monitor the performance records of the tenants so that violations of Catholic moral standards would be close to nonexistent. In case (b), an additional reason could be that the Catholic hospital already has an equity in the facilities (loan guarantee). The scandal element would have to be appraised in consultation with the diocesan bishop.

In one or both cases, the management company's negligence in assuring compliance with Catholic moral standards could lead to evidence of so many prohibited procedures performed in the facility, that the only proper means of allaying scandal might be to exercise the hospital's rights to assume charge of the office building, or to renegotiate with the management company for the outright sale of the facility. On the other hand, a sufficient reason for justifying continued material cooperation (and exercising increased vigilance over the management company's performance) could be the solid probability that the management company would react to any tampering with the original agreements by negotiating a lease agreement for an office building with the non-Catholic hospital in that two-hospital city, and thus posing a definite threat to the survival of the Catholic hospital. Furthermore, even if the Catholic hospital did survive financially, it would lose the limited and yet considerable influence it had under the land-lease agreement in limiting the number of immoral procedures (including abortions) in the area.

A Joint-Venture Medical Office Building

Two neighboring hospitals (the only two in the city) are urgently in need of a medical office building. The need is based not only on repeated requests from their staff physicians, but also on the advantage of attracting competent physicians to the area so as to increase their patient population. There is no land available in the area except a parcel of adequate size between the Catholic and the non-sectarian hospital—a parcel owned by the Catholic hospital. A long-standing atmosphere of distrust and incrimination between the two hospitals and corresponding civic groups was relaxed somewhat, when the authorities of the non-sectarian hospital approached the Catholic hospital with a

---

[733]*Canon Law Digest,* IX (Cf. note 44), pp. 42–46.

proposal for a separate corporate entity to finance, construct and manage a medical office building as a joint venture of the two hospitals.

During long months of frank and heated discussions, no secret was made of the fact that the non-sectarian hospital had been "doing abortions;" and that they had promoted a very expanded program of family planning of the Planned Parenthood variety. They realized, however, that the Catholic hospital would have to insist on written assurances, both in the lease agreement and in the management agreement, that prohibited procedures (including many aspects of their family planning program) would not be tolerated in the office building. They agreed to such written assurances, but insisted on proper regard for their good faith in so doing and refused expressly to have any type of termination clause added to the agreements (whereby verified violations of the agreements would entitle the Catholic hospital *alone* to manage the facility). They were willing, however, to begin the venture with a limited land-lease and management feature whereby either side could terminate its association with the project voluntarily after 3 years. Thereafter the project, if continued as a mutual venture, would be based on long-term agreements.

Material cooperation in such a venture would be remote, but it would also be *necessary* or indispensable in the sense that a negative response from the Catholic hospital would preclude any possibility of building the facility in such a convenient area. Provided that the ongoing discussions with the authorities of the non-sectarian hospital resulted in definite assurances that they would discontinue abortions and also discourage direct-sterilizations *in their own hospital* (as well as in the medical office bldg.), one of the reasons for giving favorable consideration to the venture could be of the "greater good to be fostered" variety—based not only on the prospect of eliminating abortions in the area, but on improved relations with non-Catholics in the area through the valid expectation of other dividends possible from collaboration in a venture based on mutual good faith and respect. Such dividends could include cost-cutting and improved-services features such as joint use of extremely-expensive equipment, sharing in medical technology, avoiding the duplication of specialized services, etc. Another reason could be the fact that the Catholic hospital lacked the finances and personnel to build and manage the office building on their own, and perhaps also a well-founded danger that the lack of an office building would threaten the very survival of the Catholic hospital.

If efforts at good will, mutual respect and collaboration fail, the Catholic hospital can take advantage of the short-term lease and management agreement to terminate the venture and attempt to proceed on their own. The ecumenical aspects of the proposal should be given due consideration also as a feature which could temper the scandal potential of the venture. The bishop of the diocese would have to have the last word. Proceeding with the proposal would also constitute alienation of Church property with the obligation of obtaining the permission of the Holy See.

A Catholic Hospital as a Member of a Three-Hospital Consortium

There are three hospitals in the city: A Catholic hospital, dedicated in every way to Catholic moral standards but definitely in danger of being forced to close in time due to the prosperity of the other two hospitals; A non-sectarian Memorial Hospital initially established to provide services which were prohibited in the other two hospitals (when both were Catholic); A formerly-Catholic hospital, now owned and managed by a group of mostly Catholic laymen with a somewhat-Catholic philosophy of health care. This hospital had to close as a Catholic apostolate five years previously because the sponsoring religious community had lost control of its dedication to Catholic moral standards.[734] All three of the hospitals will have nothing to do with abortions and euthanasia, but Memorial Hospital and the formerly-Catholic hospital offer contraceptive-sterilization procedures. A serious proposal is made to form a separately-incorporated three-hospital consortium as a unified professional management company. The rationale behind the proposal is not only the cost-control advantages (sharing equipment, avoiding duplication of specialized services, etc.), but also a well-established sentiment in the community that the continuation of the Catholic presence in health care definitely is an asset in the area. The area is about 50% Catholic.

The governing board for this consortium would have equal representation from each of the three hospitals. The proposed bylaws would state that each hospital would establish and maintain its own philosophy and standards on moral-medical issues so that religious values would not be lost. The other two hospitals would also promise in writing to discontinue direct-sterilization procedures in their hospitals and to defer to the Catholic hospital as having the only obstetrics/gynecology department of the consortium. There is an unspoken understanding, however, that the other two hospitals will establish and manage a Memorial Clinic in a building located next to Memorial Hospital which formerly housed a school for nurses. The Catholic hospital would not be associated with this Memorial Clinic in any way. It is obvious that this clinic will offer sterilization procedures and family-planning techniques which cannot be obtained at the Catholic hospital (but NOT abortions).

---

[734]This unfortunate type of alienation is known as divestiture. Cf. Maida-Cafardi, *Church Property, Church Finances, and Church Related Corporations* (cf. note 637), pp. 269 ff.

The dangers of such a remote type of material cooperation would have to be balanced against the advantages of retaining the Catholic-hospital presence in the area, and of retaining a significant influence (through its obstetrics/gynecology department) in counteracting the sterilization and family-planning activities of the clinic. If that Catholic presence in health care is eliminated in the area, the last deterrent to widespread sterilization—and perhaps also to abortions—would be eliminated as well. Expert legal and canonical advice would be required so as to guarantee the protection of the faith responsibilities of the Catholic hospital. The proposal may not be accepted without prior consultation with the bishop of the diocese (cf. quotations from the preamble of the *Catholic Hospital Directives* at the end of this chapter).

A Catholic Hospital in a Joint-Residency Program

Medical schools which do not have their own hospitals often invite area hospitals to become affiliated with them in their training programs in obstetrics and gynecology. In a two-hospital city, the only Catholic hospital in the general area which sponsors and operates its own residency program is invited to affiliate with the medical school. If the Catholic hospital responds in the negative, there is some danger that they may lose board certification for their own residency program in obstetrics and gynecology. There is evidence of a tendency in graduate medical school circles to reduce many specialized programs, and weed out the weaker or borderline programs. The loss of that residency program in this particular situation would pose a definite threat to the eventual survival of the Catholic hospital in the area.

The other non-sectarian hospital in the city also has its own residency program and has accepted the invitation to become affiliated with the medical school. If both hospitals become affiliated, each hospital could have its own director of the program with control of its own moral-medical policies. In becoming a part of a joint-residency program, however, the Catholic hospital would have to be very specific about the procedures which the residents of its own program could participate in while at the *other* hospital. Each of the Catholic residents must be wary of a contrary attitude which might endanger his medical career; yet he cannot be expected to participate in actions which are a part of an immoral procedure itself if this conflicts with his religious and ethical principles. With respect but with due conviction, therefore, every Catholic resident would be obligated to submit a formal notice to the director of the non-sectarian residency program that he may not, in conscience, take part in abortion procedures or in other immoral procedures such as direct sterilizations. Most hospitals in the U.S.A. would want to be on record as accepting and respecting such a declaration of conscience on the part of a resident.

In the event that the director of the non-sectarian residency program agrees to exempt participation in actions which are a part of the illicit procedure itself, but disagrees as to preparatory aspects of illicit surgical procedures such as administering the anesthetic before the procedure is initiated, (abortion excluded), attending to the sterilization of the surgical instruments, etc., material cooperation in such preparatory actions could be justified—but should be avoided whenever possible, and when unavoidable, performed under protest. This could not be allowed, however, with regard to actions which are a part of the illicit procedure itself.[735] The bishop of the diocese might be inclined to allow some degree of proximate material cooperation in consideration not only of the professional medical future of the Catholic residents, but also of the danger that the Catholic hospital could lose the residency program. In that event—even if the survival of the Catholic hospital is not threatened—the residency program might be assigned to a non-sectarian hospital in a nearby city where all residents, Catholic and non-Catholic, would be denied any exposure to Catholic moral-medical values and principles.

Partnership in Group Practice With an Unethical Physician

Authors agree that a Catholic physician cannot in conscience advise or recommend contraception to any patient, regardless of the patient's personal convictions. The same would apply to instructing a patient in the use of contraceptives or of referring a patient to a physician or agency for that purpose.[736] If a Catholic physician cannot understand this prohibition on the basis of material cooperation, he should still agree to comply with it on the basis of scandal.

The above observation illustrates just one aspect of the compromising position in which a Catholic physician would find himself if he enters a profes-

---

[735]Father Edwin Healy, S.J. apparently would allow a Catholic trainee, who is functioning as first assistant to the main surgeon in a prohibited procedure, to sponge and suture "given a weighty reason . . . provided scandal is avoided." *Medical Ethics* (cf. note 46), pp. 106, 107. The question is: how can scandal be avoided in a residency situation? The better solution would be: refuse to participate in such an *immediate manner*; insist on respect for your moral convictions. Cf. O'Donnell, Thomas, *Medicine and Christian Morality* (cf. note 31), pp. 33–36; Ashley-O'Rourke, *Health Care Ethics* (cf. note 80), p. 283.

[736]Cf. O'Donnell, Thomas, *Medicine and Christian Morality* (cf. note 31), pp. 36, 37; Davis, Henry, S.J., *Moral and Pastoral Theology,* I (cf. note 726), p. 351; Connell, Francis, C.SS.R., *Morals in Politics and Professions* (cf. note 725), pp. 141, 142; Healy, Edwin, S.J., *Medical Ethics* (cf. note 46), pp. 110, 111; McFadden, Charles, O.S.A., *Medical Ethics* (cf. note 17), pp. 94–97.

sional partnership with an unethical physician—or becomes associated with a group practice which includes an unethical physician. Not only does such a partnership or group relationship provide a basis for the suspicion that the association was conceived at least in part out of a design to "be all things to all men—and women," but it also puts the Catholic physician in the position of appearing to approve of the prohibited procedures which would be performed by the partner or group members.

The fact that the Catholic physician would share in the division of funds would not be, of itself, a serious concern. Many individuals receive their pay checks from pharmacological companies, for example, which engage in the research and manufacture of products which are designed for immoral uses. They do their share of the work for that company, and receive their share of profits. Other factors such as the general public's knowledge that prohibited procedures are allowed on the premises, and that the Catholic physician is put in a position of referring patients (who seek prohibited procedures) to his partner or colleagues all combine to create a situation of serious scandal. The Catholic faithful have a right to expect Catholic physicians to "stand up" for basic Catholic moral standards by avoiding such compromising professional relationships. An exception might be imagined for a father-son medical partnership, for example, where there is a basis for presuming that the father may have entered such a partnership with the prime purpose of weaning his physician-son away from liberal principles and prohibited procedures—or vice versa. In that event, however, the partnership would have to be dissolved if the noble purpose had not been realized after a prearranged and reasonably-brief period of time.

10.4 PRECAUTIONS AGAINST SCANDAL

The principal *external* sins against love of neighbor or fraternal charity are seduction, whereby one causes another to sin—scandal, whereby one provides an occasion of sin to another—and material cooperation, whereby one concurs or participates in the sin of another. Even though material cooperation in the sin of another may not be serious because it does not involve a serious sin—or because the proximity of the act of cooperation is remote in relation to the evil deed itself—or because the act of cooperation is not indispensable for the performance of the evil deed—it may still present a serious moral problem because of scandal. This should be apparent from the strong words used by the Lord Jesus with regard to giving scandal to little children (Luke,17:1 and 2). The "great care (which) must be taken against scandal and the danger of any misunderstanding" as stressed in the quotation above from the Roman Reply of 1975 is explained in the Commentary of the American Hierarchy on that quotation as follows:

> As was stated in the Roman document, the Catholic health facility must take every precaution to avoid creating misunderstanding or causing scandal to its staff, patients, or general public by offering a proper explanation when necessary. It should be made clear that the hospital disapproves of direct sterilization and that material cooperation in no way implies approval (Appendix, lines 164–170).

Scandal is defined as some word or deed (whether of omission or commission) which is in itself evil or has the appearance of evil, and provides an occasion of sin to others. The word "sin" is understood in the sense of an occasion of spiritual harm ("ruinae spiritualis") to others. For example, when the rumor spreads that Catholic Doctor X had given a talk to the senior class in a Catholic high school in which he said (without making proper distinctions), "many of you girls will have to learn how to limit your families," many young couples might interpret his remarks as an approval of contraception. His remarks were not evil, but they had the appearance of evil in the sense they could admit of an interpretation which could influence others to do wrong. Obviously if the Catholic doctor had said, "the Church is wrong in prohibiting contraceptive birth control," the message itself would have been evil. The point is, however, that even if the words or deeds have only the appearance of evil, the scandal is sinful. This applies even if others may not be enticed into sinful deeds as a consequence of such scandalous behavior.

Many examples could be given of behavior which has the appearance of evil: the married man who discusses details of marital love when adolescents are present; the Catholic farmer working his fields on Sunday; the young girls who present an occasion of sin to the young and old of the masculine gender by their frivolous style of dress, enticing manner of walking, etc. St. Paul mentions an example whereby a person's presence "reclining at table in the temple of an idol" might influence another to eat food which had been sacrificed to idols. He concludes: "Therefore, if food causes my brother to sin, I will never eat meat again, so that I may not be an occasion of sin to him" (I Cor.,8:10–13).[737]

---

[737]For a review of the traditional doctrine of the Church on scandal, cf. St. Thomas Squinas, *Summa Theologiae* (cf. note 158), II-II, q. 43, articles 1–8; Merkelbach, Henry, O.P., *Summa Theologiae Moralis,* I (cf. note 151), pp. 728–736; Prümmer, Dominic, O.P., *Handbook or Moral Theology* (cf. note 151), pp. 102, 103; Jone, Heribert, O.F.M. Cap., *Moral Theology* (cf. note 151), pp. 90–92.

A distinguished Thomistic theologian makes this helpful observation: scandal in the theological sense is not the rumor, surprise, horror or indignation associated with scandal in the common acceptance of the word, but rather the serious suspicions, rash judgments, disparaging remarks and false accusations which grow and spread among the people—even to the extent of expressions of rejoicing, approval or consent with regard to a sinful practice.[738] Translating this into a moral-medical hospital situation, it would be difficult to imagine the full extent of spiritual harm and destructive damage done to individuals and to the Church in general (enticement to personal sins, confusion over moral standards, suspicion of special exceptions for the rich and influential, loss of respect for the magisterium of the Church, etc.) when the comment is passed along (however unfair or unfounded) that "there are a lot of tubal ligations going on over at St. X Hospital."

The Narrow Limits of Lawful Scandal Situations

This discussion involves primarily *active* scandal (that is, the words or deeds as such) which is called *indirect* because the principal agent (person or institution) has no intention of leading others into sinful ways. Since as in all scandal, however, there is the *foreseen* consequence that the words or deeds in question could present an occasion of spiritual harm to others, such behavior can be allowed only if the words or deeds as such are *good or at least indifferent,* and if their omission would constitute a *serious inconvenience.* "Appearance of evil" cannot be tolerated. Of course, there would have to be a due proportion between the gravity of the inconvenience and the extent of the foreseen evil consequences. The challenge in conscience is twofold: an effective dissipation of any appearance of evil, and an honest and realistic appraisal of the gravity of the inconvenience of omitting the words or deeds altogether.

To say that *active and indirect* scandal can never be allowed to any degree due to its possible association with evil consequences would be to impose an unfair limit on an individual's potential for taking advantage of opportunities to do good. Many good and virtuous deeds would have to be omitted because of the malice, the ignorance, or the extreme sensitivities of certain individuals or groups. Most people understand that there is no pressing obligation to avoid what is known as "pharisaical" scandal, which actually can be traced to the malice of an individual who is only too ready and anxious to "take" scandal. There is an obligation, however, to take precautions in dealing with individuals who are scandalized more easily than the average person because

---

[738]Merkelbach, Henry, O.P., *Ibid.,* p. 728.

of tender age, limited education (ignorance), delicate conscience, etc. This is called "scandal of little ones" ("scandalum pusillorum" from the Latin "pusillus" which means very small, tiny, little). In speaking of such individuals, St. Thomas refers to Matthew,18:6, where Jesus is talking about little children. Many people of high moral standards but of slight education backgrounds who live more-or-less protected lives, must be included in that "easily scandalized" category.

It is important to realize, however, that it is precisely this "easily scandalized" category both among the faithful and among the general public, which is the main concern of the Church in scandal situations. Admittedly there is no obligation to omit good deeds just in order to avoid scandalizing an easily-scandalized person; for example, a priest takes advantage of a chance meeting with a militant atheist in a public lunchroom and engages him in conversation. The situation changes, however, if the *only* known reasons for cooperation in evil involve temporal goods and advantages, for example, the Catholic and the non-Catholic hospital can share some expensive facilities, cut some costs, etc. Something must be done about the scandal possibilities. St. Thomas would say that either the Catholic hospital would have to pass up such a materially-advantageous agreement with a non-Catholic hospital, or else find some way to quiet down the scandal aspects with appropriate explanations.[739] A good public-relations administrator of a Catholic hospital could dissipate the scandal possibilities by explaining that the Catholic hospital could hardly continue in operation without taking advantage of such an agreement to cut costs, etc.,—that the agreement also is viewed as an ecumenical venture, or even as a survival measure, etc.

The obligation to be on guard against scandal and its consequences rests heavily on the consciences of those who represent the Church as individuals or as Catholic institutions and agencies. Appropriately the preamble to the *Directives* speaks of the responsibility of the Catholic health facility to "reflect in its policies and practices the moral teachings of the Church," and to serve as a "courageous witness to the highest ethical and moral principles in the pursuit of excellence" (paragraph 4). If they fail in this apostolic endeavor by even appearing to compromise Catholic values and principles, the natural reaction of many of the faithful will be to say, in effect, "If they do not feel obligated to follow the rules, why should we feel obligated to do so." Add to this the undercurrents of ridicule and recrimination from the general public, and there is no doubt that all institutions and agencies which bear responsibility for promoting and reflecting Catholic values and principles in the mission

---

[739]The actual words of St. Thomas: "Tunc vel totaliter dimittenda sunt temporalia, vel aliter scandalum est sedandum, scilicet per aliquam admonitionem." *Ibid.*, II-II, q. 43, art. 8, corp.

of healing, must take the forceful and solemn warning of the Lord Jesus most seriously:

> What terrible things will come on the world through scandal! It is inevitable that scandal should occur. Nonetheless, woe to that man through whom scandal comes (Matthew, 18:7).

Dissipating the "Appearances of Evil" in Scandal Situations

It is safe to presume that most "appearances of evil" associated with scandal on the hospital front originate within the upper-echelon corridors of the hospital. First there is lack of communication—then misunderstandings—then un-checked claims and suspicions passed from one to another—then a widening of the grapevine relay from the surgical unit to the nurses' lounges, to the nurses' stations, to the corridors, to the patients, to the streets and eventually to the media. By that time, a humble remark made out of curiosity, ignorance or discontent has grown into a network of damaging suspicions, rash judgments, false accusations, etc.—even some rejoicing over the embarrassment to the Catholic hospital and the Catholic community.

Such embarrassment and scandal atmosphere can be avoided by the pre-planned application of "preventive medicine" . . . to forestall any appearances of evil. If the employees of the Catholic hospital are to be expected to defend the reputation of the hospital from "appearances of evil," they must be furnished the information-background required for *understanding* the position of the hospital. Without this prudent use of communication, *misunderstandings* will result. Any efforts to cut the lines of communication in matters of material cooperation, and to maintain a tactical conspiracy of silence (administrator, physician, surgical nurse) is bound to be counterproductive. Basic information to be furnished to all employees, should include the following:

(1) The Catholic Church cannot approve of forbidden procedures such as tubal ligations in any way if the direct purpose of the procedure is contraceptive—for example, it would be seriously sinful for a Catholic hospital to agree to "do a tubal ligation" for a woman with a serious heart condition who fears that another pregnancy would endanger her life.

(2) Such procedures can never be performed in a Catholic hospital as a service of the hospital in the sense that Catholic physicians and nurses of the staff would be assigned to actual participation in the procedure itself. This applies even though the patient can honestly say: "But I see nothing

wrong about having a tubal ligation in my case."

(3) In some rare and exceptional cases, some Catholic hospitals have had to choose between making an exception and *allowing the hospital facilities to be used by others* (not of the Catholic hospital staff) OR of facing a very real and damaging consequence for not cooperating (for example, the eventual closing of the hospital).

(4) In such rare situations, the Catholic hospital which may decide in favor of *allowing their facilities to be used* is not "doing evil," but rather cooperating reluctantly in a *material* manner (no *formal* approval given) in the performance of a merely-tolerated evil procedure so as to avoid an even greater evil to the Catholic hospital, the Catholic faith or the Catholic community.

(5) If the administration of this Catholic hospital ever encounters the need of making the choice as above in favor of such *material cooperation,* you will be informed of the essential particulars in due time so that you can be in a position to defend the reputation of this hospital from false rumors, unfounded suspicions, false accusations, etc., which could lead to serious scandal in this community. If any of the points of information above are unclear to you, please see your department head who will direct you to a source of more extensive information.

Possible means of communicating such essential information—to be repeated periodically to refresh their memories—could be one or more of the following: the administrator's bulletin to Catholic hospital personnel, memoranda furnished to all prospective hospital employees along with printed pamphlets or booklets on Catholic hospital policies, occasional bulletins from the ethics committee of the hospital, periodic "Messages from Your Chaplain," the printed hospital magazine or publication, etc.

If the "appearances of evil" do arise and advance beyond the walls of the hospital to the general public and even to the media, despite the precautions taken as above, every effort should be made to dissipate such adverse suspicions, comments, judgments, etc., by well-publicized efforts to provide an "appropriate explanation of what is really being done" (cf. *Roman Reply, 1975,* appendix, lines 59–63). The importance of consultation with the bishop of the diocese regarding both *sufficiently proportionate reasons* for contemplating material cooperation and the *serious inconvenience* in evaluating the extent of the danger of scandal cannot be overemphasized. Naturally the sufficiently proportionate reasons for contemplating material cooperation would carry a predominant weight in evaluating the gravity of the serious inconvenience. A significant factor in evaluating the gravity of the *inconvenience* could be something over and above the sufficiently proportionate reasons; for example, that a delay in proceeding with due publicity on the material cooperation decision definitely would contribute to the worsening of the scandal situation.

Ordinarily an "appropriate explanation of what is really being done" will dissipate the appearances of evil so that the hospital can apply the Principle of Material Cooperation to the exceptional situation despite the vestiges of some spiritual harm to others due to scandal. There could be situations, however, when the scandal element was so advanced and virulent that the "appearances of evil" cannot be dissipated. In such cases, the Catholic hospital administrator would have to deny the use of the hospital facilities for the tubal ligation (or other prohibited procedure). The following scandal-situations are presented as possibilities for illustration purposes: the former administrator of the hospital who had been liberal on the material cooperation issue has been replaced by a new administrator just one week before the present material-cooperation dilemma developed (hence, "on the spot"); a discontented surgical nurse who was refused information on the details of tubal ligation has spread the rumor far and wide that the woman will get her "forbidden tube tying" because she is a generous contributor to the hospital; the local newspaper is still carrying stories about a contested induced abortion at a Catholic hospital which involved a living infant, etc. In other words, there can be situations when the potential for scandal and harm to the Church cannot be dissipated simply because no appropriate explanation is possible in the current circumstances.

> *Preamble, paragraph 4:* And just as it bears responsibility to the past, so does the Catholic health facility carry special responsibility for the present and future. Any facility identified as Catholic assumes with this identification the responsibility to reflect in its policies and practices the moral teachings of the Church, under the guidance of the local bishop. Within the community the Catholic health facility is needed as a courageous witness to the highest ethical and moral principles in its pursuit of excellence.
>
> *Preamble, paragraph 8:* The moral evaluation of new scientific developments and legitimately debated questions must be finally submitted to the teaching authority of the Church in the person of the local bishop, who has the ultimate responsibility for teaching Catholic doctrine.
>
> Cf. also Vatican II's *Dogmatic Constitution on the Church,* n.27.

POSTSCRIPT: The Unifying Power of the Moral Virtue of "Pietas"

Vatican II's *Decree on Ecumenism* begins with a comment that the Lord of Ages "has begun to bestow more generously upon divided Christians remorse over their divisions and a longing for unity" (n.1). Chapter I of this book as well as chapter X provide evidence of how urgently our theologians and ethicists need that sense of "remorse over division, and longing for unity." The word "division" does not apply to commendable efforts by theologians and other scholars to search for "more suitable ways of communicating doctrine to men of their times" as mentioned in Vatican II's document, *The Church Today* (n.62). That necessary and praiseworthy process is bound to generate diverse viewpoints, various interpretations of sources, differences in the direction of scholarly research and analysis, etc., but should not result in division. The spectre of division and disunity appears when the objective is not clarification but radical change; when the magisterium of the Church is watered down by caustic innuendo; when the sources of authority are rejected or disqualified; when the family of the faithful is subjected to doubt and confusion by deliberate efforts to expand the parameters of dissent.

What is needed is a renewed sense of the "Household of the Faith" (Galatians,6:10) whereby all members of the faithful are obligated to harbor and manifest loving loyalty to our "Holy Mother, the Church"—a debt and an obligation which, in the theology of St. Thomas, can never be adequately fulfilled in an entire lifetime. Keeping differences of opinion within the family through scholarly discussion and publication is one thing; to broadcast such differences indiscriminately and even invite a personal following of adherents is a brand of divisiveness which is damaging to all that we hold dear as members of the Household of the Faith.

That damage can be averted by taking to heart three special virtues which have a separate classification under the cardinal virtue of justice insofar as no one can adequately measure up to "what is due" regardless of holiness of life or length of years. This trio is made up of the virtues of *religion* (which regulates reverence for God), *piety* (which regulates reverence for parents, family and homeland) and *respect and esteem* (which regulates reverence for those in authority, teachers, etc.).[740] Being asked to choose "which of these three is the greatest" is somewhat like choosing from among the three theological virtues of faith, hope and charity. A lack of the virtue of *religion* can alienate a person from God; a lack of *respect and esteem* can make obedience all but impossible. A lack of *piety*, however, comes closest to explaining divisiveness and disunity among theologians and ethicists today.

---

[740]*Ibid.*, II-II, q. 101, art. 1, corp., and q. 102, art. 1, corp. and ad tertium.

In order to portray that virtue of piety in its true potential, the word itself must be rescued from the *"folded hands"* stereotype. Piety has much more to do with *supporting hands.* As mentioned above, it is linked to loving loyalty to the Church. In *Cassell's Latin Dictionary,* the first meaning of the word "pius" (pious) is given as "acting dutifully." A secondary meaning is listed as "affectionate towards one's parents, benefactors, relatives, native country, etc." Similarly, in *Webster's Collegiate Dictionary,* the first-listed meaning of "pious" is "dutiful or loyal to parents, family, race, etc." A contemporary writer extolls "pietas" as follows:

> This virtue has much more to do with what we owe than with our claims. Yet if it were cultivated and practiced, it could ground the loyalty of a community's members to the traditions and institutions which give it structure and meaning, and at the same time, it could be a source of more thoughtful and measured critique of those institutions.[741]

A durable line of simple poetry comes to mind: "And though to us it seems one-sided, trouble is pretty well divided." In surveying the spectre of division and disunity as current among Catholic theologians today, the tendency often inclines to assigning the source of trouble to one side—the *other* side,—and to arrogate to oneself the only respectable mantle of loyalty. Loyalty comes in various degrees and dimensions. The first requirement of the virtue which identifies all true Christians—which is charity,—is that those especially who profess to promote and penetrate the Word of God (theologians) must persist in thinking well of those who choose to view and appreciate the traditions and institutions of the Church from another perspective or from a more critical stance. The presumption should be that their sense of remorse for any improprieties which have contributed to division or disunity is as genuine as ours; that their determination to foster the virtue of piety is as profound and authentic as our own.

The practical implications of that sense of "pietas" were expressed well by Father Val J. Peter in his address entitled "The Pastoral Approach to Magisterial Teaching" as delivered to 240 Catholic bishops of North and

---

[741]Kossel, Clifford G., "Piety: The Debts Which Precede Our Rights," in *Communio,* spring, 1985, pp. 35, 36.

Central America and the Caribbean at a workshop sponsored by the Pope John Center in February, 1984:

> Similarly we all owe Holy Mother Church this much: it is from her that any hope we may have of eternal life has been mediated to us. No matter how ill-mannered or shabby or inadequate the Church's ministers might have on occasion been in our youth, yet it was from this Church and none other that we received the hope of eternal life that burns brightly in our hearts today. *Pietas* toward Holy Mother Church is not an optional devotional practice good for pious old ladies. It is a matter of justice, something we all owe.[742]

---

[742]*Moral Theology Today* (cf. note 129), p. 91.

Appendix

REPLY OF THE SACRED CONGREGATION FOR THE DOCTRINE OF THE FAITH ON STERILIZATION IN CATHOLIC HOSPITALS
March 13, 1975

1-This sacred Congregation has diligently considered not only the prob-
2-lem of contraceptive sterilization for therapeutic purposes but also
3-the opinions indicated by different people toward a solution, and the
4-conflicts relative to requests for cooperation in such sterilizations in
5-Catholic hospitals. The Congregation has resolved to respond to
6-these questions in this way:

7-   1. Any sterilization which of itself, that is, of its own nature and
8-condition, has the sole immediate effect of rendering the generative
9-faculty incapable of procreation, is to be considered direct sterili-
10-zation, as the term is understood in the declarations of the pontifical
11-magisterium, especially of Pius XII.[1] Therefore, notwithstanding any
12-subjectively right intention of those whose actions are prompted by
13-the care or prevention of physical or mental illness which is foreseen
14-or feared as a result of pregnancy, such sterilization remains ab-
15-solutely forbidden according to the doctrine of the Church. And indeed
16-the sterilization of the faculty itself is forbidden for an even graver
17-reason than the sterilization of individual acts, since it induces a state
18-of sterility in the person which is almost always irreversible.

---

[1]Cf. especially the two allocutions to the Catholic Union of Obstetricians and to the International Society of Hematology; in AAS 43, 1951, 843–844; 50, 1958, 734–737 and in the encyclical of Paul VI, Humanae Vitae, n. 14 cf. AAS 60, 1968, 490–491.

19- Neither can any mandate of public authority, which would seek to
20-impose direct sterilization as necessary for the common good, be
21-invoked, for such sterilization damages the dignity and inviolability
22-of the human person.[2] Likewise, neither can one invoke the principle
23-of totality in this case, in virtue of which principal interference with
24-organs is justified for the greater good of the person; sterility intended
25-in itself is not oriented to the integral good of the person as rightly
26-pursued, "the proper order of goods being preserved,"[3] inasmuch
27-as it damages the ethical good of the person, which is the highest
28-good, since it deliberately deprives foreseen and freely chosen sexual
29-activity of an essential element. Thus article 20 of the medical-ethics
30-code promulgated by the Conference in 1971 faithfully reflects the
31-doctrine which is to be held, and its observance should be urged.

32- 2. The Congregation, while it confirms this traditional doctrine of
33-the Church, is not unaware of the dissent against this teaching from
34-many theologians. The Congregation, however, denies that doctrinal
35-significance can be attributed to this fact as such, so as to constitute
36-a "theological source" which the faithful might invoke and thereby
37-abandon the authentic magisterium, and follow the opinions of private
38-theologians which dissent from it.[4]

39- 3. Insofar as the management of Catholic hospitals is concerned:

40-   a) Any cooperation institutionally approved or tol-
41-   erated in actions which are in themselves, that is, by
42-   their nature and condition, directed to a contraceptive
43-   end, namely, that the natural effects of sexual actions
44-   deliberately performed by the sterilized subject be
45-   impeded, is absolutely forbidden. For the official appro-
46-   bation of direct sterilization and, a fortiori, its manage-
47-   ment and execution in accord with hospital regulations,
48-   is a matter which, in the objective order, is by its very
49-   nature (or intrinsically) evil. The Catholic hospital cannot

---

[2]Cf. Pius XI, the encyclical Casti Connubii, in AAS 22, 1930, 565.
[3]Paul VI, the encyclical Humanae Vitae, in AAS 60, 1968, 487.
[4]Cf. Vatican Council II, constitution Lumen Gentium, n. 25, 1 (in AAS, 57, 1965, 29-30);
Pius XII, Allocution to the Most Reverend Cardinals, ibid., 46, 1954, 672; the encyclical
Humani Generis, ibid., 42, 1950, 568; Paul VI, Allocution to the meeting regarding the
theology of Vatican Council II, ibid., 58, 1966, 889-896 (especially 890-894); the Allocution
to the Members of the Congregation of the Most Holy Redeemer, ibid., 59, 1967, 960-963
(especially 962).

50– cooperate with this for any reason. Any cooperation so
51– supplied is totally unbecoming the mission entrusted to
52– this type of institution and would be contrary to the
53– necessary proclamation and defense of the moral order.

54–   b) The traditional doctrine regarding material co-
55– operation, with the proper distinctions between nec-
56– essary and free, proximate and remote, remains valid,
57– to be applied with the utmost prudence, if the case
58– warrants.

59–   c) In the application of the principle of material co-
60– operation, if the case warrants, great care must be taken
61– against scandal and the danger of any misunderstand-
62– ing by an appropriate explanation of what is really being
63– done.
64–   This sacred Congregation hopes that the criteria recalled in this
65–letter will satisfy the expectations of that episcopate, in order that,
66–with the uncertainties of the faithful cleared up, the bishops might
67–more easily respond to their pastoral duty.

COMMENTARY
ON THE REPLY OF THE SACRED CONGREGATION FOR THE DOCTRINE OF THE FAITH TO NATIONAL CONFERENCE OF CATHOLIC BISHOPS ON STERILIZATION IN CATHOLIC HOSPITALS
September 15, 1977

68–In response to many requests for clarification, it is our intention here
69–to summarize key elements of the Roman document issued by the
70–Sacred Congregation for the Doctrine of the Faith, March 13, 1975,
71–as well as to make several comments on the interpretation and ap-
72–plication of the document in the American context. The purpose of
73–these remarks is to assist the local Ordinaries and Catholic health
74–care personnel in the formulation of a corporate position regarding
75–the performance of sterilization procedures.

The Congregation's Response

76– The Congregation affirmed the teaching of the magisterium that
77–"any sterilization which of itself, that is, of its own nature and
condition,
78–has the sole immediate effect of rendering the generative faculty
79–incapable of procreation," is completely forbidden. Thus, sterilization
80–may not be used as a means of contraception nor may it be used
81–as a means for the care or prevention of a physical or mental illness
82–which is foreseen or feared as a result of pregnancy. The Congre-
83–gation also affirmed that no mandate of public authority can justify
84–direct sterilization nor can the principle of totality be invoked.

85– On the other hand, procedures that induce sterility are not always
86–forbidden. The Congregation affirmed that Article 20 of the hospital
87–medical–ethical code faithfully reflects the teaching which should be
88–held and observed. As this article states, procedures that induce
89–sterility are permitted when they "(a) are immediately directed to the
90–cure, diminution, or prevention of a serious pathological condition
91–and are not directly contraceptive (that is contraception is not the
92–purpose); and (b) a simpler treatment is not reasonably available"
93–(Article 20, Ethical and Religious Directives for Catholic Health Fa-
94–cilities).

95– The document from the Sacred Congregation formulated three
96–principles that pertain to the management of Catholic hospitals and
97–sterilization procedures. For purposes of information and clarity, we
98–here reproduce these three principles as stated in the original doc-
99–ument:

100– a) Any cooperation institutionally approved or tolerated in actions
101– which are in themselves, that is, by their nature and condition,
102– directed to a contraceptive end, namely, that the natural effects
103– of sexual actions deliberately performed by the sterilized sub-
104– ject be impeded, is absolutely forbidden. The official appro-
105– bation of direct sterilization and, a fortiori, its management
106– and execution in accord with hospital regulations, is a matter
107– which, in the objective order, is by its very nature (or intrin-
108– sically) evil. The Catholic hospital therefore cannot cooperate
109– with this for any reason. Any cooperation so supplied is totally
110– unbecoming the mission entrusted to this type of institution
111– and would be contrary to the necessary proclamation and
112– defense of the moral order.

113-   b) The traditional doctrine regarding material cooperation, with
114-   the proper distinction between necessary and free, proximate
115-   and remote, remains valid, to be applied with the utmost pru-
116-   dence, if the case warrants.

117-   c) In the application of the principle of material cooperation, if
118-   the case warrants, great care must be taken against scandal
119-   and the danger of any misunderstanding by an appropriate
120-   explanation of what is really being done.

Guidelines for Hospital Policy

121- Without repeating all of the elements expressed in the Congre-
122- gation's statement, we present the following guidelines for Catholic
123- health facilities:

124-   1. As it was stated in the Roman document, the Catholic hospital
125-   can in no way approve the performance of any sterilization
126-   procedure that is directly contraceptive. Such contraceptive
127-   procedures include sterilizations performed as a means of
128-   preventing future pregnancy that one fears might aggravate
129-   a serious cardiac, renal, circulatory or other disorder. Freely
130-   approving direct sterilization constitutes formal cooperation in
131-   evil and would be "totally unbecoming the mission" of the
132-   hospital as well as "contrary to the necessary proclamation
133-   and defense of the moral order."

134-   2. The Catholic health facility has the moral responsibility (and
135-   this is legally recognized) to decide what medical procedures
136-   it will provide services for. Ordinarily, then, there will be no
137-   need or reason to provide services for objectively immoral
138-   procedures. Material cooperation will be justified only in sit-
139-   uations where the hospital because of some kind of duress
140-   or pressure cannot reasonably exercise the autonomy it has
141-   (i.e., when it will do more harm than good).

142-   3. Because of the extraordinary nature of the decision concerning
143-   material cooperation, i.e., the exception to the ethical religious
144-   directives and the potential scandal, the bishop of the diocese
145-   or his representative must be involved in the decision.

146-   4. In judging the morality of cooperation a clear distinction should
147-   be made between the reason for the sterilization and the rea-
148-   son for the cooperation. If the hospital cooperates because

424

149– of the reason for the sterilization, e.g., because it is done for
150– medical reasons, the cooperation can hardly be considered
151– material. In other words the hospital can hardly maintain under
152– these circumstances that it does not approve sterilizations
153– done for medical reasons, and this would make cooperation
154– formal. If the cooperation is to remain material, the reason for
155– the cooperation must be something over and above the reason
156– for the sterilization itself. Since, as mentioned above (n.2),
157– the hospital has authority over its own decisions, this should
158– not happen with any frequency.

159– 5. In making judgments about the morality of cooperation each
160– case must be decided on its own merits. Since hospital sit-
161– uations, and even individual cases, differ so much, it would
162– not be prudent to apply automatically a decision made in one
163– hospital, or even in one case, to another.

164– 6. As was stated in the Roman document, the Catholic Health
165– facility must take every precaution to avoid creating misun-
166– derstanding or causing scandal to its staff, patients, or general
167– public by offering a proper explanation when necessary. It
168– should be made clear that the hospital disapproves of direct
169– sterilization and that material cooperation in no way implies
170– approval.

171–Direct sterilization is a grave evil. The allowance of material coop-
172–eration in extraordinary cases is based on the danger of an even
173–more serious evil, e.g., the closing of the hospital could be under
174–certain circumstances a more serious evil.

175– This is a commentary on the response of the Sacred Congregation
176–for the Doctrine of the Faith regarding the use of material cooperation
177–on the part of Catholic health-care facilities in cases of sterilization.
178–It is not meant to be a general discussion of the application of material
179–cooperation as such, and, therefore, should not be extended to other
180–areas.

STATEMENT ON TUBAL LIGATION
July 3, 1980

181–Since we note among Catholic health care facilities a certain con-
182–fusion in the understanding and application of authentic Catholic

183-teaching with regard to the morality of tubal ligation as a means of
184-contraceptive sterilization (cf.nos.18 & 20; Ethical and Religious
185-Directives for Catholic Health Facilities) the National Conference of
186-Catholic Bishops makes the following clarification:

187- 1. The traditional teaching of the Church as reaffirmed by the
188-Sacred Congregation for the Doctrine of the Faith on March 13, 1975
189-clearly declares the objective immorality of contraceptive (direct) ster-
190-ilization even if done for medical reasons.

191- 2. The principle of totality does not apply to contraceptive steri-
192-lization and cannot be used to justify it.

193- 3. Formal cooperation in the grave evil of contraceptive sterili-
194-zation, either by approving or tolerating it for medical reasons, is
195-forbidden and totally alien to the mission entrusted by the Church to
196-Catholic health care facilities.

197- 4. The reason for justifying material cooperation as described in
198-the NCCB Commentary on the SCDF response refers not to medical
199-reasons given for the sterilization but to grave reasons extrinsic to
200-the case. Catholic health care facilities in the United States complying
201-with the Ethical and Religious Directives are protected by the First
202-Amendment from pressures intended to require medical cooperation
203-in contraceptive sterilization. In the unlikely and extraordinary situ-
204-ation in which the principle of material cooperation seems to be
205-justified, consultation with the Bishop or his delegate is required.

206- 5. The local Ordinary has responsibility for assuring that the moral
207-teachings of the Church be taught and followed in health care facilities
208-which are to be recognized as Catholic. In this important matter there
209-should be increased and continuing collaboration between the Bishop,
210-health care facilities and their sponsoring religious communities. Lo-
211-cal conditions will suggest the practical structures necessary to insure
212-this collaboration.

213- 6. The NCCB profoundly thanks the many physicians, adminis-
214-trators and personnel of Catholic health care facilities who faithfully
215-maintain the teaching and practice of the Church with regard to
216-Catholic moral principles.

Index

PLEASE NOTE the "Quick Reference" Commentary on each of the *Ethical and Religious Directives* by Father Albert Moraczewski, O.P., following this index.

427

medicine, 207, 208

spiral in cost of health care, 63, 64

Teratogenic Diseases: alcohol and pregnancy, 112; 211, 212

Terminal Condition: danger of presuming incompetency, 201, 202

definition of, 168

relative to nursing care, 178, 179

problem of how much to tell, 198–200

"useful" v. "useless" means, 162; 174; 185; 223, 224

see also mentally incompetent; nutrition/ hydration; ordinary/extraordinary means

Terminal Condition, Irreversible: antibiotics administration, 191

CPR not warranted, 165–167

does not apply to handicapped patients, 169; 183

guidelines on nutrition/hydration, 185ff.

meaning of "qualified person," 168

relative meaning of term, 186

with regard to hyperalimentation (IV), 181, 182

Testing, Diagnostic, etc.: often overdone, 167, 168

see also costs, medical

Testing, Prenatal: see obstetrics

Theologians: consulted in Directives revision process, 4ff.; 313; 375ff.

controversial issues in moral-medical field, 313, 314; 375ff.

disappointments in Directives revision process, 378–380

lawful freedom of inquiry and of expression, footnote 152, and 417, 418

represented on ethics committees, 308

see also authority in the Church; magisterium of the Church

Therapeutic: abortion terminology, 266, 267

regarding research on the unborn, 325, 326

Thomas Aquinas, St.: ensoulment doctrine, 94

example to illustrate principle of the double effect, 249ff.

principle of totality, 204; 215, 216

"scandal of the little ones," 412, 413

Tonsillectomy: not justified if elective, 226

Totality, Principle of: "anatomical" v. "functional" wholeness, 217

association with Directive 6, 91

cannot justify sterilization, 86; 91; 218, 219; 385

conditions for removal of organs, 217, 218

definition of, 204, 205; 215, 216

involved in average medical treatment, 225

"man" v. "humanity" (Pius XII), 216

principle applied by Pius XII, 218, 219

problem of the transsexual, 228–231

relationship to integrity, 205–207

see also integrity and totality, principles of

TOT Procedure (Tubal Ovum Transfer): Archbishop Pilarczyk's comments, 44

"moral union" concept, 47

pioneer efforts, 1983, 43, 44

see also GIFT procedure

Transfusions: see blood transfusions

Transplants: see organ transplants, human

Transsexualism: contrary to the principle of totality, 230

need of psychotherapy, 230, 231

question of gender ambiguity, 231, 232

see also impotence, sexual

Trophoblastic Disease: see hydatidiform mole

Trustees, Board of: "in conscience" responsibilities in re: Catholic Directives, 145

may appoint officers of ethics committee, 308

representation on the ethics committee, 308, 309

Truth in Human Relationships: extent of patient's "right to know," 198–200

Informing patient of his/her condition, 198–200; 351–353

mental reservations, 350, 351

see also physician-patient relationship

Truth, Religious: obligation to adhere to, 120, 121

Tubal Ligations: unreasonable to expect doctrinal changes, 313

see also sterilization; uterine isolation

ETHICAL AND RELIGIOUS DIRECTIVES FOR CATHOLIC HEALTH FACILITIES

(Marginal reference indicates where topic is discussed in this book)

The "Quick Reference" Commentary (following the Preamble) on each Directive was Contributed by Father Albert Moraczewski, O.P., Ph.D., Director of the Regional Office of the Pope John Center in Houston, Texas

PREAMBLE

Paragraph 1

Cf.
Chapter III
pp. 67–70

Catholic health facilities witness to the saving presence of Christ and His Church in a variety of ways: by testifying to transcendent spiritual beliefs concerning life, suffering, and death; by humble service to humanity and especially to the poor; by medical competence and leadership; and by fidelity to the Church's teachings while ministering to the good of the whole person.

Paragraph 2

Cf. Chapter II
pp. 20–22

Chapter X
pp. 391–398

The total good of the patient, which includes his higher spiritual as well as his bodily welfare, is the primary concern of those entrusted with the management of a Catholic health facility. So important is this, in fact, that if an institution could not fulfill its basic mission in this regard, it would have no justification for continuing its existence as a Catholic health facility. Trustees and administrators of Catholic health facilities should understand that this responsibility affects their relationship with every patient, regardless of religion, and is seriously binding in conscience.

Paragraph 3

A Catholic-sponsored health facility, its board of trustees, and administration face today a serious

461

Cf.
Chapter VIII
pp. 300–304

difficulty as, with community support, the Catholic health facility exists side by side with other medical facilities not committed to the same moral code, or stands alone as the one facility serving the community. However, the health facility identified as Catholic exists today and serves the community in a large part because of the past dedication and sacrifice of countless individuals whose lives have been inspired by the Gospel and the teachings of the Catholic Church.

Paragraph 4

Cf.
Chapter X
pp. 410–416

And just as it bears responsibility to the past, so does the Catholic health facility carry special responsibility for the present and future. Any facility identified as Catholic assumes with this identification the responsibility to reflect in its policies and practices the moral teachings of the Church, under the guidance of the local bishop. Within the community the Catholic health facility is needed as a courageous witness to the highest ethical and moral principles in its pursuit of excellence.

Paragraph 5

Cf.
Chapter IV
pp. 143–145

Chapter X
pp. 398–402

The Catholic-sponsored health facility and its board of trustees, acting through its chief executive officer, further, carry an overriding responsibility in conscience to prohibit those procedures which are morally and spiritually harmful. The basic norms delineating this moral responsibility are listed in these *Ethical and Religious Directives for Catholic Health Facilities*. It should be understood that patients and those who accept board membership, staff appointment or privileges, or employment in a Catholic health facility will respect and agree to abide by its policies and these Directives. Any attempt to use a Catholic health facility for procedures contrary to these norms would indeed compromise the board and administration in its responsibility to seek and protect the total good of its patients, under the guidance of the Church.

Paragraph 6

Cf.
Chapter VI
pp. 215–225

These Directives prohibit those procedures which, according to present knowledge, are recognized as clearly wrong. The basic moral absolutes which underlie these Directives are not subject to change, although particular applications might be modified as scientific investigation and theological development open up new problems or cast new light on old ones.

Paragraph 7

Cf.
Chapter VIII
pp. 313–315

In addition to consulting among theologians, physicians, and other medical and scientific personnel in local areas, the Committee on Health Affairs of the United States Catholic Conference, with the widest consultation possible, should regularly receive suggestions and recommendations from the field, and should periodically discuss any possible need for an updated revision of these Directives.

Paragraph 8

Cf.
Chapter X
pp. 410–416

The moral evaluation of new scientific developments and legitimately debated questions must be finally submitted to the teaching authority of the Church in the person of the local bishop, who has the ultimate responsibility for teaching Catholic doctrine.

Ethical and Religious Directives for Catholic Health Facilities

Directive 1

The procedures listed in these Directives as permissible require

"As permissible:" This pertains only to those medical or surgical procedures which the patient may have done or the physician may do.

the consent, at least
implied or reasonably
presumed, of the
patient or his guard-
ians. This condition
is to be understood
in all cases.

Discussed in this
book:

Chapter V
pp. 154–203

"Require consent:" It is always understood that
the patient is **(a)** capable of giving consent, and
(b) has been properly informed regarding the
benefits and risks reasonably anticipated.

"At least implied or reasonably presumed:"
The patient implies consent by some words or
sign which communicates to the physician that
the patient has implicitly given consent. If this
word of implied consent is lacking, the physician
may be able to judge from knowledge of the patient that consent would be given if, in the
proper circumstances, the consent has been requested or invited.

"Of the patient or his guardian:" The patient
has the primary right and responsibility, but if
incompetent (i.e., too young) a proxy is to give
consent, attempting to respond as the patient
would if he were capable. This presumes that the
proxy is in the position **to know** some of the
patient's mind and truly loves the patient so that
he sincerely respects the patient's wishes and
truly desires the patient's authentic well being.

Directive 2

No person may be
obliged to take part
in a medical or surgi-
cal procedure which
he judges in cons-
cience to be immoral;
nor may a health
facility or any of its
staff be obliged to
provide a medical or
surgical procedure
which violates their

"No person:" Includes physicians, nurses, technicians or other members of the staff who in
some way contribute or support the procedure in
question.

"May be obliged:" This refers to pressures
placed on the person and includes strong verbal
persuasion, threats (stated or implied) of economic loss or other undesirable consequences.

**"Which he judges in conscience to be im-
moral:"** The individual is convinced that to par-

conscience or these
Directives.

Discussed in this
book:

Chapter IV
pp. 145–148

ticipate in the procedure would violate what the
person holds to be a matter of morality; the
action would be for them morally evil.

"Health facility or any of its staff:" This includes the Board of Trustees (or equivalent), the
administration, medical, surgical, nursing, professional technical and non-technical members of
the health facility's staff.

"Their conscience or these Directives:" While
the conscience of persons is subjective and indi-
vidualized, the **Directives** represent an official,
objective statement of relevant principles and
their application to situations in the health care
facility.

Directive 3

Every patient, re-
gardless of the extent
of his physical or
psychic disability,
has a right to be
treated with a respect
consonant with his
dignity as a person.

Discussed in this
book:

Chapter II
pp. 20–33

"Every patient:" All persons admitted to the
health facility or to the emergency room, as well
as those born within the health facility. Also included are the unborn whose mother has been
admitted to the facility or emergency room.

**"Right to be treated with a respect consonant
with his dignity as a person:"** All personnel of
the health facility have the moral obligation to
deal with patients with due care and attention,
having a special regard to their current vulnera-
bility. At times of illness or injury, persons often
experience a decrease in self-esteem and thus
more readily feel themselves to be persons of no
consequence. Discussions with or about patients
should not so focus on the patient's illness or
condition so as to overlook the patient. Of particular importance are those staff discussions carried on in the presence of the patient which
should not ignore the patient as if he were
merely a piece of furniture in the room. Not to
be forgotten is that seemingly unconscious (or

sleeping) patients sometimes are not unconscious (or sleeping) and can at times hear and understand conversations in their vicinity.

Directive 4

Man has the right and the duty to protect the integrity of his body together with all of its bodily functions.

Discussed in this book:

Chapter VI pp. 204–215

"Man has the right:" A human being, as such, has a **moral** title, rooted in the natural law, which requires others to respect the integrity of his body and its functions.

"Man has . . . the duty:" A human being, as such, has the **moral** obligation to make use of those means ordinarily deemed as necessary to maintain his own life and health.

"To protect the integrity of his body:" The preservation of functional integrity and anatomical wholeness requires due respect to the subordination of structure to function and the latter to life. This means a part may be sacrificed when its removal would be required to maintain the health or life of the individual.

Directive 5

Any procedure potentially harmful to the patient is morally justified only insofar as it is designed to produce a proportionate good.

Discussed in this book:

Chapter VII pp. 247–265

"Any procedure potentially harmful:" Previous experience and knowledge permits one, e.g., the physician or patient to judge that a particular procedure may cause some injury to the patient.

"Morally justified:" The procedure is morally good, i.e., it promotes the authentic well-being of the patient.

"Designed to produce:" The objective of the procedure, e.g., surgical excision of an inflamed appendix, is to remove a pathological tissue or correct a malfunctioning organ or tissue which is an actual or imminent significant threat to the well-being of the patient.

The intention, too, of those performing the procedure is likewise directed to restoring or maintaining the health of the individual.

"Produce a proportionate good:" The good effect to be achieved must be at least equal or greater than the potential harm (the evil effect) which may result from the procedure. Granted that it is difficult to attach a quantitatively determined moral value to any object, nonetheless one can say that life is more precious than health; health than property. The loss of a limb is outweighed by the preservation of life, etc.

Directive 6

Ordinarily the proportionate good that justifies a medical or surgical procedure should be the total good of the patient himself.

Discussed in this book:

    Chapter II pp. 20–22

    Chapter VI pp. 215–225

"Ordinarily:" The principle would be applicable in most cases but allows for exceptions; for example, medical research in which the individual freely volunteers having given his informed consent.

"Should be the total good of the patient:" Total good could be the life or health of the individual, not merely the restoration of a function or part, as such.

Directive 7

Adequate consultation is recommended,

"Adequate consultation:" If the issue is a moral one, then the consultant(s) selected should

not only when there is doubt concerning the morality of some procedure, but also with regard to all procedures involving serious consequences, even though such procedures are listed here as permissible. The health facility has the right to insist on such consultations.

Discussed in this book:

Chapter VIII
pp. 304–312

not only be competent in the area of medical ethics but also be familiar with, and loyal to, the relevant official church teaching.

"but also with regard to all procedures involving serious consequences:" What is envisioned are matters such as the possibility of death or the loss of a limb or major function. Suitable medical or surgical consultants are called for, so that the patient receives the best appropriate care available in the particular circumstances.

"The health facility has the right:" To help insure that the patient admitted to the facility receives truly competent treatment and care, the health facility has the moral title to insist that its staff, who have been given the privilege to admit and care for patients on its premises, observe this requirement. Among additional reasons, the hospital needs to protect itself against lawsuits which may arise as the result of staff incompetency or negligence.

Directive 8

Everyone has the right and the duty to prepare for the solemn moment of death. Unless it is clear, therefore, that a dying patient is already well-prepared for death as regards both spiritual and temporal affairs, it is the physician's duty to inform him of his critical condition or to have some other responsible person

"Everyone has the right and duty to prepare for death:" Every human person has the moral title to the opportunity for cleansing his conscience in preparation for the moment of divine judgment. The person also has a right to whatever assistance may be necessary to bring this about. Both spiritual and temporal matters are included. For anyone to interfere with a dying person's spiritual preparation would be to commit a grave injustice.

"Everyone has the . . . duty, etc.:" Each individual has likewise a serious moral **obligation** to make the preparation mentioned above and should not hesitate to request, or seek, the help of a priest, or other religious minister if pre-

impart this information.

Discussed in this book:

Chapter V
pp. 198–201

Chapter IX,
pp. 351–353

ferred by a non-catholic, as well as to settle debts, be reconciled with family members or friends, and make such provisions so as to discharge other obligations in justice or charity.

"It is the physician's duty to inform him . . .:" Since the physician is one who knows and appreciates best the patient's medical condition, and who also, of course, has by covenant the care of the patient, he has the primary obligation to inform the patient of his condition. The physician ordinarily should personally discharge that obligation. However, if for some reasonable cause, the physician is unable, the physician still has the responsibility of delegating an individual who can suitably communicate the truth in a sensitive manner. This individual may be a nurse, a social worker, a member of the family or a person from the Pastoral Care Department.

Directive 9

The obligation of professional secrecy must be carefully fulfilled not only as regards the information on the patients' charts and records but also as regards confidential matters learned in the exercise of professional duties. Moreover, the charts and records must be duly safeguarded against inspection by those who have no right to see them.

"Obligation of professional secrecy . . .:" In order to safeguard the confidentiality of information imparted or learned during the exercise of professional duties, the keeping of such information secret is a serious moral obligation. All too often there is a tendency on the part of some health care personnel to discuss cases in the cafeteria, hallways or elevators. Sometimes personnel will pass on to the patient or family incomplete or poorly understood information so that considerable confusion arises leading to undue anxiety or unsubstantiated optimism.

Discussed in this
book:

Directive 10

The directly intended termination of any patient's life, even at his own request, is always morally wrong.

Discussed in this
book:

"Directly intended termination:" Death may sometimes result, indirectly, during a surgical procedure, e.g., cardiac arrest. Another type of **indirect** death can result from a hazardous treatment which represents a desperate effort to deal with a life-threatening condition, e.g., a heart transplant which is not successful. Still another **indirect** death is that of a fetus when it becomes an urgent necessity to remove a cancerous uterus even though the fetus is not yet viable and it is foreseen with certainty that with present technology the fetus cannot be kept alive. While in these three cases death was the result, it was not **intended;** the death of these individuals was neither the objective nor the means by which a desired good was obtained.

The **Directive** prohibits the **directly intended** death of a person. Whatever other goal may be also intended, the purpose of the procedure cannot be achieved unless the death of the individual is brought about. The prohibition is aimed at the procedure whose necessary and desired result is the death of the individual. This would be murder, euthanasia, or mercy killing.

"Even at his own request:" One may not formally cooperate with another's action which is objectively a serious moral evil, no matter how noble may be the ultimate purpose. To cooperate **formally** means that one concurs with the objectively immoral intention of the other person. To cooperate **materially** means that one does **not** concur with the other person's evil intention, but contributes either to the act itself (**immediate** material cooperation) or to some **circumstances leading** to the act (mediate material cooperation). Nor may one cooperate materially and immediately with another's action the result of which would be his death.

"Is always morally wrong:" This statement means that there are no circumstances or good intentions which could change the objective immorality of such an action. It is an example of an exceptionless moral principle.

Directive 11

From the moment of conception, life must be guarded with the greatest care. Any deliberate medical procedure, the *purpose* of which is to deprive a fetus or an embryo of its life, is immoral.

Discussed in this book:

Chapter III pp. 93–96

Chapter VII, pp. 266–299

"From the moment of conception:" Conception, is defined as the moment when the new individual is constituted from fusion of the pronuclei of egg and sperm. The resulting single diploid cell, the zygote, has now its full genetic complement and a new human life has begun its long journey to adulthood.

"life must be guarded with the greatest care:" While the Magisterium of the Church has avoided definitely asserting that a human person is present from conception onwards (see its **Declaration on Abortion,** 1974, Chapter III), it has insisted repeatedly that life is, at the very least, intrinsically directed to **full** human life and must be given all rights and respect due to a human person. However, the facts of modern science, properly evaluated, argue strongly for the existence of a human person from the first cell (the zygote) onwards. (See the Pope John Center's, **An Ethical Evaluation of Fetal Experimentation: An Interdisciplinary Study,** 1976, especially Appendix I.)

471

"Any deliberate medical procedure, the purpose of which is to deprive a fetus, or an embryo of its life, is immoral:" The notion of "deliberate" is that act which is done knowingly and freely. Furthermore, if the direct and immediate objective (i.e., the purpose) of that procedure is to terminate the life of a living human person, whether as a goal or a means to another goal, albeit a worthy one, it is objectively immoral.

Directive 12

Abortion, that is, the directly intended termination of pregnancy before viability, is never permitted nor is the directly intended destruction of a viable fetus. Every procedure whose sole immediate effect is the termination of pregnancy before viability is an abortion, which, in its moral context, includes the interval between conception and implantation of the embryo. Catholic hospitals are not to provide abortion services based upon the principle of material cooperation.

"Directly intended:" This phrase means that it is the known and specific effect or consequence of a freely chosen procedure.

"Viability:" The state of the fetus that permits him to survive outside of the mother's womb even if technological assistance is required. Because of the latter qualification, viability for any fetus will depend not only on its own physiological maturity but also on the quality of technological support available at the time, at that place.

"directed intended destruction of a viable fetus:" The practice for example, of fetal dismemberment by the use of a suction apparatus or other means, or an act whose immediate objective is to destroy the life of an otherwise viable fetus, is a form of infanticide.

"Every procedure whose sole immediate effect is the termination of pregnancy before viability:" If the procedure's immediate effect is also the excision of a life-threatening pathological uterus (which is also concurrently bearing a child), then that procedure is not, in the **moral** sense, an abortion. (Some want to call it an **indirect** abortion, but that terminology can be

Discussed in this book:

Chapter III pp. 96–105

misleading since it is a **morally** legitimate surgical procedure.)

"includes the interval between conception and implantation of the embryo:" This inclusion is the basis of calling some of the artificial contraceptive procedures "abortifacient" since physiologically the "birth control" effect is the result, in part at least, of rendering the endometrium unsuitable for implantation with the consequent loss of the young, preimplantation embryo.

"Catholic hospitals are not to provide abortion services based upon the principle of material cooperation:" That principle requires not only that the hospital not concur with the intention of those desiring and performing the abortion (formal cooperation) and that its cooperation does not flow into the sinful procedure itself, but also that there be an extrinsic reason (that is outside of the reasons for the sinful act) that is weightier than the good which is lost **by** the unlawful procedure. There can be **no** justifying reason for the deliberate and direct taking of innocent human life. Hence, there can be no justifiable material cooperation.

Directive 13

Operations, treatments, and medications, which do not directly intend termination of pregnancy but which have as their purpose the cure of a proportionately serious pathological condition of

"Do not directly intend termination of pregnancy:" The **specific** objective (and effect) of the procedure is **not** the premature removal of the fetus from its proper and natural life-support system, even if it is foreseen that the action necessarily will also result in the unintended and undesired death of the fetus.

". . . which have as their purpose the cure of a proportionately serious pathological situa-

the mother, are permitted when they cannot be safely postponed until the fetus is viable, even though they may or will result in the death of the fetus. If the fetus is not certainly dead, it should be baptized.

Discussed in this book:

Chapter VII pp. 246–265

Chapter II, pp. 21–27

tion:" The purpose of the patient (and the physician as the patient's agent) is to treat, and cure if possible, an existing pathological condition. The disorder must be such that it constitutes a real threat to the life of the mother. Moreover, it is to be understood that there are no other available means to correct the disorder or remove the life threatening condition.

"If the fetus is not certainly dead, it should be baptized:" With a very young fetus, it may be difficult to ascertain with any certitude that it is dead. Where there is a reasonable doubt about the status of the fetus, it is better to baptize the fetus conditionally, such as, "If you are able to be baptized, I baptize you, etc." (see **Directive 36**). However, if the administration of the sacrament is prevented for prudential or other reasons, those involved may rest assured that the infant is consigned to God's love and mercy.

Directive 14

Regarding the treatment of hemorrhage during pregnancy and before the fetus is viable: Procedures that are designed to empty the uterus of a living fetus still effectively attached to the mother are not permitted: procedures designed to stop hemorrhage (as distinguished from those designed precisely to expel the living and attached

"**Procedures that are designed to empty the uterus, etc.:**" The precise objective (and primary effect) of the action is to force a living fetus from its proper place, and because this would be occurring before it was viable (see **Directive 12**, explanation) the death of the fetus will inevitably follow.

"**still effectively attached to the mother . . .:**" Because of some abnormality, the situation can occur when the fetus' attachment to the mother via the placenta has so deteriorated that the fetus is no longer receiving an adequate supply of oxygen and nutrients. Without some prompt corrective measure (when possible), the death of the fetus becomes inevitably. As long as the fetus is receiving an adequate supply of oxygen and nu-

fetus) are permitted insofar as necessary, even if fetal death is inevitably a side effect.

Discussed in this book:

Chapter VII
pp. 274-277

trients in its uterine location it may not be forcibly removed.

"Are not permitted . . .:" The procedure is morally evil because it is by intention and execution a direct attack on the life of an innocent person (i.e., one who has not committed a crime worthy of death). The Principle of Double Effect requires among others, that the desired good effect, here, the preservation of the woman's life and or health, is not obtained by means of the evil effect, here, the death of the fetus. In the procedures that are morally permitted, the good effect mentioned above is attained concurrently with the unintended, undesired but foreseen evil effect the death of the fetus. The goal, no matter how good or worthy or important, may not be obtained by means of an evil effect. One may not do evil to obtain a good.

Directive 15

Cesarean section for the removal of a viable fetus is permitted, even with risk to the life of the mother, when necessary for successful delivery. It is likewise permitted, even with risk for the child, when necessary for the safety of the mother.

Discussed in this book:

Chapter VI
pp. 220-223

". . . even with risk to the life of the mother:" In most regions of developed nations, the performance of a cesarean section for the delivery of a child can be done with relatively little danger to the mother. However, there may be particular circumstances (for example, the mother's physical status may be poor) when a cesarean delivery may represent some threat to the mother's health. If the infant's life is at stake, the cesarean section may be done even if the procedure represents a risk to the mother. In this situation, the safe delivery of the infant (the good effect) results concurrently with the risk to the mother's life (the evil effect). Since the good effect (the child's safe delivery) is not out-weighed by the evil effect (the risk to mother's life) nor is the former obtained by means of the latter, performing the cesarean delivery is morally good.

"It is likewise permitted, even with the risk for the child, when necessary for the safety of the mother:" The Principle of Double Effect, applied above, is similarly applicable in the converse situation. The cesarean delivery should not be done merely for the **convenience** of patient (or physician). There must be a genuine threat to the well-being of the mother.

Clearly from this **Directive**, it is apparent that the Church does not favor the child over the mother, or vice versa. It is a matter of both being of equal basic value. When the life of either one is threatened, then appropriate steps can be taken at the risk of the other, provided the requirements of the Principle of Double Effect are observed.

Directive 16

In extrauterine pregnancy, the dangerously affected part of the mother (e.g., cervix, ovary, or fallopian tube) may be removed, even though fetal death is foreseen provided that: a. the affected part is presumed already to be so dangerously affected as to warrant its removal, and that b. the operation is not just a separation of the embryo or fetus from its site within the part (which

"**Extrauterine pregnancy . . .:**" Also known as ectopic pregnancy. The developing human being is situated in a non-natural site and has only a very small probability of developing to viability.

". . . **the affected part is presumed already to be so damaged and dangerously affected as to warrant its removal:**" The damaged part may rapidly hemorrhage which can be so severe as to lead to serious injury or death to both embryo and mother.

". . . **the operation is not just a separation of the embryo or fetus from its site . . .:**" If it is only a removal of the embryo from its ectopic site which, for the moment at least, is the source of its nourishment and oxygen, that would be a direct attack on its life. It should be mentioned, however, that some authors would argue that it is

476

would be a direct abortion from a uterine appendage); and that c. the operation cannot be postponed without notably increasing the danger to the mother.

Discussed in this book:

      Chapter VII
      pp. 267–274

possible that the procedure is not precisely to remove the embryo but the placenta which is, or has, **burrowed** itself into the maternal tissue to get access to the blood supply. They claim that it is the placenta (which is **not** part of the embryo it should be noted) that is causing the tissue damage. Hence, the objective of the surgeon's procedure is to remove the offending placenta (good effect), and only incidentally but necessarily is the embryo removed (evil effect). Hence, according to this opinion, the procedure would be morally acceptable. Morally speaking, it remains an "open question."

Directive 17

Hysterectomy, in the presence of pregnancy and even before viability, is permitted when directed to the removal of a dangerous pathological condition of the uterus of such serious nature that the operation cannot be safely postponed until the fetus is viable.

Discussed in this book:

      Chapter VII
      pp. 288–289

"Hysterectomy, is permitted when directed to the removal of a dangerous pathological condition of the uterus:" The surgical removal of a uterus when the uterus is itself normal and healthy is not permissible. But when it is in a pathological state, e.g., cancerous or severely damaged, and its presence is a threat here and now to the life or health of the woman it may be removed. This is true even if the woman is pregnant and the condition of the fetus is pre or post the point of viability. By virtue of the Principle of Double Effect this can be done because the lives of mother and infant are on a par, and the life of the mother is not preserved by the removal or death of the fetus but by the removal of the pathological uterus.

". . . cannot be safely postponed . . .:" In such a situation it is necessary that an honest judgment be made that the hysterectomy truly cannot be safely postpone any longer. Every effort should be made to take those measures which might provide some opportunity for the fetus to survive.

Directive 18

Sterilization, whether permanent or temporary, for men or for women, may not be used as a means of contraception.

Discussed in this book:

> Chapter III
> pp. 70–86
>
> Chapter I,
> pp. 9–17
>
> Chapter X,
> pp. 374–407

"Sterilization, whether permanent or temporary . . .:" In the moral sense, sterilization here is **contraceptive** sterilization. It is the knowing and deliberate intervention into the conjugal act in a manner which renders the act infecund. That intervention changes its meaning; no longer does the act of intercourse have a procreative meaning, it is not a true **conjugal** act.

"Permanent:" By **"permanent"** is meant primarily the surgical removal of the uterus and/or fallopian tubes, and/or ovaries. It can also mean simply ligation of the fallopian tubes, i.e., "tying the tubes." But since today microsurgical techniques have improved, this procedure can be reversed in some cases so that the woman can become fertile again.

"Temporary:" As the name indicates, this class of sterilization procedure is of its nature reversible. The class would include barrier devices such as condoms, diaphragms (pessaries), sponges, spermicidal jellies and foams and anovulants (if their mode of contraception is by the inhibition of ovulation). Anovulants whose primary action is by rendering the endometrium hostile to implantation would be more accurately classified as abortifacients rather than true **contraceptives** since they do not inhibit conception. IUDs also seem to prevent procreation by acting as abortifacients.

Directive 19

Similarly excluded is every action which, either in anticipation of the conjugal act, or in its accomplish-

"Similarly excluded is every action . . .:" It is objectively morally evil knowingly and freely to initiate any action of which the desired end is to prevent procreation.

ment, or in the development of its natural consequences, proposes, whether as an end or as a means, to render procreation impossible.

Discussed in this book:

Chapter III pp. 86–90

"**. . . in anticipation of the conjugal act . . .:**" These actions include the use of anovulants, spermicidal creams, suppositories, diaphragms and condoms all of which are taken prior to sexual intercourse.

"**. . . or in its accomplishment . . .:**" Such actions might be seen as including the above as well as **Coitus interuptus** (withdrawal before ejaculation).

"**. . . or in the development of its natural consequence . . .:**" Such actions "after the fact" would include the use of a douche to wash out the sperm and the taking of a "morning-after pill." The action of which prevents implantation of the blastocyst (a stage in the development of the fertilized egg). Included also are any other actions directed at eliminating a human embryo or fetus from the womb.

"**. . . proposes, whether as an end or means, to render procreation impossible:**" It is the **intention** of the couple (or individual) freely to engage in an act of intercourse with the objective of preventing a conception or of taking actions necessary to expel a living, non-viable human embryo. Such actions are morally prohibited even if they are undertaken as a means to achieve a morally good objective such as the preservation of the woman's health. The end does not justify the means.

Directive 20

Procedures that induce sterility, whether permanent or temporary, are permitted when: a.

"**Procedures that induce sterility . . .:**" The **intention** in the use of such procedures is **not** to prevent conception, although a necessary **consequence** may be sterilization.

They are immediately directed to the cure, diminution, or prevention of a serious pathological condition and are not directly contraceptive (that is contraception is not the purpose); and b. a simpler treatment is not reasonably available. Hence, for example, oophorectomy or irradiation of the ovaries may be allowed in treating carcinoma of the breast and metastasis therefrom; and orchidectomy is permitted in the treatment of carcinoma of the prostrate.

Discussed in this book:

Chapter III
pp. 90–93

". . . They are immediately directed to the cure, dimunition, or prevention of a serious pathological condition and are not directly contraceptive . . . :" In the examples given in the Directive itself, the dimunition of the pathology is brought about by the removal of the tissues (glands) which produce hormones that stimulate growth of the cancer. While these glands are necessary for reproduction, the beneficial and desired effect is not brought about precisely by the sterilization. In other words, sterility is **not the means** by which the cancerous condition is ameliorated, but it is an undesired, even if foreseen, side effect.

". . . a simpler treatment is not available:" Because of the serious side effect, namely, the loss of reproductive capacity, other less injurious means, if available, should be employed first.

Directive 21

Because the ultimate personal expression of conjugal love in the marital act is viewed as the only fitting context for the human sharing

". . . The ultimate personal expression of conjugal love in the marital act . . . :" The conjugal act, morally, is restricted exclusively to the married couple. It is the one act which is uniquely reserved to them and not only expresses and symbolizes their love, but also strengthens it and the family which the couple cooperatively generated.

480

of the divine act of creation, donor insemination and insemination that is totally artificial are morally objectionable. However, help may be given to a normally performed conjugal act to attain its purpose. The use of the sex faculty outside the legitimate use by married partners is never permitted even for medical or other laudable purpose, e.g., masturbation as a means of obtaining seminal specimens.

Discussed in this book:

Chapter II
pp. 33–61

"... donor insemination ... [is] morally objectionable:" The use of sperm from a man not the husband of the woman being inseminated, even if by artificial means, morally is, or is equivalent to, adultery. Although the **Directive** does not specifically address the topic of a donated **egg,** extension of the principle leads to the conclusion that fertilization of an egg not from the wife of the man would also morally be equivalent to adultery.

"... insemination that is totally artificial [is] morally objectionable:" The church insists in its official statements that human procreation be brought about in a manner that does not bypass, or substitute for, the conjugal act. Artificial insemination, properly so-called, substitutes for, or by-passes, the conjugal act.

"However, help may be given to a normally performed conjugal act to attain its purpose:" The church permits assisting procedures where the integrity of the conjugal act is preserved but because of some deficiency requires some help. Such assisting procedures have been termed "assisted insemination." An example of this kind of assistance would be the taking up some of the ejaculate from the vaginal pool with a syringe and propelling it closer to the cervix. Thus, the chances of achieving one of the purposes of the conjugal act, namely, fertilization, would be increased.

"The use of the sex faculty outside the legitimate use by married partners is never permitted . . .:" This statement gives recognition that genital activity within marriage may be misused. The conjugal act, for example should be by free

481

consent of both partners. Masturbation, that is, the free and deliberate procuring of an orgasm apart from the conjugal union is immoral, no matter what may be the ultimate reason—personal, medical or procreative.

Directive 22

Hysterectomy is permitted when it is sincerely judged to be a necessary means of removing some serious uterine pathological condition. In these cases, the pathological condition of each patient must be considered individually and care must be taken that a hysterectomy is not performed merely as a contraceptive measure, or as a routine procedure after any definite number of Cesarean sections.

Discussed in this book:

Chapter VI
pp. 215–222

Directive 23

For a proportionate reason, labor may be induced after the fetus is viable.

"Hysterectomy is permitted when it is sincerely judged to be a necessary means . . .:" The **Directive** is a recognition that individuals may be tempted to have, or to perform, a hysterectomy for mere convenience or for contraceptive purposes or for some trivial pathology. While the initial judgment properly belongs to the patient in conjunction with the physician as to whether there is an adequate, justifying reason for requesting a hysterectomy, the hospital may require a review of that decision in light of subsequent pathological findings in order to ensure that only morally justifiable surgery was being performed within its walls.

". . . each patient must be considered individually . . .:" Individual responses to objectively similar pathology can differ widely. Some women, apparently, can have a number of Cesarean sections without dangerously weakening the uterus. Other women who have had one or two Cesarean sections have wombs which cannot, by the honest judgment of the physician, bear another pregnancy. Continued use of the weakened uterus would constitute a serious threat to the life and health of the woman.

"For a proportionate reason . . .:" The proportion involved is concerned with the relative values of the good (the well being of the infant)

Discussed in this book:

Chapter VII
pp. 289–293

which is threatened by premature delivery, and the good (the life or health of the mother) which is the objective of the labor induction. Even though the fetus may be viable, that is, able to survive outside of the mother's womb even if some technological support is required, if it is delivered prematurely its life and health are not as secure as if it had been a full-term infant. The earlier the labor induction, the more important must be the reason, the threatened loss of a good. Thus to induce labor for the sake of convenience of the couple (or the physician) such as a forthcoming vacation, would **not** be a proportionate reason if the fetus' well being was placed in some jeopardy. Early induction can also be justified, of course, if it is for the well being of the fetus which may require some extrauterine therapy or that it be removed from a hostile environment, e.g., a diabetic mother.

". . . **after the fetus is viable** . . .:" Viability as essential requirement is partially dependent on the available facilities for supporting a premature infant as well as the actual condition of the infant. The attending physician, preferably after consultation with appropriate experts, has to make an honest judgment regarding the fetus' viability. His conclusion should then be presented to the parents with an indication of the relative risks and benefits of early induction or postponement thereof. The couple should have the final decision.

Directive 24

In all cases in which the presence of pregnancy would render some procedure illicit (e.g., curettage), the physician must make

"**In all cases in which the presence of a pregnancy would render some procedure illicit** . . .:" The presumption here is that the procedure in question would either bring about an abortion or seriously injure, perhaps fatally, the fetus. Some diagnostic procedures such as

use of such pregnancy tests and consultation as may be needed in order to be reasonably certain that the patient is not pregnant. It is to be noted that curettage of the endometrium after rape to prevent implantation of a possible embryo is morally equivalent to abortion.

Discussed in this book:

Chapter VIII, pp. 333–341

Chapter III, pp. 105–111

amniocentesis or fetoscopy may in some instances be considered illicit because of the serious threat they would pose to the health or life of the infant. Conversely, there may be times when the information only obtainable by amniocentesis or fetoscopy is of such importance for the ultimate well being of the infant, that the risk may be taken.

". . . **make use of pregnancy tests . . .:**" If it is clear that the procedure such as curettage or some therapeutic maneuver for the mother's health would inflict serious harm (or death) on the unborn infant, then appropriate tests to determine the presence of a pregnancy need to be carried out. If the results are ambiguous, normally the presence of a pregnancy should be favored.

". . . **curettage of the endometrium (D and C) after rape . . .**" Scraping (the lining) the uterine lining or the administration of a drug (e.g., "morning-after pill") which would make the implantation of the blastocyst (fertilized egg) impossible, are actions which morally are equivalent to abortion because the procedures are knowingly undertaken with the realization that the death of the unborn individual would result.

Directive 25

Radiation therapy of the mother's reproductive organs is permitted during pregnancy only when necessary to suppress a dangerous pathological condition.

"**Radiation Therapy . . .:**" This includes such forms of therapy such as x-ray, gamma ray and other forms of ionizing radiation.

"**. . . of the mother's reproductive organs:**" In particular, such radiation of the ovaries can result in sterility.

"**during pregnancy:**" The danger of radiation

Discussed in this book:

Chapter VII pp. 286–287

therapy, of course, is the injury which can be done to the unborn child. Rapidly growing tissue, that is, where active cell division is taking place, is particularly vulnerable to ionizing radiation. Depending on the energy level and the duration of the radiation therapy, the injury to the cells can result in death of the developing embryo or fetus, or it can bring about genetic mutations—some of which may lead to cancer.

". . . is permitted only when necessary to suppress a dangerous pathological condition:" The Principle of Double Effect requires, among other conditions, that the evil effect (the loss of a good, namely, life and/or physical well being of the fetus as well as the integrity of the mother's reproductive system) does not outweigh the good to be attained (preservation of the mother's life and/or health). Hence, the "dangerous pathological condition" has to be assessed carefully and the urgent need for radiation therapy be evaluated against the calculated risk.

Directive 26

Therapeutic procedures which are likely to be dangerous are morally justifiable for proportionate reasons.

Discussed in this book:

Chapter VII pp. 248–265

"Therapeutic procedures . . .:" Of this nature, therapeutic procedures are those medical activities which are directed to cure a disease, correct a malfunction, repair a part, eliminate or reduce pain and other undesirable symptoms or consequences of the condition being treated in the patient. Hence, medical (and other) procedures which are not directed to benefit this particular person, are not considered by this **Directive,** but by the next **(#27).**

". . . likely to be dangerous . . .:" In the best estimate of the responsible physician, the proposed procedure as judged from previous experience (personal or contained in the medical literature) entails a risk of injury. Included in such a judgment are the seriousness of the injury and the degree of probability that the injury will take place.

"**. . . are morally justifiable for proportionate reasons:**" The "proportionate reason" is the good which is sought by the therapeutic procedure. This good may be the preservation of life, the full or partial restoration of health, the elimination or lessening of intense pain. This desired good must be equal to or greater than the good which is being threatened, that is, the injury— loss of life or health, loss of a body part or function, loss of consciousness.

Directive 27

Experimentation on patients without due consent is morally objectionable, and even the moral right of the patient to consent is limited by his duties of stewardship.

Discussed in this book:

**Chapter VIII
pp. 321–327**

"**Experimentation on patients:**" In a medical and clinical context, experimentation refers to the use of a medical procedure on a human subject, who may or may not be a patient. For the purpose of this **Directive,** however, the subject is a patient. The procedure is deemed to be experimental because it has **not** yet been accepted by the medical community as a standard treatment for a specific disease or disorder, or for a subclass of patients, e.g., infants, the elderly. There is the presumption, of course, that established or standard modes of treatment have been tried unsuccessfully, or that the particular status of the individual has ruled out **a priori** the accepted procedures.

"**. . . without due consent is morally objectionable:**" Human dignity requires that the patient (or proxy if incompetent) gives "due consent" to the procedure. This means that the patient (or proxy) be informed of the potential risks and benefits, not only of the experimental procedure, but also of the standard alternatives, all of which must be explained to the patient in a manner intelligible to him. To the extent possible, the patient's decision, that is, the consent, should be a reasonable act which means that it proceeds with correct information and freedom. Without such a consent, the patient is being treated unjustly.

". . . **moral right of the patient to consent is limited by his duties of stewardship:**" Human beings have received from God, the sovereign Lord, a limited dominion over themselves and nature. With regards to the human person, the limitation pertains to life and the integrity of the body-soul unit. God is the master of life; he gives and he takes. The psycho-physiological integrity of the human body needs to be preserved. A part or function may not be removed or destroyed unless it is necessary to preserve the whole. A minor part or function may be sacrificed to preserve a major part or function; e.g., a gangrenous foot or hand may be amputated to save the leg or arm (which ultimately preserves the well-being and life of the individual). Stewardship, simply means that human beings, as rational creatures are accountable to the Creator for actions, knowingly and freely undertaken.

Directive 28

Euthanasia ("mercy killing") in all its forms is forbidden. The failure to supply the ordinary means of preserving life is equivalent to euthanasia. However, neither the physician nor the patient is obliged to the use of extraordinary means.

"**Euthanasia ('mercy killing') in all its forms is forbidden:**" While the **motive** may be laudable, namely, to relieve someone of severe pain or some other intolerable burden, the **intention and objective** of the act is to terminate a person's life. Whether the deliberate termination of a human life is done by an overdose of a therapeutic drug, by the administration of a poison, by the injection of air or by a weapon such as a gun, such an act is an unjust killing and as such is a grave evil.

487

"**The failure to supply ordinary means of preserving life is equivalent to euthanasia:**" In this medico-ethical context, "ordinary means" refers to procedures for maintaining life which are of some benefit and do not impose a grave burden on the patient or others. These means are also termed "proportionate means" or "ethically ordinary means." Such means are ethically obligatory. To be noted is that there is no **list** of such ordinary means because judgment must be made in each particular case in light of all the relevant circumstances. For one patient, a particular procedure might be an **acceptable** burden, for another that same procedure may truly constitute an **undue** burden. The judgment primarily pertains to the patient or proxy.

At the present time, the obligation always to provide nourishment and hydration is a controverted matter, both among theologians and the courts.

"**neither physician nor the patient is obliged to the use of extraordinary means:**" The "extraordinary means" (ethically extraordinary or disproportionate) are those procedures which are **not** ethically ordinary; they either are useless and/or they impose a grave burden on the patient or others. As mentioned above, the patient has the primary responsibility for the decision (with physician input) with respect to which the physician may follow with clear conscience.

These ethically extraordinary means are therefore ethically non-obligatory; they are optional, one may or may not choose to use them.

It should be noted here that sometimes what is morally acceptable may not be so legally, and conversely. The course of action actually taken will take into account both spheres, the moral and the legal.

Directive 29

It is not euthanasia to give a dying person sedatives and analgesics for the alleviation of pain, when such a measure is judged necessary, even though they may deprive the patient of the use of reason, or shorten his life.

Discussed in this book:

Chapter III
pp. 118, 119

"It is not euthanasia to give a dying person sedatives and analgesics for the alleviation of pain:" The motive is the reduction or elimination of pain. The purpose (or objective) of the act (the administration of the analgesic) is the alleviation of pain, not the killing of the patient. The one act has two effects, the elimination or alleviation of pain (the good effect) and, possibly, the loss of consciousness and/or shortening of life (the evil effect). The good effect does result from the evil effect, but rather is morally concurrent with it.

Prolonged pain, especially when unremitting and/or intense, can make the attainment of spiritual values more difficult. It is difficult to converse with family or friends, to pray, to trust God when the individual is in constant, intolerable pain.

". . . when such a measure is judged necessary." Because of the condition of the patient, the physician may be tempted to make the decision unilaterally. Yet, if circumstances permit, the patient should be consulted to make sure that the patient desires such medication. It can happen that for reasons known only to the patient, he may wish to tolerate some level of pain for a time or for the duration of his disease. Ideally, the pain control should be monitored daily to make sure that no more or no less medication is used than needed and desired by the patient. It is a sort of medical scandal, that more than half of the patients in the United States experience less than adequate pain control.

Directive 30

The transplantation of organs from living

"The transplantation of organs from living donors is morally permissible . . .:" Only

donors is morally permissible when the anticipated benefit to the recipient is proportionate to the harm done to the donor, provided that the loss of such organ(s) does not deprive the donor of life itself nor of the functional integrity of his body.

Discussed in this book:

Chapter VIII
pp. 315–321

those **organs** which are paired, such as the kidneys, are potentially able to be transplanted. **Tissues** such as blood and bone marrow, of course, can also be removed and given to another person—with appropriate informed consent.

At one time, there was an apparent moral objection to organ transplants from living donors because, the loss of an organ was not compensated by a proportionate gain for the donor, as would be required by the Principle of Totality. But motivated by love of neighbor, a person can, within limits, donate an organ.

". . . when the anticipated benefit to the recipient is proportionate to the harm done to the donor . . .:" If an individual has no functioning kidney, receiving a good kidney is a clear benefit and does outweigh the loss of the one kidney by the donor since the one kidney can carry out normal renal function for the donor. Yet, of course, with only one kidney there is no backup in case of disease or accident. Also to be considered are the anesthetic and surgical risks.

". . . provided the loss of such organ(s) does not deprive the donor of life itself nor the functional integrity of his body:" The donor still has a more fundamental obligation to preserve, namely, his or her own life and functional integrity. Thus, the life of the donor could not be sacrificed by the donation of a heart so that another could live whose life was about to be taken by disease (or injury) and not deliberately by the action of a free agent. (In the latter case, a person could die in the place of another as a manifest sign of Christian faith and love.)

A single kidney can be donated providing that the remaining kidney is healthy and capable of carrying the renal load of the donor's body. The donor has not been deprived of **functional** integrity of the body even if he has lost **structural** integrity.

Directive 31

Post-mortem examinations must not be begun until death is morally certain. Vital organs, that is, organs necessary to sustain life, may not be removed until death has taken place. The determination of the time of death must be made in accordance with responsible and commonly accepted scientific criteria. In accordance with current medical practice, to prevent any conflict of interest, the dying patient's doctor or doctors should ordinarily be distinct from the transplant team.

Discussed in this book:

Chapter VIII pp. 327–333

". . . until death is morally certain . . .:" When the dying process is gradual, such as is found among terminal stages of cancer patients, it is sometimes difficult to ascertain the precise moment of death. When in doubt, it is generally better to wait until the evidence is more secure. Even then only moral certitude is required, not the certitude of a mathematical proof or of a proof in physics or chemistry. That certitude is based on reasonably available evidence interpreted by the standards of the medical profession.

"The determination of death must be in accordance with responsible and commonly accepted medical criteria:" Normally, it is the physician who ascertains and declares the person to be dead. The time honored criteria are the permanent cessation of spontaneous respiration and of the heartbeat. However, there are times when the patient is being supported by a mechanical respirator and other life-support systems. Under these conditions, it is very difficult to determine whether there is a cessation of spontaneous respiration and heartbeat. Currently, a generally accepted alternative method is what is called "brain-related criteria"—the total and irreversible cessation of all brain function, including brain stem. This is brain death, the death of the person.

". . . The dying patient's doctor or doctors should ordinarily be distinct from the trans-

plant team:" The decision that the patient has died is made by his physicians. Once that is made, the transplant team can begin their work, and since the viability of the desired organs is of the utmost importance, perfusion of the body with appropriate fluids will generally be continued or reinstituted promptly.

After the flurry of heart transplants of the late sixties and early seventies, the frequency of failures resulted in a reduction of heart transplants. However, lessons were learned about the rejection phenomenon and patient selection so that in certain medical centers (e.g., Stanford) the failure rate is much more acceptable. The kidney transplant program is older and has had notable success over the years. Transplantation of livers is now beginning to be done more frequently with some success.

Directive 32

Ghost surgery, which implies the calculated deception of the patient as to the identity of the operating surgeon, is morally objectionable.

Discussed in this book:

Chapter VIII
pp. 341–343

"Ghost surgery . . . :" This is a surgical procedure performed by a person who is not the surgeon whom the patient believes is doing the surgery.

If the surgeon is, in addition, not competent to perform the surgery properly, there is an added injustice. The substitute may be a surgical resident for whom the attending physician wishes to provide some experience. In that situation, it is imperative that the legally responsible physician inform, and obtain consent of, the patient. But if the resident is merely **assisting** the principle surgeon, that would not be "ghost surgery." In the present legal atmosphere, "ghost surgery" is much less likely to occur.

". . . which implies calculated deception of the patient . . . :" The attending physician/surgeon agrees to do the surgery, but deliberately without telling the patient, he retains another physician/surgeon to perform the surgery. The patient has no knowledge of the switch prior or subsequent to the surgery. If, however, a last minute switch had been necessary because of some emergency, for example, the surgeon suddenly became incapacitated and the surgery could not prudently be postponed, then this would not be "ghost surgery," providing that later at an appropriate time, the patient was informed.

Directive 33

Unnecessary procedures, whether diagnostic or therapeutic, are morally objectionable. A procedure is unnecessary when no proportionate reason justifies it. A fortiori, any procedure that is contraindicated by sound medical standards is unnecessary.

Discussed in this book:

Chapter VI
pp. 243–245

"Unnecessary procedures, whether diagnostic or therapeutic, are morally objectionable:" Diagnostic procedures are those tests employed to assist the physician make a diagnosis, determine the severity of the condition and assess the medical status of the patient. The contemporary physician has a plethora of diagnostic tests available, some of which such as CAT scans and MRI can be quite expressive. To assert that a particular procedure is unnecessary may be difficult to substantiate.

Surgical procedures of late have come under particular scrutiny. Among the surgical procedures concerning which questions have been raised are coronary vessel by-pass surgery and hysterectomy. Surgeons and those responsible for reviewing a hospital's surgical procedure may need to be especially vigilant in their respective areas.

"A procedure is unnecessary when no proportionate reason justifies it:" The proportion is between the expected good to be derived from

493

the procedure (diagnostic or therapeutic) and the potential loss or harm which may result. This "harm" could include additional expense, longer stay in the hospital, exposure to the risk of general anesthesia, injury from surgery, false hope for recovery or cure, etc. If the additional diagnostic tests do not provide useful additional information, or the therapeutic procedure cannot, of its nature and the actual condition of the patient, notably improve his status, these procedures may be deemed unnecessary and perhaps even injurious.

Directive 34

The administration should be certain that patients in a health facility receive appropriate spiritual care.

Discussed in this book:

Chapter II
pp. 27–31

Chapter IV,
pp. 120–140

"**Administration should be certain . . .:**" This **Directive** places responsibility on the hospital's administration to provide the means by which patients are able to receive the spiritual care they need. Most often this is done by establishing, adequately funding and competently staffing a pastoral care department.

"**. . . that patients in a health facility receive appropriate spiritual care:**" Although in a Catholic health facility, the primary religious concern will be to provide for Catholic patients, those of other religious faiths are not to be overlooked or ignored. Especially since Vatican Council II, there has been an awareness of the rights of persons belonging to other religious groups.

In practice, the religious composition of the patient population—which can differ greatly from region to region—should be considered in staffing the pastoral care department. Clearly, provision cannot be made on staff for the great variety of religious affiliations found in the patient population. For these, and indeed for all patients,

494

some protocol should be established which would permit easy access of the patients to their respective clergy person and vice versa.

Directive 35

Except in cases of emergency (i.e., danger of death), all requests for baptism made by adults or for infants should be referred to the chaplain of the health facility.

Discussed in this book:

Chapter II
pp. 21–27

"Except in cases of emergency (i.e., danger of death) . . .:" Canon 867, 2 states: "If the infant is in danger of death, it is to be baptized without any delay." Hence, if the chaplain cannot be reached expeditiously, then someone else may confer baptism (see the following **Directive 36**).

". . . all requests for baptism should be referred to the chaplain of the health facility:" This **Directive** presupposes that a **request** for baptism has been made, either by the patient himself or by the parent (or guardian) of a noncompetent person (e.g., a child). However, Canon 868, 2 specifies that "An infant of Catholic parents, indeed even of non-Catholic parents, may in danger of death be baptized even if the parents are opposed to it." It should be noted that the canon says "**may** . . . be baptized" (emphasis added), it does **not require** that baptism be conferred in such cases. Prudence should be exercised in deciding whether or not to baptize such a child.

Directive 36

If a priest is not available, anyone having the use of reason and proper intention can baptize. The ordinary method of conferring

"If a priest is not available, anyone having the use of reason and proper intention can baptize:" The priest, along with the Bishop or a deacon, are the regular ministers of Baptism. Along with these three categories, anyone else can administer the sacrament of Baptism. The individual need not be a catholic or even a chris-

495

emergency baptism is as follows: **The person baptizing pours water on the head in such a way that it will flow on the skin, and, while the water is being poured, must pronounce these words audibly:** <u>I baptize you in the name of the Father, and of the Son, and of the Holy Spirit</u>. **The same person who pours the water must pronounce the words.**

Discussed in this book:

Chapter II pp. 21–27

tian; it is sufficient that he or she actually have the use of reason **(so that it is a human act)** and have the proper intention, namely, to administer the sacrament of Baptism according to what the church intends and desires.

"The ordinary method of conferring emergency baptism . . .:" This procedure is only to be used in an emergency when the appropriate liturgical rite cannot be followed.

Since the sacrament symbolizes "washing," it is important that the action be suggestive of or symbolize, washing. Hence, in pouring water it should flow over at least the principal part of the body (if the whole body is not immersed), namely, the head, and not the hair, but over the skin.

"I baptize you in the name of the Father, and of the Son, and the Holy Spirit:" These words follow the instruction of Jesus as contained in the Scriptures, namely, Matthew 28:19. All three Divine Persons should be named. In order for the words and action to be compatible, the same person pours the water who says the words.

Directive 37

When emergency baptism is conferred, the chaplain should be notified.

Discussed in this book:

Chapter II pp. 21–27

"Emergency baptism:" "An adult in danger of death may be baptized if, with some knowleuge of the principal truths of the faith, he or she has in some manner manifested the intention to receive baptism and promises to observe the requirements of the christian religion" (Canon 865, 2).

"If the infant is in danger of death, it is to be baptized without any delay" (Canon 867, 2).

"... The chaplain should be notified:" Since he is the official representative of the church, the guardian of the sacraments, he needs to be informed so that an appropriate record can be kept. Should the child survive, it would be important for his future that access to records be available. Were he to enter marriage or become a religious priest, his baptismal status would be vital.

This notification, best made in writing, should include all relevant information: name, place, time, reason for the emergency baptism, who performed the baptism and who were other witnesses.

Directive 38

It is the mind of the Church that the sick should have the widest possible liberty to receive the sacraments frequently. The generous cooperation of the entire staff and personnel is requested for this purpose.

Discussed in this book:

Chapter IV
pp. 131–136

"It is the mind of the church ...:" Her mind, her desires are reflected especially in those parts of the Code of Canon Law which are concerned with the sacraments as well as in her liturgical prescriptions and papal writings and allocutions.

"... sick should have the widest possible liberty to receive the sacraments frequently:" In the Code of Canon Law, for example, the fasting requirements for the reception of the Eucharist by the sick and the elderly are mitigated (see Canon 919, 3) so as to encourage frequent reception. In addition, the church encourages frequent reception of the Sacrament of Penance. To meet the special needs of the seriously sick and dying, the church provides the Sacrament of the Anointing of the sick.

"The generous cooperation of the entire staff and personnel is requested for this purpose:" The administration needs to provide a chapel or oratory where the blessed sacrament can be reserved and a Pastoral Care Department which would have the particular responsibility of meeting the spiritual needs of the patients. Other staff members should willingly forward requests of the patient (or family) for spiritual care to the appropriate person. As much as possible, the medical care of the patient should make room for spiritual care; and those who approach the patient to minister spiritually, especially in response to a patient's request, should not be prohibited or made to feel unwanted or in the way. If such persons are legitimately present and are observing reasonable rules for the discharging of their spiritual ministry, they should be welcomed.

Directive 39

While providing the sick abundant opportunity to receive Holy Communion, there should be no interference with the freedom of the faithful to communicate or not to communicate.

Discussed in this book:

"While providing the sick abundant opportunity to receive Holy Communion . . .:" As indicated in the previous Directive (38), the administration and staff in their respective roles strive to make access to the sacraments, and indeed, to spiritual care in general, convenient for the sick—with due respect to the proper order of medical activities.

". . . there should be no interference with the freedom of the faithful to communicate or not to communicate:" Two excesses are to be avoided:

1) Making it difficult for the patient to communicate because of unreasonable insistence on hospital routine, or

2) insistent urging of the patient to receive the Eucharist and overlooking the patient's desire **not** to communicate at this time. It is **not**

proper for the staff to inquire why the individual does not wish to communicate. This kind of situation requires great sensitivity and spiritual discernment, and ordinarily would be best handled by the priest-chaplain. Not to be overlooked is that the **Directive** refers to the "faithful" as the persons involved. Generally, Holy Communion would be given to those who are members of the Roman Catholic Church (see Canon 844, 1), but may be given upon request, and under certain conditions, to members of the Eastern Church "not in full communion with the catholic church (see Canon 844, 3), or, in danger of death to members of christian churches not in full communion with Rome (see Canon 844, 4).

Directive 40

In wards and semi-private rooms, every effort should be made to provide sufficient privacy for confession.

Discussed in this book:

Chapter IV pp. 131–132

"**In wards and semi-private rooms . . .:**" This statement presupposes that the room (or ward) is in fact occupied by more than one person. If not, then there should not be a problem.

"**. . . to provide sufficient privacy for confession:**" In some situations, a conference room or other staff room which can be used temporarily may provide the desired privacy. If the patient is sufficiently ambulatory, sometimes a walk to an outside quiet spot or to a visiting area may be possible. A screen or curtain around the bed, unfortunately, does not usually provide adequate **acoustic** privacy even if there is visual isolation. At times, opportunity can be taken if the "roommate" is temporarily absent from the vicinity. When all else fails, the confessor and patient will have to lower their voices (if possible), speak close to the other's ear, and resort to minimum, but essential words.

Directive 41

Special care and concern should be shown that those who are seriously ill or are dangerously ill due to sickness or old age receive the Sacrament of Anointing. A prudent or probable judgment about the seriousness of the sickness is sufficient. If necessary a doctor may be consulted, although there should be no reason for scruples.

A sick person should be anointed before surgery whenever a dangerous illness is the reason for the surgery. Old people may be anointed if they are in weak condition although no dangerous illness is present. Sick children may be anointed if they have sufficient use of reason to be comforted by this sacrament.

The sacrament may be repeated if the sick person recovers after anointing, or

". . . Those who are seriously ill or are dangerously ill due to sickness or old age . . .:" No longer called "Extreme Unction," this sacrament is for those faithful who are in some danger (of death) because of some **intrinsic** reason such as a disease, injury or old age. It does not apply to a person who is threatened by an **external** cause such as a fireman fighting a dangerous fire, a soldier about to go into battle, or a person about to be executed. It is a sacrament for the sick.

"A sick person should be anointed before surgery whenever a dangerous illness is the reason for the surgery:" The qualification re-emphasizes that this is a sacrament for the sick (understood to include injuries from accidents and debilitation from old age). Thus, surgery done for a minor illness, e.g., to straighten a crooked finger, or for cosmetic reasons (e.g., a face-life) would **not** be the occasion for administering this sacrament. Even if surgery represents a danger, it is an **external** threat, not an illness.

"Normally the sacrament is celebrated when the sick person is fully conscious:" The presumption in this **Directive** is that the individual has asked for the sacrament or has indicated acceptance when it was offered, and is suitably disposed to receive it. Canon 1007 puts forth a caveat: "The anointing of the sick is not to be conferred upon those who obstinately persist in a manifestly grave sin."

during the same illness, the danger becomes more serious.

Normally the sacrament is celebrated when the sick person is fully conscious. It may be conferred upon the sick who have lost consciousness or the use of reason, if, as Christian believers, they would have asked for it if they were in control of their faculties.

Discussed in this book:

Chapter IV
pp. 139–141

Directive 41a

All baptized Christians who can receive communion are bound to receive viaticum. Those in danger of death from any cause are obliged to receive communion. The administration of this sacrament is not to be delayed for the

"All baptized Christians who can receive communion are bound to receive viaticum:" Canon 912 states that "Any baptized person who is not forbidden by law may and must be admitted to holy communion."

Persons, for example, "upon whom the penalty of excommunication or interdict has been declared, and others who obstinately persist in manifest grave sin, are not to be admitted to holy communion" (Canon 915). Non-catholic christians in danger of death could receive viati-

faithful are to be nourished by it while still in full possession of their faculties.

Discussed in this book:

Chapter IV
pp. 136–139

Chapter II
pp. 27–31

cum if they belong to the Eastern Church or accept the basic teaching of the catholic church with regard to the Eucharist. The circumstances and conditions are stated in Canon 844, nn. 3 and 4.

"The administration of this sacrament is not to be delayed . . ." When the danger of death is proximate from any cause (it need not be due to sickness), the individual should be given the opportunity to receive viaticum even if the person had previously received on the same day. This would occur if, for example, the individual had received communion at a morning Mass and later in the day was seriously injured in an automobile accident.

Directive 41b

For special cases, when sudden illness or some other cause has unexpectedly placed one of the faithful in danger of death, the continuous rite should be used by which the sick person may be given the sacraments of penance, anointing, and eucharist as viaticum in one service.

Discussed in this book:

Chapter IV
pp. 136–139

"For special cases, when sudden illness or some other cause has unexpectedly placed one of the faithful in danger of death . . .:" In modern times, this is most likely to be encountered in the emergency room, although an unforeseen cardiac arrest or other dire emergency situation can arise while the patient is in the hospital for some other condition.

". . . the continuous rite should be used by which the sick person may be given the sacraments of penance, anointing, and eucharist as viaticum in one service:" While this is the desired manner of proceeding, the emergency situation may be of such a nature that the medical ministrations allow no room (in space or time) for the chaplain to approach the patient. He may give, if appropriate, an "emergency" absolution, or choose to wait until he can more readily have access to the patient. It is possible, too, that the individual is physically unable to receive viaticum, in which case it is omitted for the present. The sacrament of penance and the sacrament of anointing are then administered successively.

Directive 42

Personnel of a Catholic health facility should make every effort to satisfy the spiritual needs and desires of non-Catholics. Therefore, in hospitals and similar institutions conducted by Catholics, the authorities in charge should, with the consent of the patient, promptly advise ministers of other communions of the presence of their communicants and afford them every facility for visiting the sick and giving them spiritual and sacramental ministrations.

Discussed in this book:

Chapter IV
pp. 141, 142

Chapter II
pp. 27–31

"Personnel of a Catholic health facility should make every effort to satisfy the spiritual needs and desires of non-Catholics." A policy and protocol should be established by the Board and administration so that all personnel would be alerted to the need and be aware of what steps, e.g., who to notify when they become aware of the spiritual needs of a non-Catholic patient.

". . . the authorities in charge, should with the consent of the patient, promptly advise ministers of other communions . . .:" This provision underlines the need for a protocol as to who does the notification. It may be the administration, but more often it may be the Director of the Pastoral Care Department, or one delegated for that task. Having a designated procedure and persons will avoid duplication of notifications or their omission because of the lack of clear responsibility.

". . . and afford them every facility for visiting the sick . . .:" The visiting clergy should be made to feel welcome. If at all possible, appropriate parking facilities should be designated, e.g., "Visiting Clergy." Parking should be gratis. Unless there is a special reason, their visits should not be restricted with regard to time.

Directive 43

If there is a reasonable cause present for not burying a fetus or member of the human body, these may be cremated in a manner consonant with the dignity of the deceased human body.

Discussed in this book:

**Chapter IV
pp. 149–151**

"If there is a reasonable cause . . .:" The church prefers that her faithful members including fetuses and amputated limbs be buried in a catholic cemetery or other suitable place. So long as the reason for cremation is not a way of denying the Resurrection, the church is not opposed to cremation. Hence, a "reasonable cause" could be expense, danger of contagion, or convenience as long as the circumstances would not convey a lack of due respect for the human remains. With regards to a fetus, the parent's wishes should not be ignored.

". . . these may be cremated in a manner consonant with the dignity of the deceased human body:" It is important that the dead fetus or amputated limbs are not simply incinerated with garbage or other hospital trash. Human remains should be cremated separately from trash and in a manner that bespeaks of respect for the dead human body. A special protocol should be issued for this purpose.

APPENDIX II

Instruction of the Congregation for the Doctrine of the Faith, Feb. 22, 1987

PLEASE NOTE

When the following Instruction of the Congregation for the Doctrine of the Faith was released for publication on March 10, 1987, the publication process of this book was too far advanced to warrant references to this important Instruction within the text or footnotes of *Catholic Identity in Health Care*. The following listing will assist the reader, however, in associating the responses to the 14 questions proposed in the Instruction with the corresponding discussion of those questions in this book.

IN THE CDF INSTRUCTION:

IN THIS BOOK:

1) Respect Due to the Human Embryo—Chapter I, n.1

"Safeguarding Human Life," pp. 93–98

2) Morality of Prenatal Diagnosis, Ch.I, n.2

"Discrimination Against Human Life," pp. 105–111

3) Therapeutic Procedures on the Human Embryo, Ch.I, n.3

"Clinical Research on the Unborn," pp. 325–327

4) Research and Experimentation on Human Embryos, Ch.I, n.4

"Moral Guidance in Human Experimentation," pp. 323–325; "Postmortem Examinations," pp. 327, 328; "Religious Freedom and Cremation," pp. 149–151

5) "In Vitro" Research on Human Embryos," Ch.I, n.5

"Fertility Procedures which Must be Regarded as Immoral," pp. 56–59

6) Other Techniques of Manipulating Human Embryos," Ch.I, n.6

"Possible and Pending Genetic Techniques," pp. 61–62

7) Why Human Procreation Must Take Place in Marriage, Ch.II, Section A, n.1

"The Priority of Personhood," p. 32; "Allowing Life to Begin," pp. 70–73

8) Heterologous Artificial Insemination and Christian Marriage, Ch.II, Sec.A., n.2

"Fertility Procedures Which Must be Regarded as Immoral," pp. 55–61

9) Morality of Surrogate Motherhood, Ch.II, Sec.A, n.3

"The Morality of Surrogate Motherhood," pp. 59–61

10) Required Connection Between Procreation and the Conjugal Act, Ch.II, Sec.B, n.4

"Pope Pius XII on the Subject of Artificial Insemination," pp. 41–43; "The Case Against Contraception," pp. 72, 73; "Procedures that Induce Sterility, pp. 90–93

11) Morality of Homologous "In Vitro" Fertilization, Ch.II, Sec.B., n.5

"Pope Pius XII on the Subject of Artificial Insemination," pp. 41, 42; "Artificial Insemination by the Husband," p. 55

12) Morality of Homologous Artificial Insemination, Ch.II, Sec.B, n.6

"Moral Considerations," pp. 35, 36; "Other Promising Approaches to Human Fertility," pp. 40–51

13) Medical Intervention in Human Procreation, Ch.II, Sec.B, n.7

"The Principle of Human Dignity," pp. 20, 21; "The Priority of Personhood," p. 32; "The Principles of Integrity and Totality," pp. 204–206

CONGREGATION FOR THE DOCTRINE OF THE FAITH

INSTRUCTION
ON
RESPECT FOR HUMAN LIFE IN ITS ORIGIN
AND ON THE DIGNITY OF PROCREATION
REPLIES TO CERTAIN QUESTIONS OF THE DAY

FOREWORD

The Congregation for the Doctrination of the Faith has been approached by various Episcopal Conferences or individual Bishops, by theologians, doctors and scientists, concerning biomedical techniques which make it possible to intervene in the initial phase of the life of a human being and in the very processes of procreation and their conformity with the principles of Catholic morality. The present Instruction, which is the result of wide consultation and in particular of a careful evaluation of the declarations made by Episcopates, does not intend to repeat all the Church's teaching on the dignity of human life as it originates and on procreation, but to offer, in the light of the previous teaching of the Magisterium, some specific replies to the main questions being asked in this regard.

The exposition is arranged as follows: an introduction *will recall the fundamental principles, of an anthropological and moral character, which are necessary for a proper evaluation of the problems and for working out replies to those questions; the* first *part will have as its subject respect for the human being from the first moment of his or her existence; the* second *part will deal with the moral questions raised by technical interventions on human procreation; the* third *part will offer some orientations on the relation-*

ships between moral law and civil law in terms of the respect due to human embryos and foetuses* and as regard the legitimacy of techniques of artificial procreation.

INTRODUCTION

1.
BIOMEDICAL RESEARCH AND THE TEACHING
OF THE CHURCH

The gift of life which God the Creator and Father has entrusted to man calls him to appreciate the inestimable value of what he has been given and to take responsibility for it: this fundamental principle must be placed at the centre of one's reflection in order to clarify and solve the moral problems raised by artificial interventions on life as it originates and on the processes of procreation.

Thanks to the progress of the biological and medical sciences, man has at his disposal ever more effective therapeutic resources; but he can also acquire new powers, with unforeseeable consequences, over human life at its very beginning and in its first stages. Various procedures now make it possible to intervene not only in order to assist but also to dominate the processes of procreation. These techniques can enable man to "take in hand his own destiny", but they also expose him "to the temptation to go beyond the limits

---

*The terms "zygote", "pre-embryo", "embryo" and "foetus" can indicate in the vocabulary of biology successive stages of the development of a human being. The present Instruction makes free use of these terms, attributing to them an identical ethical relevance, in order to designate the result (whether visible or not) of human generation, from the first moment of its existence until birth. The reason for this usage is clarified by the text (cf I, 1).

of a reasonable dominion over nature".[1] They might constitute progress in the service of man, but they also involve serious risks. Many people are therefore expressing an urgent appeal that in interventions on procreation the values and rights of the human person be safeguarded. Requests for clarification and guidance are coming not only from the faithful but also from those who recognize the Church as "an expert in humanity"[2] with a mission to serve the "civilization of love"[3] and of life.

The Church's Magisterium does not intervene on the basis of a particular competence in the area of the experimental sciences; but having taken account of the data of research and technology, it intends to put forward, by virtue of its evangelical mission and apostolic duty, the moral teaching corresponding to the dignity of the person and to his or her integral vocation. It intends to do so by expounding the criteria of moral judgment as regards the applications of scientific research and technology, especially in relation to human life and its beginnings. These criteria are the respect, defence and promotion of man, his "primary and fundamental right" to life,[4] his dignity as a person who is endowed with a spiritual soul and with moral responsibility[5] and who is called to beatific communion with God.

The Church's intervention in this field is inspired also by the love which she owes to man, helping him to recognize and respect his rights and duties. This love draws from the fount of Christ's love: as she contemplates the mystery of the Incarnate Word, the Church also comes to understand the "mystery of man";[6] by proclaiming the Gospel of salvation, she reveals to man his dignity and invites him to discover fully the truth of his own being. Thus the Church once more puts forward the divine law in order to accomplish the work of truth and liberation.

For it is out of goodness—in order to indicate the path of life—that God gives human beings his commandments and the grace to observe them: and it is likewise out of goodness—in order to help them persevere along the same

---

[1]Pope John Paul II, *Discourse to those taking part in the 81st Congress of the Italian Society of Internal Medicine and the 82nd Congress of the Italian Society of General Surgery,* 27 October 1980: *AAS* 72 (1980) 1126.

[2]Pope Paul VI, *Discourse to the General Assembly of the United Nations Organization,* 4 October 1965; *AAS* 57 (1965) 878; Encyclical *Populorum Progressio,* 13: *AAS* 59 (1967) 263.

[3]Pope Paul VI, *Homily during the Mass closing the Holy Year,* 25 December 1975: *AAS* 68 (1976) 145; Pope John Paul II, Encyclical *Dives in Misericordia,* 30: *AAS* 72 (1980) 1224.

[4]Pope John Paul II, *Discourse to those taking part in the 35th General Assembly of the World Medical Association,* 29 October 1983: *AAS* 76 (1984) 390.

[5]Cf. Declaration *Dignitatis Humanae,* 2.

[6]Pastoral Constitution *Gaudium et Spes,* 22; Pope John Paul II, Encyclical *Redemptor Hominis,* 8: *AAS* 71 (1979) 270–272.

path—that God always offers to everyone his forgiveness. Christ has compassion on our weaknesses: he is our Creator and Redeemer. May his spirit open men's hearts to the gift of God's peace and to an understanding of his precepts.

2.
SCIENCE AND TECHNOLOGY
AT THE SERVICE OF THE HUMAN PERSON

God created man in his own image and likeness: "male and female he created them" (*Gen* 1:27), entrusting to them the task of "having dominion over the earth" (*Gen* 1:28). Basic scientific research and applied research constitute a significant expression of this dominion of man over creation. Science and technology are valuable resources for man when placed at his service and when they promote his integral development for the benefit of all; but they cannot of themselves show the meaning of existence and of human progress. Being ordered to man, who initiates and develops them, they draw from the person and his moral values the indication of their purpose and the awareness of their limits.

It would on the one hand be illusory to claim that scientific research and its applications are morally neutral; on the other hand one cannot derive criteria for guidance from mere technical efficiency, from research's possible usefulness to some at the expense of others, or, worse, still, from prevailing ideologies. Thus science and technology require, for their own intrinsic meaning, an unconditional respect for the fundamental criteria of the moral law: that is to say, they must be at the service of the human person, of his inalienable rights and his true and integral good according to the design and will of God.[7]

The rapid development of technological discoveries gives greater urgency to this need to respect the criteria just mentioned: science without conscience can only lead to man's ruin. "Our era needs such wisdom more than bygone ages if the discoveries made by man are to be further humanized. For the future of the world stands in peril unless wiser people are forthcoming".[8]

---

[7]Cf. Pastoral Constitution *Gaudium et Spes*, 35.

[8]Pastoral Constitution *Gaudium et Spes*, 15; cf. also Pope Paul VI, Encyclical *Populorum Progressio*, 20: *AAS* 59 (1967) 267; Pope John Paul II, Encyclical *Redemptor Hominis*, 15: *AAS* 71 (1979) 286–289; Apostolic Exhortation *Familiaris Consortio*, 8: *AAS* 74 (1982) 89.

3.
ANTHROPOLOGY AND PROCEDURES
IN THE BIOMEDICAL FIELD

Which moral criteria must be applied in order to clarify the problems posed today in the field of biomedicine? The answer to this question presupposes a proper idea of the nature of the human person in his bodily dimension.

For it is only in keeping with his true nature that the human person can achieve self-realization as a "unified totality":[9] and this nature is at the same time corporal and spiritual. By virtue of its substantial union with a spiritual soul, the human body cannot be considered as a mere complex of tissues, organs and functions, nor can it be evaluated in the same way as the body of animals; rather it is a constitutive part of the person who manifests and expresses himself through it.

The natural moral law expresses and lays down the purposes, rights and duties which are based upon the bodily and spiritual nature of the human person. Therefore this law cannot be thought of as simply a set of norms on the biological level; rather it must be defined as the rational order whereby man is called by the Creator to direct and regulate his life and actions and in particular to make use of his own body.[10]

A first consequence can be deduced from these principles: an intervention on the human body affects not only the tissues, the organs and their functions but also involves the person himself on different levels. It involves, therefore, perhaps in an implicit but nonetheless real way, a moral significance and responsibility. Pope John Paul II forcefully reaffirmed this to the World Medical Association when he said: "Each human person, in his absolutely unique singularity, is constituted not only by his spirit, but by his body as well. Thus, in the body and through the body, one touches the person himself in his concrete reality. To respect the dignity of man consequently amounts to safeguarding this identity of the man '*corpore et anima unus*', as the Second Vatican Council says (*Gaudium et Spes*, 14, par. 1). It is on the basis of this anthropological vision that one is to find the fundamental criteria for decision-making in the case of procedures which are not strictly therapeutic, as, for example, those aimed at the improvement of the human biological condition".[11]

---

[9]Pope John Paul II, Apostolic Exhortation *Familiaris Consortio*, 11: *AAS* 74 (1982) 92.

[10]Cf. Pope Paul VI, Encyclical *Humanae Vitae*, 10: *AAS* 60 (1968) 487–488.

[11]Pope John Paul II, *Discourse to the members of the 35th General Assembly of the World Medical Association*, 29 October 1983: *AAS* 76 (1984) 393.

Applied biology and medicine work together for the integral good of human life when they come to the aid of a person stricken by illness and infirmity and when they respect his or her dignity as a creature of God. No biologist or doctor can reasonably claim, by virtue of his scientific competence, to be able to decide on people's origin and destiny. This norm must be applied in a particular way in the field of sexuality and procreation, in which man and woman actualize the fundamental values of love and life.

God, who is love and life, has inscribed in man and woman the vocation to share in a special way in his mystery of personal communion and in his work as Creator and Father.[12] For this reason marriage possesses specific goods and values in its union and in procreation which cannot be likened to those existing in lower forms of life. Such values and meanings are of the personal order and determine from the moral point of view the meaning and limits of artificial interventions on procreation and on the origin of human life. These interventions are not to be rejected on the grounds that they are artificial. As such, they bear witness to the possibilities of the art of medicine. But they must be given a moral evaluation in reference to the dignity of the human person, who is called to realize his vocation from God to the gift of love and the gift of life.

4.
FUNDAMENTAL CRITERIA FOR A MORAL JUDGMENT

The fundamental values connected with the techniques of artificial human procreation are two: the life of the human being called into existence and the special nature of the transmission of human life in marriage. The moral judgment on such methods of artificial procreation must therefore be formulated in reference to these values.

Physical life, with which the course of human life in the world begins, certainly does not itself contain the whole of a person's value, nor does it represent the supreme good of man who is called to eternal life. However it does constitute in a certain way the "fundamental" value of life, precisely because upon this physical life all the other values of the person are based and developed.[13] The inviolability of the innocent human being's right to life

---

[12]Cf. Pope John Paul II, Apostolic Exhortation *Familiaris Consortio*, 11: *AAS* 74 (1982) 91-92; cf. also Pastoral Constitution *Gaudium et Spes*, 50.

[13]Sacred Congregation for the Doctrine of the Faith, *Declaration on Procured Abortion*, 9, *AAS* 66 (1974) 736- 737.

"from the moment of conception until death"[14] is a sign and requirement of the very inviolability of the person to whom the Creator has given the gift of life.

By comparison with the transmission of other forms of life in the universe, the transmission of human life has a special character of its own, which derives from the special nature of the human person. "The transmission of human life is entrusted by nature to a personal and conscious act and as such is subject to the all-holy laws of God: immutable and inviolable laws which must be recognized and observed. For this reason one cannot use means and follow methods which could be licit in the transmission of the life of plants and animals.".[15]

Advances in technology have now made it possible to procreate apart from sexual relations through the meeting *in vitro* of the germ-cells previously taken from the man and the woman. But what is technically possible is not for that very reason morally admissible. Rational reflection on the fundamental values of life and of human procreation is therefore indispensable for formulating a moral evaluation of such technological interventions on a human being from the first stages of his development.

5.
TEACHINGS OF THE MAGISTERIUM

On its part, the Magisterium of the Church offers to human reason in this field too the light of Revelation: the doctrine concerning man taught by the Magisterium contains many elements which throw light on the problems being faced here.

From the moment of conception, the life of every human being is to be respected in an absolute way because man is the only creature on earth that God has "wished for himself"[16] and the spiritual soul of each man is "immediately created" by God;[17] his whole being bears the image of the Creator. Human life is sacred because from its beginning it involves "the creative

---

[14]Pope John Paul II, *Discourse to those taking part in the 35th General Assembly of the World Medical Association*, 29 October 1983: *AAS* 76 (1984) 390.

[15]Pope John XXIII, Encyclical *Mater et Magistra*, III: *AAS* 53 (1961) 447.

[16]Pastoral Constitution *Gaudium et Spes*, 24.

[17]Cf. Pope Pius XII, Encyclical *Humani Generis: AAS* 42 (1950) 575; Pope Paul VI, *Professio Fidei: AAS* 60 (1968) 436.

action of God"[18] and it remains forever in a special relationship with the Creator, who is its sole end.[19] God alone is the Lord of life from its beginning until its end: no one can, in any circumstance, claim for himself the right to destroy directly an innocent human being.[20]

Human procreation requires on the part of the spouses responsible collaboration with the fruitful love of God;[21] the gift of human life must be actualized in marriage through the specific and exclusive acts of husband and wife, in accordance with the laws inscribed in their persons and in their union.[22]

I
RESPECT FOR HUMAN EMBRYOS

Careful reflection on this teaching of the Magisterium and on the evidence of reason, as mentioned above, enables us to respond to the numerous moral problems posed by technical interventions upon the human being in the first phases of his life and upon the processes of his conception.

1. WHAT RESPECT IS DUE TO THE HUMAN EMBRYO, TAKING INTO ACCOUNT HIS NATURE AND IDENTITY?

---

[18]Pope John XXIII, Encyclical *Mater et Magistra*, III: *AAS* 53 (1961) 447; cf. Pope John Paul II, *Discourse to priests participating in a seminar on "Responsible Procreation"*, 17 September 1983, *Insegnamenti di Giovanni Paolo II*, VI, 2 (1983) 562: "At the origin of each human person there is a creative act of God: no man comes into existence by chance; he is always the result of the creative love of God".

[19]Cf. Pastoral Constitution *Gaudium et Spes*, 24.

[20]Cf. Pope Pius XII, *Discourse to the Saint Luke Medical-Biological Union*, 12 November 1944: *Discorsi e Radiomessaggi* VI (1944-1945) 191-192.

[21]Cf. Pastoral Constitution *Gaudium et Spes*, 50.

[22]Cf. Pastoral Constitution *Gaudium et Spes*, 51: "When it is a question of harmonizing married love with the responsible transmission of life, the moral character of one's behaviour does not depend only on the good intention and the evaluation of the motives: the objective criteria must be used, criteria drawn from the nature of the human person and human acts, criteria which respect the total meaning of mutual self-giving and human procreation in the context of true love.".

The human being must be respected—as a person—from the very first instant of his existence.

The implementation of procedures of artificial fertilization has made possible various interventions upon embryos and human foetuses. The aims pursued are of various kinds: diagnostic and therapeutic, scientific and commercial. From all of this, serious problems arise. Can one speak of a right to experimentation upon human embryos for the purpose of scientific research? What norms or laws should be worked out with regard to this matter? The response to these problems presupposes a detailed reflection on the nature and specific identity—the word "status" is used—of the human embryo itself.

At the Second Vatican Council, the Church for her part presented once again to modern man her constant and certain doctrine according to which: "Life once conceived, must be protected with the utmost care; abortion and infanticide are abominable crimes".[23] More recently, the *Charter of the Rights of the Family*, published by the Holy See, confirmed that "Human life must be absolutely respected and protected from the moment of conception".[24]

This Congregation is aware of the current debates concerning the beginning of human life, concerning the individuality of the human being and concerning the identity of the human person. The Congregation recalls the teachings found in the *Declaration on Procured Abortion*: "From the time that the ovum is fertilized, a new life is begun which is neither that of the father nor of the mother; it is rather the life of a new human being with his own growth. It would never be made human if it were not human already. To this perpetual evidence . . . modern genetic science brings valuable confirmation. It has demonstrated that, from the first instant, the programme is fixed as to what this living being will be: a man, this individual-man with his characteristic aspects already well determined. Right from fertilization is begun the adventure of a human life, and each of its great capacities requires time . . . to find its place and to be in a position to act".[25] This teaching remains valid and is further confirmed, if confirmation were needed, by recent findings of human biological science which recognize that in the zygote* resulting from fertilization the biological identity of a new human individual is already constituted.

---

[23]Pastoral Constitution *Gaudium et Spes*, 51.

[24]Holy See, *Charter of the Rights of the Family*, 4: *L'Osservatore Romano,* 25 November 1983.

[25]Sacred Congregation for the Doctrine of the Faith, Declaration on Procured Abortion, 12–13: *AAS* 66 (1974) 738.

*The zygote is the cell produced when the nuclei of the two gametes have fused.

Certainly no experimental datum can be in itself sufficient to bring us to the recognition of a spiritual soul; nevertheless, the conclusions of science regarding the human embryo provide a valuable indication for discerning by the use of reason a personal presence at the moment of this first appearance of a human life: how could a human individual not be a human person? The Magisterium has not expressly committed itself to an affirmation of a philosophical nature, but it constantly reaffirms the moral condemnation of any kind of procured abortion. This teaching has not been changed and is unchangeable.[26]

Thus the fruit of human generation, from the first moment of its existence, that is to say from the moment the zygote has formed, demands the unconditional respect that is morally due to the human being in his bodily and spiritual totality. The human being is to be respected and treated as a person from the moment of conception; and therefore from that same moment his rights as a person must be recognized, among which in the first place is the inviolable right of every innocent human being to life.

This doctrinal reminder provides the fundamental criterion for the solution of the various problems posed by the development of the biomedical sciences in this field: since the embryo must be treated as a person, it must also be defended in its integrity, tended and cared for, to the extent possible, in the same way as any other human being as far as medical assistance is concerned.

2. IS PRENATAL DIAGNOSIS MORALLY LICIT?

If prenatal diagnosis respects the life and integrity of the embryo and the human foetus and is directed towards its safeguarding or healing as an individual, then the answer is affirmative.

For prenatal diagnosis makes it possible to know the condition of the embryo and of the foetus when still in the mother's womb. It permits, or makes it possible to anticipate earlier and more effectively, certain therapeutic, medical or surgical procedures.

Such diagnosis is permissible, with the consent of the parents after they have been adequately informed, if the methods employed safeguard the life and integrity of the embryo and the mother, without subjecting them to dis-

---

[26]Cf. Pope Paul VI, *Discourse to participants in the Twenty-third National Congress of Italian Catholic Jurists*, 9 December 1972: *AAS* 64 (1972) 777.

proportionate risks.[27] But this diagnosis is gravely opposed to the moral law when it is done with the thought of possibly inducing an abortion depending upon the results: a diagnosis which shows the existence of a malformation or a hereditary illness must not be the equivalent of a death-sentence. Thus a woman would be committing a gravely illicit act if she were to request such a diagnosis with the deliberate intention of having an abortion should the results confirm the existence of a malformation or abnormality. The spouse or relatives or anyone else would similarly be acting in a manner contrary to the moral law if they were to counsel or impose such a diagnostic procedure on the expectant mother with the same intention of possibly proceeding to an abortion. So too the specialist would be guilty of illicit collaboration if, in conducting the diagnosis and in communicating its results, he were deliberately to contribute to establishing or favouring a link between prenatal diagnosis and abortion.

In conclusion, any directive or programme of the civil and health authorities or of scientific organizations which in any way were to favour a link between prenatal diagnosis and abortion, or which were to go as far as directly to induce expectant mothers to submit to prenatal diagnosis planned for the purpose of eliminating foetuses which are affected by malformations or which are carriers of hereditary illness, is to be condemned as a violation of the unborn child's right to life and as an abuse of the prior rights and duties of the spouses.

3. ARE THERAPEUTIC PROCEDURES CARRIED OUT ON THE HUMAN EMBRYO LICIT?

As with all medical interventions on patients, *one must uphold as licit procedures carried out on the human embryo which respect the life and integrity of the embryo and do not involve disproportionate risks for it but are directed towards its healing, the improvement of its condition of health, or its individual survival.*

---

[27]The obligation to avoid disproportionate risks involves an authentic respect for human beings and the uprightness of therapeutic intentions. It implies that the doctor "above all . . . must carefully evaluate the possible negative consequences which the necessary use of a particular exploratory technique may have upon the unborn child and avoid recourse to diagnostic procedures which do not offer sufficient guarantees of their honest purpose and substantial harmlessness. And if, as often happens in human choices, a degree of risk must be undertaken, he will take care to assure that it is justified by a truly urgent need for the diagnosis and by the importance of the results that can be achieved by it for the benefit of the unborn child himself" (Pope John Paul II, *Discourse to Participants in the Pro-Life Movement Congress*, 3 December 1982: *Insegnamenti di Giovanni Paolo II*, V, 3 [1982] 1512). This clarification concerning "proportionate risk" is also to be kept in mind in the following sections of the present Instruction, whenever this term appears.

Whatever the type of medical, surgical or other therapy, the free and informed consent of the parents is required, according to the deontological rules followed in the case of children. The application of this moral principle may call for delicate and particular precautions in the case of embryonic or foetal life.

The legitimacy and criteria of such procedures have been clearly stated by Pope John Paul II: "A strictly therapeutic intervention whose explicit objective is the healing of various maladies such as those stemming from chromosomal defects will, in principle, be considered desirable, provided it is directed to the true promotion of the personal well-being of the individual without doing harm to his integrity or worsening his conditions of life. Such an intervention would indeed fall within the logic of the Christian moral tradition".[28]

4. HOW IS ONE TO EVALUATE MORALLY RESEARCH AND EXPERIMENTATION* ON HUMAN EMBRYOS AND FOETUSES?

Medical research must refrain from operations on live embryos, unless there is a moral certainty of not causing harm to the life or integrity of the unborn child and the mother, and on condition that the parents have given their free and informed consent to the procedure. It follows that all research, even when limited to the simple observation of the embryo, would become illicit were it to involve risk to the embryo's physical integrity or life by reason of the methods used or the effects induced.

As regards experimentation, and presupposing the general distinction between experimentation for purposes which are not directly therapeutic and experimentation which is clearly therapeutic for the subject himself, in the case in point one must also distinguish between experimentation carried out on embryos which are still alive and experimentation carried out on embryos

---

[28]Pope John Paul II, *Discourse to the Participants in the 35th General Assembly of the World Medical Association*, 29 October 1983: *AAS* 76 (1984) 392.

*Since the terms "research" and "experimentation" are often used equivalently and ambiguously, it is deemed necessary to specify the exact meaning given them in this document.

1)By *research* is meant any inductive-deductive process which aims at promoting the systematic observation of a given phenomenon in the human field or at verifying a hypothesis arising from previous observations.

2) By *experimentation* is meant any research in which the human being (in the various stages of his existence: embryo, foetus, child or adult) represents the object through which or upon which one intends to verify the effect, at present unknown or not sufficiently known, of a given treatment (e.g. pharmacological, teratogenic, surgical, etc.).

which are dead. *If the embryos are living, whether viable or not, they must be respected just like any other human person; experimentation on embryos which is not directly therapeutic is illicit.*[29]

No objective, even though noble in itself, such as a foreseeable advantage to science, to other human beings or to society, can in any way justify experimentation on living human embryos or foetuses, whether viable or not, either inside or outside the mother's womb. The informed consent ordinarily required for clinical experimentation on adults cannot be granted by the parents, who may not freely dispose of the physical integrity or life of the unborn child. Moreover, experimentation on embryos and foetuses always involves risk, and indeed in most cases it involves the certain expectation of harm to their physical integrity or even their death.

To use human embryos or foetuses as the object or instrument of experimentation constitutes a crime against their dignity as human beings having a right to the same respect that is due to the child already born and to every human person.

The *Charter of the Rights of the Family* published by the Holy See affirms: "Respect for the dignity of the human being excludes all experimental manipulation or exploitation of the human embryo".[30] The practice of keeping alive human embryos *in vivo* or *in vitro* for experimental or commercial purposes is totally opposed to human dignity.

In the case of experimentation that is clearly therapeutic, namely, when it is a matter of experimental forms of therapy used for the benefit of the embryo itself in a final attempt to save its life, and in the absence of other reliable forms of therapy, recourse to drugs or procedures not yet fully tested can be licit.[31]

The corpses of human embryos and foetuses, whether they have been deliberately aborted or not, must be respected just as the remains of other human beings. In particu-

---

[29]Cf. Pope John Paul II, *Address to a Meeting of the Pontifical Academy of Sciences*, 23 October 1982: *AAS* 75 (1983) 37: "I condemn, in the most explicit and formal way, experimental manipulations of the human embryo, since the human being, from conception to death, cannot be exploited for any purpose whatsoever".

[30]Holy See, *Charter of the Rights of the Family*, 4b: *L'Osservatore Romano*, 25 November 1983.

[31]Cf. Pope John Paul II, Address to the Participants in the Convention of the Pro-Life Movement, 3 December 1982: *Insegnamenti di Giovanni Paolo II*, V, 3 (1982) 1511: "Any form of experimentation on the foetus that may damage its integrity or worsen its condition is unacceptable, except in the case of a final effort to save it from death". Sacred Congregation for the Doctrine of the Faith, *Declaration on Euthanasia*, 4: *AAS* 72 (1980) 550: "In the absence of other sufficient remedies, it is permitted, with the patient's consent, to have recourse to the means provided by the most advanced medical techniques, even if these means are still at the experimental stage and are not without a certain risk".

lar, they cannot be subjected to mutilation or to autopsies if their death has not yet been verified and without the consent of the parents or of the mother. Furthermore, the moral requirements must be safeguarded that there be no complicity in deliberate abortion and that the risk of scandal be avoided. Also, in the case of dead foetuses, as for the corpses of adult persons, all commercial trafficking must be considered illicit and should be prohibited.

5. HOW IS ONE TO EVALUATE MORALLY THE USE FOR RESEARCH PURPOSES OF EMBRYOS OBTAINED BY FERTILIZATION 'IN VITRO'?

Human embryos obtained *in vitro* are human beings and subjects with rights: their dignity and right to life must be respected from the first moment of their existence. *It is immoral to produce human embryos destined to be exploited as disposable "biological material".*

In the usual practice of *in vitro* fertilization, not all of the embryos are transferred to the woman's body; some are destroyed. Just as the Church condemns induced abortion, so she also forbids acts against the life of these human beings. *It is a duty to condemn the particular gravity of the voluntary destruction of human embryos obtained 'in vitro' for the sole purpose of research, either by means of artificial insemination or by means of "twin fission".* By acting in this way the researcher usurps the place of God; and, even though he may be unaware of this, he sets himself up as the master of the destiny of others inasmuch as he arbitrarily chooses whom he will allow to live and whom he will send to death and kills defenceless human beings.

Methods of observation or experimentation which damage or impose grave and disproportionate risks upon embryos obtained *in vitro* are morally illicit for the same reasons. Every human being is to be respected for himself, and cannot be reduced in worth to a pure and simple instrument for the advantage of others. *It is therefore not in conformity with the moral law deliberately to expose to death human embryos obtained 'in vitro'.* In consequence of the fact that they have been produced *in vitro*, those embryos which are not transferred into the body of the mother and are called "spare" are exposed to an absurd fate, with no possibility of their being offered safe means of survival which can be licitly pursued.

6. WHAT JUDGMENT SHOULD BE MADE ON OTHER PROCEDURES OF MANIPULATING EMBRYOS CONNECTED WITH THE "TECHNIQUES OF HUMAN REPRODUCTION"?

Techniques of fertilization *in vitro* can open the way to other forms of biological and genetic manipulation of human embryos, such as attempts or plans for fertilization between human and animal gametes and the gestation of human embryos in the uterus of animals, or the hypothesis or project of constructing artificial uteruses for the human embryo. *These procedures are contrary to the human dignity proper to the embryo, and at the same time they are contrary to the right of every person to be conceived and to be born within marriage and from marriage.*[32] *Also, attempts or hypotheses for obtaining a human being without any connection with sexuality through "twin fission", cloning or parthenogenesis are to be considered contrary to the moral law, since they are in opposition to the dignity both of human procreation and of the conjugal union.*

The freezing of embryos, even when carried out in order to preserve the life of an embryo—cryopreservation—*constitutes an offence against the respect due to human beings* by exposing them to grave risks of death or harm to their physical integrity and depriving them, at least temporarily, of maternal shelter and gestation, thus placing them in a situation in which further offences and manipulation are possible.

Certain attempts to influence chromosomic or genetic inheritance are not therapeutic but are aimed at producing human beings selected according to sex or other predetermined qualities. These manipulations are contrary to the personal dignity of the human being and his or her integrity and identity. Therefore in no way can they be justified on the grounds of possible beneficial consequences for future humanity.[33] Every person must be respected for himself: in this consists the dignity and right of every human being from his or her beginning.

---

[32]No one, before coming into existence, can claim a subjective right to begin to exist; nevertheless, it is legitimate to affirm the right of the child to have a fully human origin through conception in conformity with the personal nature of the human being. Life is a gift that must be bestowed in a manner worthy both of the subject receiving it and of the subjects transmitting it. This statement is to be borne in mind also for what will be explained concerning artificial human procreation.

[33]Cf. Pope John Paul II, *Discourse to those taking part in the 35th General Assembly of the World Medical Association*, 29 October 1983: *AAS* 76 (1984) 391.

II
INTERVENTIONS UPON HUMAN PROCREATION

By "artificial procreation" or "artificial fertilization" are understood here the different technical procedures directed towards obtaining a human conception in a manner other than the sexual union of man and woman. This Instruction deals with fertilization of an ovum in a test-tube (*in vitro* fertilization) and artificial insemination through transfer into the woman's genital tracts of previously collected sperm.

A preliminary point for the moral evaluation of such technical procedures is constituted by the consideration of the circumstances and consequences which those procedures involve in relation to the respect due the human embryo. Development of the practice of *in vitro* fertilization has required innumerable fertilizations and destructions of human embryos. Even today, the usual practice presupposes a hyperovulation on the part of the woman: a number of ova are withdrawn, fertilized and then cultivated *in vitro* for some days. Usually not all are transferred into the genital tracts of the woman; some embryos, generally called "spare", are destroyed or frozen. On occasion, some of the implanted embryos are sacrificed for various eugenic, economic or psychological reasons. Such deliberate destruction of human beings or their utilization for different purposes to the detriment of their integrity and life is contrary to the doctrine on procured abortion already recalled.

The connection between *in vitro* fertilization and the voluntary destruction of human embryos occurs too often. This is significant: through these procedures, with apparently contrary purposes, life and death are subjected to the decision of man, who thus sets himself up as the giver of life and death by decree. This dynamic of violence and domination may remain unnoticed by those very individuals who, in wishing to utilize this procedure, become subject to it themselves. The facts recorded and the cold logic which links them must be taken into consideration for a moral judgment on IVF and ET (*in vitro* fertilization and embryo transfer): the abortion-mentality which has made this procedure possible thus leads, whether one wants it or not, to man's domination over the life and death of his fellow human beings and can lead to a system of radical eugenics.

Nevertheless, such abuses do not exempt one from a further and thorough ethical study of the techniques of artificial procreation considered in themselves, abstracting as far as possible from the destruction of embryos produced *in vitro*.

The present Instruction will therefore take into consideration in the first place the problems posed by heterologous artificial fertilization (II, 1–3),* and subsequently those linked with homologous artificial fertilization (II, 4–6).**

Before formulating an ethical judgment on each of these procedures, the principles and values which determine the moral evaluation of each of them will be considered.

A
HETEROLOGOUS ARTIFICIAL FERTILIZATION

1. WHY MUST HUMAN PROCREATION TAKE PLACE IN MARRIAGE?

Every human being is always to be accepted as a gift and blessing of God. However, from the moral point of view a truly responsible procreation vis-à-vis the unborn child must be the fruit of marriage.

For human procreation has specific characteristics by virtue of the personal dignity of the parents and of the children: the procreation of a new person, whereby the man and the woman collaborate with the power of the Creator, must be the fruit and the sign of the mutual self-giving of the spouses, of their love and of their fidelity.[34] *The fidelity of the spouses in the unity of marriage involves reciprocal respect of their right to become a father and a mother only through each other.*

---

*By the term *heterologous artificial fertilization* or *procreation*, the Instruction means techniques used to obtain a human conception artificially by the use of gametes coming from at least one donor other than the spouses who are joined in marriage. Such techniques can be of two types:

a) Heterologous IVF and ET: the technique used to obtain a human conception through the meeting *in vitro* of gametes taken from at least one donor other than the two spouses joined in marriage.

b) Heterologous artificial insemination: the technique used to obtain a human conception through the transfer into the genital tracts of the woman of the sperm previously collected from a donor other than the husband.

**By *artificial homologous fertilization or procreation*, the Instruction means the technique used to obtain a human conception using the gametes of the two spouses joined in marriage. Homologous artificial fertilization can be carried out by two different methods:

a) Homologous IVF and ET: the technique used to obtain a human conception through the meeting *in vitro* of the gametes of the spouses joined in marriage.

b) Homologous artificial insemination: the technique used to obtain a human conception through the transfer into the genital tracts of a married woman of the sperm previously collected from her husband.

[34]Cf. Pastoral Constitution on the Church in the Modern World, *Gaudium et Spes*, 50.

The child has the right to be conceived, carried in the womb, brought into the world and brought up within marriage: it is through the secure and recognized relationship to his own parents that the child can discover his own identity and achieve his own proper human development.

The parents find in their child a confirmation and completion of their reciprocal self-giving: the child is the living image of their love, the permanent sign of their conjugal union, the living and indissoluble concrete expression of their paternity and maternity.[35]

By reason of the vocation and social responsibilities of the person, the good of the children and of the parents contributes to the good of civil society; the vitality and stability of society require that children come into the world within a family and that the family be firmly based on marriage.

The tradition of the Church and anthropological reflection recognize in marriage and in its indissoluble unity the only setting worthy of truly responsible procreation.

2. DOES HETEROLOGOUS ARTIFICIAL FERTILIZATION CONFORM TO THE DIGNITY OF THE COUPLE AND TO THE TRUTH OF MARRIAGE?

Through IVF and ET and heterologous artificial insemination, human conception is achieved through the fusion of gametes of at least one donor other than the spouses who are united in marriage. *Heterologous artificial fertilization is contrary to the unity of marriage, to the dignity of the spouses, to the vocation proper to parents, and to the child's right to be conceived and brought into the world in marriage and from marriage.*[36]

---

[35]Cf. Pope John Paul II, Apostolic Exhortation *Familiaris Consortio*, 14: *AAS* 74 (1982) 96.

[36]Cf. Pope Pius XII, *Discourse to those taking part in the 4th International Congress of Catholic Doctors*, 29 September 1949: *AAS* 41 (1949) 559. According to the plan of the Creator, "A man leaves his father and his mother and cleaves to his wife, and they become one flesh" (*Gen* 2:24). The unity of marriage, bound to the order of creation, is a truth accessible to natural reason. The Church' Tradition and Magisterium frequently make reference to the Book of Genesis, both directly and through the passages of the New Testament that refer to it: *Mt* 19:4-6; *Mk* 10:5-8; *Eph* 5:31. Cf. Athenagoras, *Legatio pro christianis*, 33: *PG* 6, 965-967; St. Chrysostom, *In Matthaeum homiliae*, LXII, 19, 1: *PG* 58 597; St Leo the Great, *Epist. ad Rusticum*, 4: *PL* 54, 1204; Innocent III, Epist. *Gaudemus in Domino: DS* 778; Council of Lyons II, *IV Session: DS* 860; Council of Trent, *XXIV Session: DS* 1798. 1802; Pope Leo XIII, Encyclical *Arcanum Divinae Sapientiae: ASS* 12 (1879/80) 388-391; Pope Pius XI, Encyclical *Casti Connubii: AAS* 22 (1930) 546-547; Second Vatican Council, *Gaudium et Spes*, 48; Pope John Paul II, Apostolic Exhortation *Familiaris Consortio*, 19: *AAS* 74 (1982) 101-102; *Code of Canon Law*, Can. 1056.

Respect for the unity of marriage and for conjugal fidelity demands that the child be conceived in marriage; the bond existing between husband and wife accords the spouses, in an objective and inalienable manner, the exclusive right to become father and mother solely through each other.[37] Recourse to the gametes of a third person, in order to have sperm or ovum available, constitutes a violation of the reciprocal commitment of the spouses and a grave lack in regard to that essential property of marriage which is its unity.

Heterologous artificial fertilization violates the rights of the child; it deprives him of his filial relationship with his parental origins and can hinder the maturing of his personal identity. Furthermore, it offends the common vocation of the spouses who are called to fatherhood and motherhood: it objectively deprives conjugal fruitfulness of its unity and integrity; it brings about and manifests a rupture between genetic parenthood, gestational parenthood and responsibility for upbringing. Such damage to the personal relationships within the family has repercussions on civil society: what threatens the unity and stability of the family is a source of dissension, disorder and injustice in the whole of social life.

These reasons lead to a negative moral judgment concerning heterologous artificial fertilization: consequently fertilization of a married woman with the sperm of a donor different from her husband and fertilization with the husband's sperm of an ovum not coming from his wife are morally illicit. Furthermore, the artificial fertilization of a woman who is unmarried or a widow, whoever the donor may be, cannot be morally justified.

The desire to have a child and the love between spouses who long to obviate a sterility which cannot be overcome in any other way constitute understandable motivations; but subjectively good intentions do not render heterologous artificial fertilization conformable to the objective and inalienable properties of marriage or respectful of the rights of the child and of the spouses.

---

[37]Cf. Pope Pius XII, *Discourse to those taking part in the 4th International Congress of Catholic Doctors*, 29 September 1949: *AAS* 41 (1949) 560; *Discourse to those taking part in the Congress of the Italian Catholic Union of Midwives*, 29 October 1951: *AAS* 43 (1951) 850; *Code of Canon Law*, Can. 1134.

3. Is "SURROGATE"* MOTHERHOOD MORALLY LICIT?

No, for the same reasons which lead one to reject heterologous artificial fertilization: for it is contrary to the unity of marriage and to the dignity of the procreation of the human person.

Surrogate motherhood represents an objective failure to meet the obligations of maternal love, of conjugal fidelity and of responsible motherhood; it offends the dignity and the right of the child to be conceived, carried in the womb, brought into the world and brought up by his own parents; it sets up, to the detriment of families, a division between the physical, psychological and moral elements which constitute those families.

B
HOMOLOGOUS ARTIFICIAL FERTILIZATION

Since heterologous artificial fertilization has been declared unacceptable, the question arises of how to evaluate morally the process of homologous artificial fertilization: IVF and ET and artificial insemination between husband and wife. First a question of principle must be clarified.

4. WHAT CONNECTION IS REQUIRED FROM THE MORAL POINT OF VIEW BETWEEN PROCREATION AND THE CONJUGAL ACT?

a) The Church's teaching on marriage and human procreation affirms the "inseparable connection, willed by God and unable to be broken by man on his own initiative, between the two meanings of the conjugal act: the unitive meaning and the procreative meaning. Indeed, by its intimate structure, the conjugal act, while most closely uniting husband and wife, capacitates them for the generation of new lives, according to laws inscribed in the very being of man and of woman".[38] This principle, which is based upon the

---

*By "surrogate mother" the Instruction means:

a) the woman who carries in pregnancy an embryo implanted in her uterus and who is genetically a stranger to the embryo because it has been obtained through the union of the gametes of "donors". She carries the pregnancy with a pledge to surrender the baby once it is born to the party who commissioned or made the agreement for the pregnancy.

b) the woman who carries in pregnancy an embryo to whose procreation she has contributed the donation of her own ovum, fertilized through insemination with the sperm of a man other than her husband. She carries the pregnancy with a pledge to surrender the child once it is born to the party who commissioned or made the agreement for the pregnancy.

[38]Pope Paul VI, Encyclical Letter *Humanae Vitae*, 12: *AAS* 60 (1968) 488–489.

nature of marriage and the intimate connection of the goods of marriage, has well-known consequences on the level of responsible fatherhood and motherhood. "By safeguarding both these essential aspects, the unitive and the procreative, the conjugal act preserves in its fullness the sense of true mutual love and its ordination towards man's exalted vocation to parenthood".[39]

The same doctrine concerning the link between the meanings of the conjugal act and between the goods of marriage throws light on the moral problem of homologous artificial fertilization, since "it is never permitted to separate these different aspects to such a degree as positively to exclude either the procreative intention or the conjugal relation".[40]

Contraception deliberately deprives the conjugal act of its openness to procreation and in this way brings about a voluntary dissociation of the ends of marriage. Homologous artificial fertilization, in seeking a procreation which is not the fruit of a specific act of conjugal union, objectively effects an analogous separation between the goods and the meanings of marriage.

Thus, *fertilization is licitly sought when it is the result of a "conjugal act which is per se suitable for the generation of children to which marriage is ordered by its nature and by which the spouses become one flesh".[41] But from the moral point of view procreation is deprived of its proper perfection when it is not desired as the fruit of the conjugal act, that is to say of the specific act of the spouses' union.*

b) The moral value of the intimate link between the goods of marriage and between the meanings of the conjugal act is based upon the unity of the human being, a unity involving body and spiritual soul.[42] Spouses mutually express their personal love in the "language of the body", which clearly involves both "sponsal meanings" and parental ones.[43] The conjugal act by which the couple mutually express their self-gift at the same time expresses openness to the gift of life. It is an act that is inseparably corporal and spiritual. It is in their bodies and through their bodies that the spouses consummate their marriage and are able to become father and mother. In order to respect the language of their bodies and their natural generosity, the conjugal union must take place with respect for its openness to procreation; and the

---

[39]*Loc. cit., ibid.,* 489.

[40]Pope Pius XII, *Discourse to those taking part in the Second Naples World Congress on Fertility and Human Sterility,* 19 May 1956: *AAS* 48 (1956) 470.

[41]*Code of Canon Law,* Can. 1061. According to this Canon, the conjugal act is that by which the marriage is consummated if the couple "have performed (it) between themselves in a human manner".

[42]Cf. Pastoral Constitution *Gaudium et Spes,* 14.

[43]Cf. Pope John Paul II, *General Audience on 16 January 1980: Insegnamenti di Giovanni Paolo II,* III, 1 (1980) 148- 152.

procreation of a person must be the fruit and the result of married love. The origin of the human being thus follows from a procreation that is "linked to the union, not only biological but also spiritual, of the parents, made one by the bond of marriage".[44] Fertilization achieved outside the bodies of the couple remains by this very fact deprived of the meanings and the values which are expressed in the language of the body and in the union of human persons.

c) Only respect for the link between the meanings of the conjugal act and respect for the unity of the human being make possible procreation in conformity with the dignity of the person. In his unique and irrepeatable origin, the child must be respected and recognized as equal in personal dignity to those who give him life. The human person must be accepted in his parents' act of union and love; the generation of a child must therefore be the fruit of that mutual giving[45] which is realized in the conjugal act wherein the spouses cooperate as servants and not as masters in the work of the Creator who is Love.[46]

In reality, the origin of a human person is the result of an act of giving. The one conceived must be the fruit of his parents' love. He cannot be desired or conceived as the product of an intervention of medical or biological techniques; that would be equivalent to reducing him to an object of scientific technology. No one may subject the coming of a child into the world to conditions of technical efficiency which are to be evaluated according to standards of control and dominion.

The moral relevance of the link between the meanings of the conjugal act and between the goods of marriage, as well as the unity of the human being and the dignity of his origin, demand that the procreation of a human person be brought about as the fruit of the conjugal act specific to the love between spouses. The link between procreation and the conjugal act is thus shown to be of great importance on the anthropological and moral planes, and it throws light on the positions of the Magisterium with regard to homologous artificial fertilization.

5. Is homologous 'in vitro' fertilization morally licit?

The answer to this question is strictly dependent on the principles just mentioned. Certainly one cannot ignore the legitimate aspirations of sterile couples. For some, recourse to homologous IVF and ET appears to be the only way of fulfilling their sincere desire for a child. The question is asked

---

[44]Pope John Paul II, *Discourse to those taking part in the 35th General Assembly of the World Medical Association*, 29 October 1983: *AAS* 76 (1984) 393.

[45]Cf. Pastoral Constitution *Gaudium et Spes*, 51.

[46]Cf. Pastoral Constitution *Gaudium et Spes*, 50.

whether the totality of conjugal life in such situations is not sufficient to ensure the dignity proper to human procreation. It is acknowledged that IVF and ET certainly cannot supply for the absence of sexual relations[47] and cannot be preferred to the specific acts of conjugal union, given the risks involved for the child and the difficulties of the procedure. But it is asked whether, when there is no other way of overcoming the sterility which is a source of suffering, homologous *in vitro* fertilization may not constitute an aid, if not a form of therapy, whereby its moral licitness could be admitted.

The desire for a child—or at the very least an openness to the transmission of life—is a necessary prerequisite from the moral point of view for responsible human procreation. But this good intention is not sufficient for making a positive moral evaluation of *in vitro* fertilization between spouses. The process of IVF and ET must be judged in itself and cannot borrow its definitive moral quality from the totality of conjugal life of which it becomes part nor from the conjugal acts which may precede or follow it.[48]

It has already been recalled that, in the circumstances in which it is regularly practised, IVF and ET involves the destruction of human beings, which is something contrary to the doctrine on the illicitness of abortion previously mentioned.[49] But even in a situation in which every precaution were taken to avoid the death of human embryos, homologous IVF and ET dissociates from the conjugal act the actions which are directed to human fertilization. For this reason the very nature of homologous IVF and ET also must be taken into account, even abstracting from the link with procured abortion.

Homologous IVF and ET is brought about outside the bodies of the couple through actions of third parties whose competence and technical activity determine the success of the procedure. Such fertilization entrusts the life and identity of the embryo into the power of doctors and biologists and establishes the domination of technology over the origin and destiny of the human person. Such a relationship of domination is in itself contrary to the dignity and equality that must be common to parents and children.

Conception *in vitro* is the result of the technical action which presides over fertilization. *Such fertilization is neither in fact achieved nor positively willed as the expression and fruit of a specific act of the conjugal union. In homologous IVF and ET,*

---

[47]Cf. Pope Pius XII, *Discourse to those taking part in the 4th International Congress of Catholic Doctors*, 29 September 1949: *AAS* 41 (1949) 560: "It would be erroneous . . . to think that the possibility of resorting to this means (artificial fertilization) might render valid a marriage between persons unable to contract it because of the *impedimentum impotentiae*".

[48]A similar question was dealt with by Pope Paul VI, Encyclical *Humanae Vitae*, 14: *AAS* 60 (1968) 490–491.

[49]Cf. *supra*: I, 1 ff.

therefore, even if it is considered in the context of 'de facto' existing sexual relations, the generation of the human person is objectively deprived of its proper perfection: namely, that of being the result and fruit of a conjugal act in which the spouses can become "cooperators with God for giving life to a new person".[50]

These reasons enable us to understand why the act of conjugal love is considered in the teaching of the Church as the only setting worthy of human procreation. For the same reasons the so- called "simple case", i.e. a homologous IVF and ET procedure that is free of any compromise with the abortive practice of destroying embryos and with masturbation, remains a technique which is morally illicit because it deprives human procreation of the dignity which is proper and connatural to it.

Certainly, homologous IVF and ET fertilization is not marked by all that ethical negativity found in extra-conjugal procreation; the family and marriage continue to constitute the setting for the birth and upbringing of the children. Nevertheless, in conformity with the traditional doctrine relating to the goods of marriage and the dignity of the person, *the Church remains opposed from the moral point of view to homologous 'in vitro' fertilization. Such fertilization is in itself illicit and in opposition to the dignity of procreation and of the conjugal union, even when everything is done to avoid the death of the human embryo.*

Although the manner in which human conception is achieved with IVF and ET cannot be approved, every child which comes into the world must in any case be accepted as a living gift of the divine Goodness and must be brought up with love.

6. How is homologous artificial insemination to be evaluated from the moral point of view?

Homologous artificial insemination within marriage cannot be admitted except for those cases in which the technical means is not a substitute for the conjugal act but serves to facilitate and to help so that the act attains its natural purpose.

The teaching of the Magisterium on this point has already been stated.[51] This teaching is not just an expression of particular historical circumstances but is based on the Church's doctrine concerning the connection between the

---

[50]Pope Paul II, Apostolic Exhortation *Familiaris Consortio* 14: *AAS* 74 (1982) 96.

[51]Cf. *Response of the Holy Office*, 17 March 1897: *DS* 3323; Pope Pius XII, *Discourse to those taking part in the 4th International Congress of Catholic Doctors*, 29 September 1949: *AAS* 41 (1949) 560: *Discourse to the Italian Catholic Union of Midwives*, 29 October 1951: *AAS* 43 (1951) 850: *Discourse to those taking part in the Second Naples World Congress on Fertility and Human Sterility*, 19 May 1956: *AAS* 48 (1956) 471–473; *Discourse to those taking part in the 7th International Congress of the International Society of Haematology*, 12 September 1958: *AAS* 50 (1958) 733; Pope John XXIII, Encyclical *Mater et Magistra*, III: *AAS* 53 (1961) 447.

conjugal union and procreation and on a consideration of the personal nature of the conjugal act and of human procreation. "In its natural structure, the conjugal act is a personal action, a simultaneous and immediate cooperation on the part of the husband and wife, which by the very nature of the agents and the proper nature of the act is the expression of the mutual gift which, according to the words of Scripture, brings about union 'in one flesh' ".[52] Thus moral conscience "does not necessarily proscribe the use of certain artificial means destined solely either to the facilitating of the natural act or to ensuring that the natural act normally performed achieves its proper end".[53] If the technical means facilitates the conjugal act or helps it to reach its natural objectives, it can be morally acceptable. If, on the other hand, the procedure were to replace the conjugal act, it is morally illicit.

Artificial insemination as a substitute for the conjugal act is prohibited by reason of the voluntarily achieved dissociation of the two meanings of the conjugal act. Masturbation, through which the sperm is normally obtained, is another sign of this dissociation: even when it is done for the purpose of procreation, the act remains deprived of its unitive meaning: "It lacks the sexual relationship called for by the moral order, namely the relationship which realizes 'the full sense of mutual self-giving and human procreation in the context of true love' ".[54]

7. What moral criterion can be proposed with regard to medical intervention in human procreation?

The medical act must be evaluated not only with reference to its technical dimension but also and above all in relation to its goal which is the good of persons and their bodily and psychological health. The moral criteria for medical intervention in procreation are deduced from the dignity of human persons, of their sexuality and of their origin.

Medicine which seeks to be ordered to the integral good of the person must respect the specifically human values of sexuality.[55] *The doctor is at the service of persons and of*

---

[52]Pope Pius XII, *Discourse to the Italian Catholic Union of Midwives*, 29 October 1951: *AAS* 43 (1951) 850.

[53]Pope Pius XII, *Discourse to those taking part in the 4th International Congress of Catholic Doctors*, 29 September 1949: *AAS* 41 (1949) 560.

[54]Sacred Congregation for the Doctrine of the Faith, *Declaration on Certain Questions Concerning Sexual Ethics*, 9: *AAS* 68 (1976) 86, which quotes the Pastoral Constitution *Gaudium et Spes*, 51. Cf. *Decree of the Holy Office*, 2 August 1929: *AAS* 21 (1929) 490; Pope Pius XII, *Discourse to those taking part in the 26th Congress of the Italian Society of Urology*, 8 October 1953: *AAS* 45 (1953) 678.

[55]Cf. Pope John XXIII, Encyclical *Mater et Magistra*, III: *AAS* 53 (1961) 447.

human procreation. He does not have the authority to dispose of them or to decide their fate. A medical intervention respects the dignity of persons when it seeks to assist the conjugal act either in order to facilitate its performance or in order to enable it to achieve its objective once it has been normally performed".[56]

On the other hand, it sometimes happens that a medical procedure technologically replaces the conjugal act in order to obtain a procreation which is neither its result nor its fruit. In this case the medical act is not, as it should be, at the service of conjugal union but rather appropriates to itself the procreative function and thus contradicts the dignity and the inalienable rights of the spouses and of the child to be born.

The humanization of medicine, which is insisted upon today by everyone, requires respect for the integral dignity of the human person first of all in the act and at the moment in which the spouses transmit life to a new person. It is only logical therefore to address an urgent appeal to Catholic doctors and scientists that they bear exemplary witness to the respect due to the human embryo and to the dignity of procreation. The medical and nursing staff of Catholic hospitals and clinics are in a special way urged to do justice to the moral obligations which they have assumed, frequently also, as part of their contract. Those who are in charge of Catholic hospitals and clinics and who are often Religious will take special care to safeguard and promote a diligent observance of the moral norms recalled in the present Instruction.

8. The suffering caused by infertility in marriage

The suffering of spouses who cannot have children or who are afraid of bringing a handicapped child into the world is a suffering that everyone must understand and properly evaluate.

On the part of the spouses, the desire for a child is natural: it expresses the vocation to fatherhood and motherhood inscribed in conjugal love. This desire can be even stronger if the couple is affected by sterility which appears incurable. Nevertheless, marriage does not confer upon the spouses the right to have a child, but only the right to perform those natural acts which are *per se* ordered to procreation.[57]

---

[56]Cf. Pope Pius XII, *Discourse to those taking part in the 4th International Congress of Catholic Doctors,* 29 September 1949: *AAS* 41 (1949), 560.

[57]Cf. Pope Pius XII, *Discourse to the taking part in the Second Naples World Congress on Fertility and Human Sterility,* 19 May 1956: *AAS* 48 (1956) 471–473.

A true and proper right to a child would be contrary to the child's dignity and nature. The child is not an object to which one has a right, nor can he be considered as an object of ownership: rather, a child is a gift, "the supreme gift"[58] *and the most gratuitous gift of marriage, and is a living testimony of the mutual giving of his parents. For this reason, the child has the right, as already mentioned, to be the fruit of the specific act of the conjugal love of his parents; and he also has the right to be respected as a person from the moment of his conception.*

Nevertheless, whatever its cause or prognosis, sterility is certainly a difficult trial. The community of believers is called to shed light upon and support the suffering of those who are unable to fulfill their legitimate aspiration to motherhood and fatherhood. Spouses who find themselves in this sad situation are called to find in it an opportunity for sharing in a particular way in the Lord's Cross, the source of spiritual fruitfulness. Sterile couples must not forget that "even when procreation is not possible, conjugal life does not for this reason lose its value. Physical sterility in fact can be for spouses the occasion for other important services to the life of the human person, for example, adoption, various forms of educational work, and assistance to other families and to poor or handicapped children".[59]

Many researchers are engaged in the fight against sterility. While fully safeguarding the dignity of human procreation, some have achieved results which previously seemed unattainable. Scientists therefore are to be encouraged to continue their research with the aim of preventing the causes of sterility and of being able to remedy them so that sterile couples will be able to procreate in full respect for their own personal dignity and that of the child to be born.

III.
MORAL AND CIVIL LAW

THE VALUES AND MORAL OBLIGATIONS
THAT CIVIL LEGISLATION
MUST RESPECT AND SANCTION IN THIS MATTER

The inviolable right to life of every innocent human individual and the rights of the family and of the institution of marriage constitute fundamental

---

[58]Pastoral Constitution *Gaudium et Spes*, 50.
[59]Pope John Paul II, Apostolic Exhortation *Familiaris Consortio*, 14: *AAS* 74 (1982) 97.

moral values, because they concern the natural condition and integral vocation of the human person; at the same time they are constitutive elements of civil society and its order.

For this reason the new technological possibilities which have opened up in the field of biomedicine require the intervention of the political authorities and of the legislator, since an uncontrolled application of such techniques could lead to unforeseeable and damaging consequences for civil society. Recourse to the conscience of each individual and to the self-regulation of researchers cannot be sufficient for ensuring respect for personal rights and public order. If the legislator responsible for the common good were not watchful, he could be deprived of his prerogatives by researchers claiming to govern humanity in the name of the biological discoveries and the alleged "improvement" processes which they would draw from those discoveries. "Eugenism" and forms of discrimination between human beings could come to be legitimized: this would constitute an act of violence and a serious offense to the equality, dignity and fundamental rights of the human person.

The intervention of the public authority must be inspired by the rational principles which regulate the relationships between civil law and moral law. The task of the civil law is to ensure the common good of people through the recognition of and the defence of fundamental rights and through the promotion of peace and of public morality.[60] In no sphere of life can the civil law take the place of conscience or dictate norms concerning things which are outside its competence. It must sometimes tolerate, for the sake of public order, things which it cannot forbid without a greater evil resulting. However, the inalienable rights of the person must be recognized and respected by civil society and the political authority. These human rights depend neither on single individuals nor on parents; nor do they represent a concession made by society and the State: they pertain to human nature and are inherent in the person by virtue of the creative act from which the person took his or her origin.

Among such fundamental rights one should mention in this regard: a) every human being's right to life and physical integrity from the moment of conception until death; b) the rights of the family and of marriage as an institution and, in this area, the child's right to be conceived, brought into the world and brought up by his parents. To each of these two themes it is necessary here to give some further consideration.

In various States certain laws have authorized the direct suppression of innocents: the moment a positive law deprives a category of human beings of the protection which civil legislation must accord them, the State is denying

---

[60]Cf. Declaration *Dignitatis Humanae*, 7.

the equality of all before the law. When the State does not place its power at the service of the rights of each citizen, and in particular of the more vulnerable, the very foundations of a State based on law are undermined. The political authority consequently cannot give approval to the calling of human beings into existence through procedures which would expose them to those very grave risks noted previously. The possible recognition by positive law and the political authorities of techniques of artificial transmission of life and the experimentation connected with it would widen the breach already opened by the legalization of abortion.

As a consequence of the respect and protection which must be ensured for the unborn child from the moment of his conception, the law must provide appropriate penal sanctions for every deliberate violation of the child's rights. The law cannot tolerate—indeed it must expressly forbid—that human beings, even at the embryonic stage, should be treated as objects of experimentation, be mutilated or destroyed with the excuse that they are superfluous or incapable of developing normally.

The political authority is bound to guarantee to the institution of the family, upon which society is based, the juridical protection to which it has a right. From the very fact that it is at the service of people, the political authority must also be at the service of the family. Civil law cannot grant approval to techniques of artificial procreation which, for the benefit of third parties (doctors, biologists, economic or governmental powers), take away what is a right inherent in the relationship between spouses; and therefore civil law cannot legalize the donation of gametes between persons who are not legitimately united in marriage.

Legislation must also prohibit, by virtue of the support which is due to the family, embryo banks, *post mortem* insemination and "surrogate motherhood".

It is part of the duty of the public authority to ensure that the civil law is regulated according to the fundamental norms of the moral law in matters concerning human rights, human life and the institution of the family. Politicians must commit themselves, through their interventions upon public opinion, to securing in society the widest possible consensus on such essential points and to consolidating this consensus wherever it risks being weakened or is in danger of collapse.

In many countries, the legalization of abortion and juridical tolerance of unmarried couples makes it more difficult to secure respect for the fundamental rights recalled by this Instruction. It is to be hoped that States will not become responsible for aggravating these socially damaging situations of injustice. It is rather to be hoped that nations and States will realize all the cultural, ideological and political implications connected with the techniques of artificial procreation and will find the wisdom and courage necessary for issuing laws which are more just and more respectful of human life and the institution of the family.

The civil legislation of many states confers an undue legitimation upon certain practices in the eyes of many today; it is seen to be incapable of guaranteeing that morality which is in conformity with the natural exigencies of the human person and with the "unwritten laws" etched by the Creator upon the human heart. All men of good will must commit themselves, particularly within their professional field and in the exercise of their civil rights, to ensuring the reform of morally unacceptable civil laws and the correction of illicit practices. In addition, "conscientious objection" vis-à-vis such laws must be supported and recognized. A movement of passive resistence to the legitimation of practices contrary to human life and dignity is beginning to make an ever sharper impression upon the moral conscience of many, especially among specialists in the biomedical sciences.

CONCLUSION

The spread of technologies of intervention in the processes of human procreation raises very serious moral problems in relation to the respect due to the human being from the moment of conception, to the dignity of the person, of his or her sexuality, and of the transmission of life.

With this Instruction the Congregation for the Doctrine of the Faith, in fulfilling its responsibility to promote and defend the Church's teaching in so serious a matter, addresses a new and heartfelt invitation to all those who, by reason of their role and their commitment, can exercise a positive influence and ensure that, in the family and in society, due respect is accorded to life and love. It addresses this invitation to those responsible for the formation of consciences and of public opinion, to scientists and medical professionals, to jurists and politicians. It hopes that all will understand the incompatibility between recognition of the dignity of the human person and contempt for life and love, between faith in the living God and the claim to decide arbitrarily the origin and fate of a human being.

In particular, the Congregation for the Doctrine of the Faith addresses an invitation with confidence and encouragement to theologians, and above all to moralists, that they study more deeply and make ever more accessible to the faithful the contents of the teaching of the Church's Magisterium in the light of a valid anthropology in the matter of sexuality and marriage and in the context of the necessary interdisciplinary approach. Thus they will make it possible to understand ever more clearly the reasons for and the validity of this teaching. By defending man against the excesses of his own power, the Church of God reminds him of the reasons for his true nobility; only in this way can the possibility of living and loving with that dignity and liberty which derive from respect for the truth be ensured for the men and women of tomorrow. The precise indications which are offered in the present Instruction therefore are not meant to halt the effort of reflection but rather to give it a renewed impulse in unrenounceable fidelity to the teaching of the Church.

In the light of the truth about the gift of human life and in the light of the moral principles which flow from that truth, everyone is invited to act in the area of responsibility proper to each and, like the good Samaritan, to recognize as a neighbour even the littlest among the children of men (Cf. *Lk* 10:29–37). Here Christ's words find a new and particular echo: "What you do to one of the least of my brethren, you do unto me" (*Mt* 25:40).

During an audience granted to the undersigned Prefect after the plenary session of the Congregation for the Doctrine of the Faith, the Supreme Pontiff, John Paul II, approved this Instruction and ordered it to be published.

Given at Rome, from the Congregation for the Doctrine of the Faith, February 22, 1987, the Feast of the Chair of St. Peter, the Apostle.

JOSEPH Card. RATZINGER
Prefect

ALBERTO BOVONE
Titular Archbishop of Caesarea in Numidia
Secretary